MONOGRAPHS ON
STATISTICS AND APPLIED PROBABILITY

General Editors

D.R. Cox, D.V. Hinkley, D. Rubin and B.W. Silverman

(Full details concerning this series are available from the publishers)

Design and Analysis of Cross-Over Trials

BYRON JONES

The University of Kent

and

MICHAEL G. KENWARD

The University of Reading

CHAPMAN AND HALL

LONDON • NEW YORK • TOKYO • MELBOURNE • MADRAS

UK	Chapman and Hall, 2–6 Boundary Row, London SE1 8HN
USA	Chapman and Hall, 29 West 35th Street, New York NY10001
JAPAN	Chapman and Hall Japan, Thomson Publishing Japan, Hirakawacho Nemoto Building, 7F, 1-7-11 Hirakawa-cho, Chiyoda-ku, Tokyo 102
AUSTRALIA	Chapman and Hall Australia, Thomas Nelson Australia, 480 La Trobe Street, PO Box 4725, Melbourne 3000
INDIA	Chapman and Hall India, R. Sheshadri, 32 Second Main Road, CIT East, Madras 600 035

First edition 1989
Reprinted 1990

© 1989 Chapman and Hall

Typeset in 10/12 Times by Thomson Press (India) Ltd,
New Delhi
Printed in Great Britain by
St Edmundsbury Press Ltd, Bury St Edmunds, Suffolk

ISBN 0 412 30000 1 (HB)

Library of Congress Cataloging-in-Publication Data

Jones, Byron, 1951–
   Design and analysis of cross-over trials / Byron Jones and
Michael G. Kenward.
   p.   cm. — (Monographs on statistics and applied
probability)
   Includes indexes.
   ISBN 0-412-30000-1 (U.S.)
   1. Crossover trials.   I. Kenward, Michael G., 1956–
II. Title.   III. Series.
R853.C76J66   1989
614.5'07—dc20   89-31952
                                             CIP

To Hilary, Charlotte and Alexander
and to Pirkko

Contents

Preface

This book is concerned with a particular sort of comparative trial known as the cross-over trial in which the subjects receive different sequences of treatments. Such trials are widely used in clinical and medical research and in other diverse areas such as veterinary science, psychology, sports science, dairy science and agriculture. The book is the first to be entirely devoted to the cross-over trial and aims to provide a reasonably comprehensive and unified account of the subject. Up until now the large and continually growing literature has been spread widely, both in statistical and in subject-matter journals. This book should be suitable to the newcomer to cross-over trials and to the experienced statistician. Whenever possible we have put the more elementary material at the beginning of each chapter in order to make the methods of design and analysis available to the practitioner who does not want to get into the more detailed theory. The book has been written from a practical point of view and we have only included details of theory where these are essential or are needed to describe current research topics which look likely to be of practical importance in the future. The reader who requires a more academic treatment should also find much useful material in the book. Final-year and postgraduate students who are taking either specialized courses in the design of experiments or more general courses on clinical trials should also find much to interest them, certainly in the earlier chapters.

We have been fortunate during the writing of this book to have received helpful comments and advice from a number of friends and colleagues. We are particularly grateful to John Matthews who, on behalf of Chapman and Hall, carefully read each chapter as it was written. Others who were kind enough to read and comment on early draft sections and single chapters were Andy Grieve, Matthew Law and Hans Hockey. We are grateful to the following for letting us see, at various stages in the writing of this book, pre-publication copies of papers they had written: David Fletcher, Peter Freeman, Andy Grieve, Matthew Koch, Sue Lewis, John Matthews and Harji Patel. For giving us access to their unpublished data we are grateful to Peter Blood, Ed Bryant, Arend Heyting, John Lewis, Jorgen Seldrup and Robert Woodfield. For permission to use their data we are grateful to Ciba-Geigy Pharmaceuticals, ICI Pharmaceuticals, Duphar B.V., the Ortho Pharmaceuticals Corporation and the Upjohn Company. We are also grateful to Philip North for allowing us access to the many cross-over data sets analysed by his Applied Statistics Research Unit. Prior to and during the writing of the book we were fortunate to belong to a working group organized by Peter Armitage. He and the other members of the group, Sir David Cox, John Matthews, John Lewis and Alan Ebbutt, were always a source of useful advice and comment. The calculations in the book were done for the most part in the Genstat language. We are grateful to Hans Hockey for sharing his knowledge of Genstat. The drafts of the book were typed by us at a computer terminal using the *troff* system. We are grateful to Mike Bremner and Eryl Bassett, for their help with using that system. We thank George Dyke for providing the historical information on the Rothamstead field trials. Finally, we wish to thank Elizabeth Johnston, senior editor at Chapman and Hall, for her help and patience during the writing of this book. Naturally, of course, we take full responsibility for any inaccuracies that remain in the text.

Byron Jones
Canterbury

Michael G. Kenward
Reading

November 1988

CHAPTER 1

Introduction

1.1 What is a cross-over trial?

At different phases in their development, drugs and other treatments for disease are compared using clinical trials. A good general introduction to clinical trials is given by Pocock (1983). In the sort of trials with which we are concerned the drugs are usually assessed by comparing their effects in human subjects. In a **cross-over trial** each experimental subject receives two or more different treatments. The order in which each subject receives the treatments depends on the particular design chosen for the trial. The simplest design is the one known as the 2 × 2 design. In this design each subject receives two different treatments, which we conventionally label as A and B. Half the subjects receive A first and then, after a suitably chosen period of time, **cross over** to B. The remaining subjects receive B first and then cross over to A. A typical example of such a trial is given in Example 1.1.

Example 1.1

The aim of this trial was to compare an oral mouthwash (treatment A) with a placebo mouthwash (treatment B). The 41 subjects who took part in the trial were healthy volunteers.

The trial, which lasted 15 weeks, was divided into two treatment periods of 6 weeks each, with a 'wash-out' period of 3 weeks in between. One variable of interest was a subject's plaque score after using each of the two different mouthwashes. Prior to the first treatment period an average plaque score was obtained for each subject.

Some data obtained from the trial described in Example 1.1 will be analysed in Chapter 2, which is devoted to the 2 × 2 trial. The definition of a wash-out period and the reasons for including such periods will be given in Section 1.3.

An example of a cross-over trial which compared more than two treatments is given in Example 1.2.

Example 1.2

The aims of this trial were to compare the effects of four treatments A, B, C and D on muscle blood flow and cardiac output in patients with intermittent claudication. Fourteen subjects took part in the trial and their treatment sequences are shown in Table 1.1. The seven weeks that the trial lasted were divided into four one-week treatment periods with a one-week wash-out period separating each pair of treatment periods.

A notable feature of the trial described in Example 1.2 is that every subject received the treatments in a different order. If 16 subjects could have been used then an alternative design for four treatments might have used only four different treatment sequences, with four subjects on each sequence. With more than two treatments there are clearly many more cross-over designs to choose from. This is the

Table 1.1 *Treatment sequences used in Example 1.2*

Subject	Period			
	1	2	3	4
1	B	D	C	A
2	A	C	B	D
3	C	A	D	B
4	D	B	A	C
5	B	A	D	C
6	A	D	C	B
7	C	B	A	D
8	D	C	B	A
9	B	C	D	A
10	C	D	A	B
11	C	A	B	D
12	A	C	D	B
13	B	D	A	C
14	A	B	D	C

topic of Chapter 5, where we also analyse some data from the trial described in Example 1.2.

1.2 With which sort of cross-over trial are we concerned?

As might be guessed from the examples just given, the emphasis in this book is on cross-over trials as used in medical and pharmaceutical research, particularly research as undertaken within the pharmaceutical industry. With very few exceptions, all the data sets we describe and analyse were obtained as part of trials undertaken by clinicians and statisticians working in the pharmaceutical industry. However, the theory, methods and practice we describe are applicable in almost any situation where cross-over trials are deemed appropriate. Such situations include, for example, veterinary research, animal feeding trials, sports science and psychological experiments. Parkes (1982), for example, has described the use of a cross-over trial to investigate occupational stress, and Raghavarao (1989) has described a potential application of cross-over trials in (non-pharmaceutical) industry. Readers from these and other subject matter areas should have no difficulty in applying the contents of this book to their own individual situations.

1.3 Why do cross-over trials need special consideration?

The feature that distinguishes the cross-over trial from other trials which compare treatments is that measurements on different treatments are obtained from each subject. This feature brings with it advantages and disadvantages.

The main advantage is that the treatments are compared 'within subjects'. That is, every subject provides a direct comparison of the treatments he or she has received. In Example 1.1, for example, each subject provides two measurements: one on A and one on B. The difference between these measurements removes any 'subject effect' from the comparison. Of course, this within-subject difference could also be thought of as a comparison between the two treatment periods. That is, even if the two treatments were identical, a large difference between the two measurements on a subject might be obtained if, for some reason, the measurements in one treatment period were significantly higher or lower than those in the other treatment period. The possibility of such a period difference has not been overlooked: it is the reason that one group of subjects received the treatments in the order AB and the other group received the treatments in the order BA. As we shall see in Chapter 2, any period difference can be allowed for when estimating the treatment difference.

The main aim of the cross-over trial is therefore to remove from the treatment (and period) comparisons any component that is related to the differences between the subjects. In clinical trials it is usually the case that the variability of measurements taken on different subjects is far greater than the variability of repeated measurements taken on the same subject. The cross-over trial aims to exploit this feature by making sure that whenever possible, important comparisons of interest are estimated using differences obtained from the within-subject measurements. This is to be contrasted with another popular design: the 'parallel group trial'. In this latter trial each subject receives only one of the possible treatments. The subjects are randomly divided into groups and each group is assigned one of the treatments being compared. Estimates of treatment differences are obtained from comparisons between the subject groups, i.e. are based on between-subject information.

Although the use of repeated measurements on the same subject brings with it great advantages, it also brings a potential disadvantage. We stress 'potential' because, as we hope to demonstrate, this disadvantage can be overcome virtually entirely if three or more treatment periods are used, and is only serious in the most basic form of the 2×2 trial. The disadvantage to which we refer is the possibility that the effect of a treatment given in one period might still be present at the start of the following period. This 'carry-over' effect, as it is known, can arise in a number of ways, as we will discuss in Chapter 2. The wash-out periods used in the trials described in Examples 1.1 and 1.2 were included to allow the effect of a treatment given in one period to be 'washed out' of the system before each subject began the next period of treatment. The measurements taken on the subjects during the treatment periods are usually also taken during the wash-out periods. These measurements, along with any 'baseline' measurements taken prior to the start of the trial, can be of value at the data analysis stage. In order to make it clear to which sort of treatment effect we are referring to in the following, we refer to the effect that a treatment has during the period in which it is administered as the **direct treatment effect**. The effect of a treatment that persists after the end of the treatment period is referred to as the **carry-over effect**. Carry-over effects which last no more than one period after the treatment has been stopped are known as **first-order** carry-over effects. More generally, carry-over effects which last up to and including k periods after the treatment has been stopped are known as **kth-order** carry-over effects. The baseline measurements mentioned above can sometimes be useful for deciding if carry-over effects are present.

Quite often the trial is preceded by a 'run-in' period which is used to familiarize subjects with the procedures they will follow during the trial and is also sometimes used as a screening period to ensure only eligible subjects proceed to the treatment periods. Also, it is quite usual for the trial to be 'double-blind'; that is, neither the subjects nor anyone concerned with the evaluation of the treatments knows which treatment a subject has received in any period.

The differences between the treatments as measured in one period might also be different from those measured in a later period because of a direct treatment-by-period interaction. That is, for some reason, the conditions present in the different periods are such that the difference between a particular pair of treatments depends on the period in which they were administered. Such an interaction might also be the result of treatments possessing different amounts of carry-over. Although in any well-planned trial the chance of treatments interacting with periods will be small, it is clearly preferable to use a design that permits the interaction to be detected and if possible to identify whether it is the result of carry-over or not. Generally, designs for more than two treatments can be constructed in such a way that they allow the interaction and carry-over to be estimated separately. Designs for two treatments however, require special attention and we consider these in Chapter 4.

1.4 Where are cross-over trials used?

In order to give some idea of where cross-over trials have been used in clinical and medical research, we looked through each issue of the *British Medical Journal* that was published during the period January 1980 to April 1988. Of the trials reported there, over 80 used the cross-over principle. Although the diseases/conditions studied in these trials were quite diverse, over half the trials were concerned with hypertension, diabetes, angina and asthma. Not unexpectedly, with such a wide variety of trials overall, the length of the treatment periods used in the different trials varied from as little as a day or a week to as much as a month or six months. The design used in most of these trials was the standard 2×2 design. A survey (Fava and Patel, 1986) of 12 large pharmaceutical companies in the USA revealed a not too dissimilar view. Out of 72 cross-over trials conducted by these companies over a five-year period, over half of the trials used the 2×2 design. Among the next most popular were designs for three and four treatments which used three or four periods, respectively. Among the areas studied using cross-over designs were acid secretion, analgesics, antiarhythmics, angina, asthma and bronchoconstriction.

A detailed comparison of 13 cross-over trials reported in the *New England Journal of Medicine* during 1978–79 was given by Louis, Lavori, Bailar and Polansky (1984). The diseases and conditions studied in these trials were again quite diverse, although they again included asthma (three trials), angina (two trials) and diabetes (two trials).

1.5 A brief history

Although our concern is with cross-over designs as used in clinical trials, the earliest uses of such designs were most likely in agriculture. Indeed, what may well have been the first cross-over trial was started in 1852 and, in a much modified form, still exists today. It originated in one of the great nineteenth-century scientific controversies. John Bennett Lawes of Rothamsted, Hertfordshire, England, and Baron Justus von Liebig of Giessen, in Germany (now West Germany) disagreed about the nutrition of crop plants. Both were somewhat vague in classifying plant nutrients as either 'organic' or 'mineral' and Liebig sometimes contradicted himself. But in 1847 he wrote (Liebig, 1847) that cultivated plants received enough nitrogen from the atmosphere 'for the purposes of agriculture', though it might be necessary for the farmer to apply 'minerals'. Lawes, a more practically minded man, but with no scientific qualification, and much junior to Liebig, knew from the results of the first few seasons of his field experimental work that the yield of wheat was greatly improved by the application of 'ammoniacal salts'. He noticed that yields varied greatly between seasons, but whenever one of his plots of wheat received 'ammoniacal salts' it gave a good yield, but when 'minerals' (i.e. phosphates, potash, etc.) were given the yield was much less. To separate the real effects of the manures from the large differences between seasons, and to clinch his refutation of Liebig's argument, he allocated two plots to an alternation of treatments which continued until long after his death. Each year one plot received ammonia without minerals, the other minerals without ammonia; the following season the applications were interchanged. The result was a total success: ammonia (after minerals in the preceding season) gave a full yield (practically equal to that given by the plot that received both every year) but minerals following ammonia gave about half as much (very little more than the plot that received minerals without ammonia every year). But Liebig never admitted his mistake.

Lawes and his co-worker J.H. Gilbert seem also to be the first to have been explicitly concerned with carry-over effects. Lawes (page 10 of a pamphlet published in 1846) gave advice on the use of artificial manures: 'Let the artificial manures be applied in greater abundance to the green crops, and the residue of these will manure the corn.' Their interest in carry-over effects is further evident from Section II of Lawes and Gilbert (1864), entitled 'Effects of the unexhausted residue from previous manuring upon succeeding crops'. The data collected in these classic experiments were among the first to occupy R.A. Fisher and his co-workers in the Statistics Department at Rothamsted. This department was created in 1919.

The particular design problems associated with long-term rotation experiments were considered by Cochran (1939). He seems to have been one of the first to formally separate out the two sorts of treatments effects (direct and carry-over) when considering which experimental plan to use.

Early interest in administering different treatments to the same experimental unit was not confined to agricultural experiments, however. Simpson (1938) described a number of cross-over trials which compared different diets given to children. In one trial he compared four different diets using 24 children. The plan of the trial was such that all possible permutations of the four diets were used, each child receiving one of the 24 different treatment sequences. He was aware of the possibility of carry-over effects and suggested that this might be allowed for by introducing a wash-out period between each pair of treatment periods. Yates (1938) considered in more detail one of the other designs suggested by Simpson (1938) and considered the efficiency of estimation of the direct, carry-over and cumulative (direct + carry-over) effects of three different sets of sequences for three treatments administered over three periods.

Cross-over trials have been used extensively in animal husbandry experiments, since at least the 1930s. Indeed, some of the most important contributions to the design theory came from workers like W.G. Cochran, H.D. Patterson and H.L. Lucas who had an interest in this area.

Brandt (1938) described the analysis of designs which compared two treatments using two groups of cattle. Depending on the number of periods, the animals in one group received the treatments in the order ABAB..., and the animals in the other group received the treatments in the order BABA.... This type of design is usually referred to as the **switchback** or **reversal** design. In a now classic paper, Cochran, Autrey and Cannon (1941) described a trial on Holstein cows which compared three treatments over three periods using two orthogonal Latin squares. They seem to have been the first to formally describe the least squares estimation of the direct and carry-over treatment effects. The design they used had the property of balance, which has been studied extensively ever since. Williams (1949, 1950) showed how balanced designs which used the minimum number of subjects could be constructed. He quoted an example taken from the milling of paper in which different pulp suspensions were compared using six different mills. We describe balanced and other sorts of design in Chapter 5.

Another early use of cross-over designs took place in the area of biological assay. Fieller (1940) described a 2×2 trial which used rabbits to compare the effects of different doses of insulin. Fieller also cites a very early paper (Marks, 1925) which described an application of the 2×2 design. Finney (1956) described the design and analysis of a number of different cross-over designs for use in biological assay. One sort of cross-over design with which we are not concerned here is when the whole trial is conducted on a single subject. These designs have also been used in biological assay. For further details see Finney and Outhwaite (1955, 1956) and Sampford (1957).

In this section we have given only a brief description of some of the early uses of cross-over trials that we are aware of. For a more comprehensive review of the uses of cross-over trials see Bishop and Jones (1984) and Hedayat and Afsarinejad (1975).

1.6 Notation and models

We assume that there are s different groups of subjects. Each group receives the t treatments in a different order and the trial is to last for p treatment periods. So for example, in a trial to compare three treatments using three periods there might be six groups of subjects corresponding to the six different treatment orderings: ABC, ACB, BAC, BCA, CAB, CBA. Each subject in group 1 would receive the treatments in the order ABC, each subject in group 2 would receive the treatments in the order ACB,..., and each subject in group 6 would receive the treatments in the order CBA. The response observed on the kth subject in period j of group i we denote by y_{ijk}.

We suppose that y_{ijk} is the observed value of a random variable Y_{ijk} which can be modelled, for example, as:

$$Y_{ijk} = \mu + s_{ik} + \pi_j + \tau_{d[i,j]} + \lambda_{d[i,j-1]} + e_{ijk}$$

The terms in this model are:

μ: a general mean
s_{ik}: the effect of subject k in group $i, i = 1, 2, \ldots, s, k = 1, 2, \ldots, n_i$
π_j: the effect of period $j, j = 1, 2, \ldots, p$
$\tau_{d[i,j]}$: the direct effect of the treatment administered in period j of group i
$\lambda_{d[i,j-1]}$: the effect of the carry-over of the treatment administered in period $j-1$ of group i, where $\lambda_{[i,0]} = 0$
e_{ijk}: a random error for subject k in period j in group i.

So, for example, the model terms for the three responses observed on the kth subject in each of groups 1 and 2 of our six-group example would be:

$$\text{Group 1: } Y_{11k} = \mu + s_{1k} + \pi_1 + \tau_1 + e_{11k}$$
$$Y_{12k} = \mu + s_{1k} + \pi_2 + \tau_2 + \lambda_1 + e_{12k}$$
$$Y_{13k} = \mu + s_{1k} + \pi_3 + \tau_3 + \lambda_2 + e_{13k}$$
$$\text{Group 2: } Y_{21k} = \mu + s_{2k} + \pi_1 + \tau_1 + e_{21k}$$
$$Y_{22k} = \mu + s_{2k} + \pi_2 + \tau_3 + \lambda_1 + e_{22k}$$
$$Y_{23k} = \mu + s_{2k} + \pi_3 + \tau_2 + \lambda_3 + e_{23k}$$

Where appropriate, we will also include second-order carry-over effects and/or direct treatment-by-period interaction effects in the model.

It is important to realize that in the above form of the model the subject effects are taken to be fixed rather than random. This we assume throughout the book, except in Chapter 2 when analysing data from the 2×2 trial without baseline values. There we assume, out of necessity, that the subject effects are random. The errors e_{ijk} are for most of this book assumed to be independent, identically distributed normal random variables with mean zero and variance σ^2. In Chapter 7 however, we consider the implications of relaxing this assumption.

The total of a set of data will be identified using the 'dot' notation. That is, a dot ($\cdot$) will replace a subscript to indicate that the data have been summed over that subscript. So for example,

$$y_{ij\cdot} = \sum_{k=1}^{n_i} y_{ijk}, \qquad y_{i\cdot\cdot} = \sum_{j=1}^{p} y_{ij\cdot}, \qquad y_{\cdot\cdot\cdot} = \sum_{i=1}^{s} y_{i\cdot\cdot}$$

The corresponding mean values will be denoted, respectively as

$$\bar{y}_{ij\cdot} = \frac{y_{ij\cdot}}{n_i}, \qquad \bar{y}_{i\cdot\cdot} = \frac{y_{i\cdot\cdot}}{pn_i}, \qquad \bar{y}_{\cdot\cdot\cdot} = \frac{y_{\cdot\cdot\cdot}}{p\sum_{i=1}^{s} n_i}$$

The transpose of a matrix or vector $\mathbf{a}$ will be denoted by $\mathbf{a}^{\mathrm{T}}$.

1.7 Model fitting

Our general principle is to fit models in a sequential manner using ordinary least squares or, where appropriate, generalized least squares. So, for example, we might fit the following models to the data obtained from the six-group example used in Section 1.6:

Model 1: $Y_{ijk} = \mu + s_{ik} + e_{ijk}$

Model 2: $Y_{ijk} = \mu + s_{ik} + \pi_j + e_{ijk}$

Model 3: $Y_{ijk} = \mu + s_{ik} + \pi_j + \tau_{d[i,j]} + e_{ijk}$

Model 4: $Y_{ijk} = \mu + s_{ik} + \pi_j + \tau_{d[i,j]} + \lambda_{d[i,j-1]} + e_{ijk}$

By comparing the regression sums of squares from these models we obtain the additional sum of squares that each new set of parameters accounts for after allowing for the contribution of parameters already in the model. Therefore, for our six-group example we would calculate:

1. the between-subject sum of squares (SS)
2. the additional SS for periods (after fitting μ and the s_{ik})
3. the additional SS for direct treatments (after fitting μ, the s_{ik} and the π_j)
4. the additional SS for carry-over (after fitting μ, the s_{ik}, the π_j and the $\tau_{d[i,j]}$).

The residual SS, for use in testing hypotheses, is taken as the residual after fitting the largest of our models, i.e. Model 4 in our example, above. If, in our example there were five subjects in each group, the skeleton form of the corresponding analysis-of-variance table would be as given in Table 1.2. The skeleton form contains only columns for the source of variation (Source) and degrees of freedom (d.f.).

Table 1.2 *Skeleton analysis of variance for six-group example*

Source	d.f.
Between subjects	29
Within subjects:	
Periods	2
Direct Treatments	2
Carry-over	2
Residual	54
Total	89

1.8 Some important concepts

Here we briefly give some definitions and define some important concepts that will be used in later chapters.

A direct treatment **contrast** is a linear combination $c_1\tau_1 + c_2\tau_2 + \cdots + c_t\tau_t$, where $c_1 + c_2 + \cdots + c_t = 0$. With two treatments there is only one such contrast and that is $\tau_2 - \tau_1$. The coefficients of this simple contrast are $c_1 = -1$ and $c_2 = 1$. With more than two treatments, however, a number of different sets of contrasts may be of interest. For example, for three treatments one set of contrasts is (a) $\tau_2 - \tau_1$ and $2\tau_3 - \tau_2 - \tau_1$, and another is (b) $\tau_2 - \tau_1$, $\tau_2 - \tau_3$ and $\tau_3 - \tau_1$. One contrast, $c_1\tau_1 + c_2\tau_2 + \cdots + c_t\tau_t$ is **orthogonal** to another $d_1\tau_1 + d_2\tau_2 + \cdots + d_t\tau_t$ if $c_1 d_1 + c_2 d_2 + \cdots + c_t d_t = 0$. The contrasts in set (a) are orthogonal but those in set (b) are not. In general we can always write down a set which includes up to $t - 1$ orthogonal contrasts. If sets of parameters in our model, when defined in terms of contrasts, are not orthogonal then the order in which these sets are sequentially added to our model, as described in the previous section, will be important. The significance of a set of parameters will depend on whether the other sets which are not orthogonal to it are included in the model or not. Only if the sets are orthogonal will the order be unimportant.

When modelling cross-over data it is very important to realize that one or more sets of parameters in our model may be intrinsically **aliased** with one or more other sets of parameters in our model. A formal definition of intrinsic aliasing is given in McCullagh and Nelder (1983, Section 3.5). Put simply, two sets of parameters are aliased if the design of the trial does not allow the data to provide separate estimates of each set of parameters. In the basic form of the 2×2 trial to be described in Chapter 2, for example, we cannot obtain separate estimates of (1) the difference between the two groups of subjects, (2) the difference between the carry-over effects, and (3) the direct treatment-by-period interaction. To obtain an unaliased estimate of the carry-over difference we must assume that there is no difference between the groups and no direct treatment-by-period interaction. The problem of aliasing is eased somewhat if run-in and wash-out baseline values are available or if more treatment periods are used.

Another important concept is **marginality**. Again the reader is referred to McCullagh and Nelder (1983, Section 3.5) for a fuller explanation of this concept. If we consider the usual linear model arrangement where we relate the parameters in the model to the response using a 'model' or 'design' matrix, then if the space spanned by the columns of the model matrix corresponding to a set of parameters S_1, say, is a subspace of the space spanned by the columns corresponding to another set of parameters, S_2, say, then S_1 is marginal to S_2. So, for example, in the basic form of the 2×2 trial the direct treatment and period effects are marginal to the direct treatment-by-period interaction. Therefore, it would not be sensible, in general, to test for the absence of the direct treatment and period effects in the presence of the direct treatment-by-period interaction. However, because of the aliasing described above, the position is not so clear regarding the carry-over effects. If the interaction can unequivocally be identified as carry-over, then estimating the direct treatment effects in the presence of the carry-over effects (i.e. in the presence of a particular type of interaction) is not unreasonable.

1.9   Aims of this book

It is the purpose of this book to provide a thorough coverage of the statistical aspects of the design and analysis of cross-over trials. We have tried to maintain a practical perspective and to avoid those topics that are of largely academic interest. The distinction is, of course, a difficult one and we have included some of the more abstract or speculative features of the subject where we consider that these may have more importance in the future. Although our approach is practically oriented, we mean this in a statistical sense. The topic is a vast one and embraces planning, ethics, recruitment, administration, reporting, and so on. Some, occasionally all, of these aspects will have a statistical component but it must be borne in mind throughout this book that the statistical features of the design and analysis are but one aspect of the overall trial. Other authors are far better equipped to write on the non-statistical aspects (accepting that there will be some overlap) and we refer to these for further reading on such topics. (See, for example, Gore and Altman, 1982; Faulder, 1985; Pocock, 1983; Friedman *et al.*, 1981.) There are also particular areas of research in which the cross-over trial plays a special and important role. Examples are bioequivalence testing and dairy science. We have not attempted to tackle the aspects that are special to these areas because we believe that such discussions belong more properly in the particular subject areas and because, again, others are better able to answer such questions. For more on bioequivalence testing see, for example, Westlake (1974, 1975, 1976, 1979a, 1979b); Mandallaz and Mau (1981); Kirkwood (1981); Selwyn and Hall (1984, 1985). For more on dairy science applications see, for example, Hoekstra (1987); Seeger (1980); Taylor and Armstrong (1953); Castle and Watson (1984); Broster and Broster (1984); Broster *et al.* (1981).

We have attempted to compromise in the level of statistical sophistication. Most of the 2×2 trial, which at the moment is by far the most commonly used in practice, is dealt with at a fairly elementary and discursive level that we hope will be accessible to those with limited statistical experience, including those whose primary role is not that of a statistician. The same is true of the introductory sections on multi-period (or higher-order) designs. To avoid over-lengthening the book however, we have been somewhat briefer in the other sections, and have expected more of the reader. This is particularly true of Chapter 7 where the most advanced material is to be found. We do not believe, however, that any of the material should prove taxing to statisticians with some experience of the design and analysis of experiments.

There is a continuing debate on the appropriate approach to statistical inference and this has found its way into some of the writing on cross-over trials. Also, unsurprisingly, there are features of the analysis of cross-over trial data about which there is disagreement, even within a particular inferential viewpoint.

We have adopted in general a fairly conventional approach to analysis, even in situations where, personally, we may be moving away from such a position. We feel it is fairest to try and reflect as best we can the currently accepted approaches in the overall viewpoint. Convention does of course tend to lag behind current developments and we have therefore made a point of reviewing critically, at the appropriate moments, some of the more recent developments and disagreements. There is little doubt that conventions will change in the future to a greater or lesser degree and such changes will develop out of current debates.

1.10 Structure of the book

In the next chapter we cover in some detail the 2×2 cross-over trial with continuous observations. This trial is by far the most commonly used in practice and this is reflected in the size of Chapter 2, which constitutes almost one-quarter of the book. We continue with the 2×2 trial in Chapter 3, where we consider binary and categorical observations. In this chapter we also develop methods that can be applied to binary and categorical observations from trials with more than two periods. Chapters 4 and 5 cover the remaining core of the cross-over material, dealing with two-treatment designs other than the 2×2 and with multi-treatment designs. The remaining two chapters are more specialized. A brief account is given in Chapter 6 of methods for the analysis of data from cross-over trials in which sequences of observations, or so-called **repeated measurements**, are collected from each subject from within each period. Finally, in Chapter 7 we discuss more recent developments in the subject in which more general models are considered for the random, or error, component of the observations. This chapter is at the moment of less practical relevance than the remainder of the book but it does give an idea of current research in the field, some of which may have an influence on future practice.

We do not formally describe methods of determining the number of subjects to be included in a cross-over trial. For an introduction to such methods see Fleiss (1986a), Lachin (1981) and Machin and Campbell (1987) for example.

CHAPTER 2

The 2 × 2 cross-over trial with continuous data

2.1 Introduction

In this chapter we consider data obtained from the 2 × 2 trial with and without run-in and wash-out periods. We assume that the response measured in each period of the trial has been recorded on a continuous scale. The analysis of binary and categorical data will be described in Chapter 3.

After introducing an example we describe two useful methods of plotting cross-over data. A linear model for the data is then introduced and used to derive two-sample t-tests for testing hypotheses about the direct treatment and carry-over effects. In addition, point and interval estimates of the differences between the treatments and between the carry-over effects are defined. A third useful plot is then described. Although all the hypothesis testing necessary for the 2 × 2 trial can be done using t-tests, we take the opportunity to describe the appropriate analysis-of-variance table for the 2 × 2 trial. Following the analysis of variance we then define the residuals from our model and use them to check the assumptions made about our model. Some inherent difficulties associated with modelling 2 × 2 data without baseline measurements are then discussed and some ways of overcoming these difficulties are described. Next the nonparametric form of the analysis is described and the chapter continues with sections on the use of run-in and wash-out baselines and on the analysis of covariance. This is then followed with a short section on how to deal with missing data and a section which describes a Bayesian analysis of the 2 × 2 trial. The chapter ends with a critical review of the 2 × 2 cross-over.

Example 2.1

To illustrate the various ways of analysing 2×2 cross-over data we will use the data listed in Table 2.1. These data, which were originally given by Patel (1983), were obtained in a trial involving subjects with mild to acute bronchial asthma. The treatments were single doses of two active drugs and we will label them as A and B, respectively. The response of interest was the forced expired volume in one second (FEV_1). Table 2.1 contains four FEV_1 values (in litres) for each subject and these are labelled as x_1, y_1, x_2 and y_2, respectively. It will be noted that we have deviated slightly from the notation defined in Chapter 1 in order to distinguish between the responses observed in the run-in and wash-out periods and the active treatment periods.

Although Patel gave no details of the trial, we will assume that half of the available subjects were to receive the treatments in the order AB and the other half were to receive the treatments in the order BA. However, not all subjects completed the trial and so the final set of results contains measurements on 8 subjects who received the treatments in the order AB and 9 subjects who received the treatments in the reverse order. The baseline FEV_1 measurement x_1 was taken during the run-in period immediately prior to giving the first treatment. Then 2 and 3 hours later FEV_1 measurements were taken again and the average of these is the y_1 value given in Table 2.1. A suitable period of time was then left before a second (wash-out) baseline measurement x_2 was taken. The second treatment was then administered and measurements taken at 2 and 3 hours to give the average value y_2.

For the moment, we will consider only the data collected during the active treatment periods, i.e. the y_1 and y_2 values. The inclusion of the baseline values x_1 and x_2 will be considered in Section 2.9. The values of y_1 and y_2 for each subject are given again in Table 2.2 along with their corresponding totals $(y_1 + y_2)$ and their differences $(y_1 - y_2)$. These totals and differences will be used in later sections.

The general notation to be used in this chapter is as follows. The subjects are divided into two groups of sizes n_1 and n_2. The n_1 subjects in group 1 receive the treatments in the order AB and the n_2 subjects in group 2 receive the treatments in the order BA. As defined in Chapter 1, the response on subject k in period j of group

Table 2.1 Patel's (1983) data – FEV_1 measurements

	Group 1 (AB)					Group 2 (BA)			
Subject	Run-in x_1	Period 1 y_1	Wash-out x_2	Period 2 y_2	Subject	Run-in x_1	Period 1 y_1	Wash-out x_2	Period 2 y_2
1	1·09	1·28	1·24	1·33	1	1·74	3·06	1·54	1·38
2	1·38	1·60	1·90	2·21	2	2·41	2·68	2·13	2·10
3	2·27	2·46	2·19	2·43	3	3·05	2·60	2·18	2·32
4	1·34	1·41	1·47	1·81	4	1·20	1·48	1·41	1·30
5	1·31	1·40	0·85	0·85	5	1·70	2·08	2·21	2·34
6	0·96	1·12	1·12	1·20	6	1·89	2·72	2·05	2·48
7	0·66	0·90	0·78	0·90	7	0·89	1·94	0·72	1·11
8	1·69	2·41	1·90	2·79	8	2·41	3·35	2·83	3·23
					9	0·96	1·16	1·01	1·25

Reprinted from Patel (1983), p. 2704, courtesy of Marcell Dekker, Inc.

Table 2.2 Data from active treatment periods – Patel's data

	Group 1 (AB)					Group 2 (BA)			
Subject	Period 1 y_1	Period 2 y_2	Total $y_1 + y_2$	Difference $y_1 - y_2$	Subject	Period 1 y_1	Period 2 y_2	Total $y_1 + y_2$	Difference $y_1 - y_2$
1	1·28	1·33	2·61	−0·05	1	3·06	1·38	4·44	1·68
2	1·60	2·21	3·81	−0·61	2	2·68	2·10	4·78	0·58
3	2·46	2·43	4·89	0·03	3	2·60	2·32	4·92	0·28
4	1·41	1·81	3·22	−0·40	4	1·48	1·30	2·78	0·18
5	1·40	0·85	2·25	0·55	5	2·08	2·34	4·42	−0·26
6	1·12	1·20	2·32	−0·08	6	2·72	2·48	5·20	0·24
7	0·90	0·90	1·80	0·00	7	1·94	1·11	3·05	0·83
8	2·41	2·79	5·20	−0·38	8	3·35	3·23	6·58	0·12
					9	1·16	1·25	2·41	−0·09

Table 2.3   *The group-by-period means for Patel's data*

Group	Period 1	Period 2	Mean
1(AB) $n_1 = 8$	$\bar{y}_{11\cdot} = 1\cdot57$	$\bar{y}_{12\cdot} = 1\cdot69$	$\bar{y}_{1\cdot\cdot} = 1\cdot63$
2(BA) $n_2 = 9$	$\bar{y}_{21\cdot} = 2\cdot34$	$\bar{y}_{22\cdot} = 1\cdot95$	$\bar{y}_{2\cdot\cdot} = 2\cdot14$
Mean	$\bar{y}_{\cdot1\cdot} = 1\cdot98$	$\bar{y}_{\cdot2\cdot} = 1\cdot83$	$\bar{y}_{\cdot\cdot\cdot} = 1\cdot90$

i is denoted by y_{ijk}, where $i = 1, 2, j = 1, 2$ and $k = 1, 2, \ldots, n_i$. The group-by-period means for Patel's data are given in Table 2.3.

2.2   Plotting the data

As with the analysis of any set of data, it is always good practice to begin by producing and inspecting graphs. A 'feel' for the data can then be obtained and any outstanding features identified. For the 2 × 2 cross-over trial two very informative types of graph can be produced by the following methods:

1. Plotting, for each group, the change in each subject's response over the two treatment periods. That is, for each subject k, in group i, the pairs of points y_{i1k} and y_{i2k} are plotted against the period labels and joined up. We refer to this plot as the **subject profiles** plot.
2. Plotting against the period labels the four group-by-period means $\bar{y}_{11\cdot}, \bar{y}_{12\cdot}, \bar{y}_{21\cdot}$ and $\bar{y}_{22\cdot}$, and joining them up. On the graph it is convenient to label these means in terms of the group and treatment they represent, i.e. as 1A, 1B, 2B, 2A, respectively. It is also convenient to join 1A with 2A and 2B with 1B. We refer to this plot as the **groups-by-periods** plot.

In both of these plots the vertical axis represents the response or mean response and the horizontal axis represents the periods.

For the data in Table 2.2 the plots obtained using method (1) are given in Figure 2.1 and the plot obtained using method (2) is given in Figure 2.2. One disadvantage of plot (1) is that if there is a large number of subjects the plotted lines become difficult to distinguish. A third useful plot will be described in Section 2.4 below.

It is clear from Figure 2.1 that there is a tendency for the FEV$_1$ values to be higher on treatment B, although some subjects have

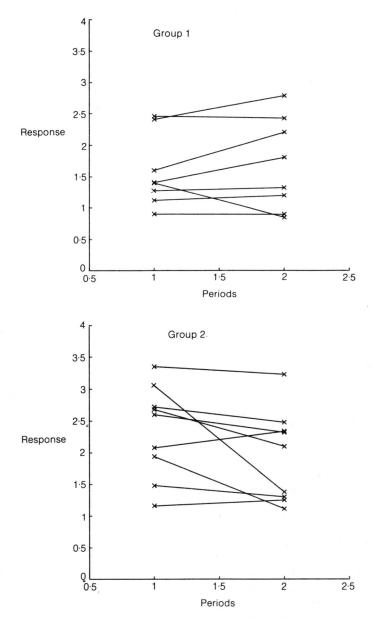

Figure 2.1 *Subject profiles for Patel's data.*

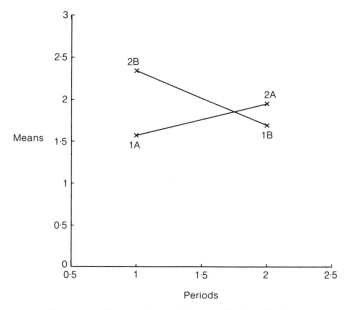

Figure 2.2 *Groups-by-periods plot for Patel's data.*

higher values on treatment A. Also, subject 1 in group 2 exhibits an unusually large drop in value between the two periods.

Figure 2.2 suggests that in the first period B gives the higher response, but in the second period it is A. The difference between the means of B and A is 0·77 in period 1 and is −0·26 in period 2. The statistical significance of these features will be considered in the next section.

Some general guidelines for interpreting the graph obtained by method (2) will be given in Section 2.7.

2.3   The analysis using *t*-tests

The linear model we assume for our data is as defined in Section 1.6 of Chapter 1 with $s = 2$, $p = 2$ and s_{ik} a *random* subject effect.

The fixed effects associated with each subject in each period in each of the two groups are displayed in Table 2.4, where τ_1 and τ_2 are the direct treatment effects of treatments A and B, respectively and λ_1 and λ_2 are the corresponding carry-over effects.

Table 2.4 *The fixed effects in the full model*

Group	Period 1	Period 2
1(AB)	$\mu + \pi_1 + \tau_1$	$\mu + \pi_2 + \tau_2 + \lambda_1$
2(BA)	$\mu + \pi_1 + \tau_2$	$\mu + \pi_2 + \tau_1 + \lambda_2$

The subject effects, s_{ik}, are assumed to be independent and identically distributed (i.i.d.) with mean 0 and variance σ_s^2. Similarly, the random errors are assumed to be i.i.d. with mean 0 and variance σ^2. In order to derive hypothesis tests it will be further assumed, unless stated otherwise, that the observed data are a random sample from a normal (Gaussian) distribution.

The linear model contains parameters to account for possible differences between the carry-over effects, if these exist, but no parameters to account for any direct treatment-by-period interaction. This interaction would occur if the difference between the direct treatment effects was not the same in each period. The reason we have omitted the interaction parameters is that, as there are only four sample means $\bar{y}_{11.}, \bar{y}_{12.}, \bar{y}_{21.}$ and $\bar{y}_{22.}$, we can include only three parameters at most to account for the differences between the means. Of the three degrees of freedom between the means, two are associated with differences between the periods and direct treatments, leaving only one to be associated with the carry-over and interaction. In other words, the carry-over and the direct-by-period interaction parameters are intrinsically aliased with each other. Indeed, there is a third possibility, that of including a parameter to account for the difference between the two groups of subjects. If this parameter is included, however, it too will be found to be aliased with the carry-over and direct-by-period interaction. This is one disadvantage of the 2×2 cross-over trial: several important effects are aliased with each other. This point will be taken up again in Section 2.7. For the moment however, we will present our analyses in terms of the model given previously, which includes the carry-over effect parameters λ_1 and λ_2.

In the remainder of this section we will describe how data from a 2×2 trial may be analysed using two-sample t-tests. This approach was first suggested by Hills and Armitage (1979) (see also Chassan, 1964). It will be noted that these t-tests are valid whatever the covariance structure of y_1 and y_2, the two measurements taken on each subject during the active treatment periods.

Testing $\lambda_1 = \lambda_2$

The first test we consider is the test of equality of the carry-over effects. We note that although we may wish to test the more specific hypothesis that $\lambda_1 = \lambda_2 = 0$, this cannot be done if the period effects are retained in the model.

In order to derive a test of the null hypothesis that $\lambda_1 = \lambda_2$, we note that the subject totals

$$t_{1k} = y_{11k} + y_{12k} \qquad \text{for the } k\text{th subject in group 1}$$

and

$$t_{2k} = y_{21k} + y_{22k} \qquad \text{for the } k\text{th subject in group 2}$$

have expectations

$$E[t_{1k}] = 2\mu + \pi_1 + \pi_2 + \tau_1 + \tau_2 + \lambda_1$$

and

$$E[t_{2k}] = 2\mu + \pi_1 + \pi_2 + \tau_1 + \tau_2 + \lambda_2$$

If $\lambda_1 = \lambda_2$ these two expectations are equal. Consequently, to test if $\lambda_1 = \lambda_2$ we can apply the familiar two-sample t-test to the subject totals. With this in mind we define $\lambda_d = \lambda_1 - \lambda_2$ and $\hat{\lambda}_d = \bar{t}_1. - \bar{t}_2.$ and note that

$$E[\hat{\lambda}_d] = \lambda_d$$

$$V[\hat{\lambda}_d] = 2(2\sigma_s^2 + \sigma^2)\left(\frac{1}{n_1} + \frac{1}{n_2}\right)$$

$$= \sigma_T^2 m, \quad \text{say,}$$

where

$$\sigma_T^2 = 2(2\sigma_s^2 + \sigma^2) \qquad \text{and} \qquad m = \frac{n_1 + n_2}{n_1 n_2}$$

To estimate σ_T^2 we use

$$\hat{\sigma}_T^2 = \sum_{i=1}^{2} \sum_{k=1}^{n_i} (t_{ik} - \bar{t}_{i.})^2 / (n_1 + n_2 - 2)$$

the pooled sample variance which has $(n_1 + n_2 - 2)$ degrees of freedom (d.f.)

On the null hypothesis that $\lambda_1 = \lambda_2$ the statistic

$$T_\lambda = \frac{\hat{\lambda}_d}{(\hat{\sigma}_T^2 m)^{1/2}}$$

has Student's t-distribution on $(n_1 + n_2 - 2)$ d.f.

In order to illustrate this test, let us refer back to Example 2.1 and the data displayed in Table 2.2. Using these data we obtain $\bar{t}_{1.} = 3\cdot2625$, $\bar{t}_{2.} = 4\cdot2867$ and $\hat{\lambda}_d = -1\cdot024$. Also $\sum_{k=1}^{8}(t_{1k} - \bar{t}_{1.})^2 = 11\cdot1823$ and $\sum_{k=1}^{9}(t_{2k} - \bar{t}_{2.})^2 = 14\cdot1006$. The pooled estimate of σ_T^2 is $\hat{\sigma}_T^2 = (11\cdot1823 + 14\cdot1006)/15 = 1\cdot6855$ and the t-statistic is

$$T_\lambda = \frac{-1\cdot024}{\left(\dfrac{17}{72} \times 1\cdot6855\right)^{1/2}} = -1\cdot623 \text{ on 15 d.f.}$$

As this is a preliminary test, prior to testing for a treatment difference, it is usual practice to follow the advice of Grizzle (1965) and to test the null hypothesis at the 10% two-sided level, rather than at the more conventional 5% level. His advice stemmed from results given by Larson and Bancroft (1963), who considered preliminary testing for multiple regression models. Some remarks on this advice will be made later in Sections 2.7 and 2.13.

There is insufficient evidence ($P = 0\cdot13$, where P is the significance level), to reject the null hypothesis. We can therefore proceed to test the null hypothesis of equal direct effects.

Testing $\tau_1 = \tau_2$ (assuming $\lambda_1 = \lambda_2$)
If we can assume that $\lambda_1 = \lambda_2$, then the period differences

$$d_{1k} = y_{11k} - y_{12k} \qquad \text{for the } k\text{th subject in group 1}$$
and
$$d_{2k} = y_{21k} - y_{22k} \qquad \text{for the } k\text{th subject in group 2}$$

have expectations

$$E[d_{1k}] = \pi_1 - \pi_2 + \tau_1 - \tau_2$$
and
$$E[d_{2k}] = \pi_1 - \pi_2 + \tau_2 - \tau_1$$

On the null hypothesis that $\tau_1 = \tau_2$ these two expectations are equal and so we can test the null hypothesis by applying the two-sample t-test to the period differences.

In particular, if we define $\tau_d = \tau_1 - \tau_2$ then $\hat{\tau}_d = \frac{1}{2}[\bar{d}_1. - \bar{d}_2.]$ is such that

$$E[\hat{\tau}_d] = \tau_d$$

and

$$V[\hat{\tau}_d] = \frac{2\sigma^2}{4}\left(\frac{1}{n_1} + \frac{1}{n_2}\right)$$

$$= \frac{\sigma_D^2}{4}m, \quad \text{say},$$

where

$$\sigma_D^2 = 2\sigma^2.$$

The pooled estimate of σ_D^2 is

$$\hat{\sigma}_D^2 = \sum_{i=1}^{2}\sum_{k=1}^{n_i}(d_{ik} - \bar{d}_{i.})^2/(n_1 + n_2 - 2)$$

On the null hypothesis that $\tau_1 = \tau_2$ the statistic

$$T_\tau = \frac{\hat{\tau}_d}{(\hat{\sigma}_D^2 m/4)^{1/2}}$$

has Student's t-distribution on $(n_1 + n_2 - 2)$ d.f.

Continuing our analysis of the data in Table 2.2, we obtain $\bar{d}_1. = -0.1175$, $\bar{d}_2. = 0.3956$ and $\hat{\tau}_d = -0.256$. Also $\sum_{k=1}^{8}(d_{1k} - \bar{d}_1.)^2 = 0.8783$ and $\sum_{k=1}^{9}(d_{2k} - \bar{d}_2.)^2 = 2.6980$. Therefore $\hat{\sigma}_D^2 = (0.8783 + 2.6980)/15 = 0.2384$ on 15 d.f. (The value of the SS for group 2 is somewhat larger than the SS for group 1 and this casts some doubt on the usefulness of the pooled estimate. We will ignore this for the moment, however, but will reconsider it in Section 2.6.)

The t-statistic is

$$T_\tau = \frac{-0.256}{\left(\frac{17}{72} \times \frac{0.2384}{4}\right)^{1/2}} = -2.158 \text{ on 15 d.f.}$$

There is some evidence ($P = 0.05$) to reject the null hypothesis at the (two-sided) 5% level.

A $(1 - \alpha)\%$ confidence interval for the treatment difference $\tau_d = \tau_1 - \tau_2$ is

$$\hat{\tau}_d \pm t_{\alpha/2, (n_1 + n_2 - 2)}\left(\frac{m\hat{\sigma}_D^2}{4}\right)^{1/2}$$

where $t_{\alpha/2,(n_1+n_2-2)}$ is the upper $(\alpha/2)\%$ point of the t-distribution on $(n_1 + n_2 - 2)$ d.f.

Putting in our observed values and a t-value of $2\cdot131$, we have that $(-0\cdot509 \leqslant \tau_d \leqslant -0\cdot003)$ is a 95% confidence interval for τ_d.

If it is of interest to test for a difference between the period effects we proceed as follows.

Testing $\pi_1 = \pi_2$ (assuming $\lambda_1 = \lambda_2$)
In order to test the null hypothesis that $\pi_1 = \pi_2$ we use the 'cross-over' differences

$$c_{1k} = d_{1k} = y_{11k} - y_{12k} \qquad \text{for the } k\text{th subject in group 1}$$

and

$$c_{2k} = -d_{2k} = y_{22k} - y_{21k} \qquad \text{for the } k\text{th subject in group 2}$$

If $\lambda_1 = \lambda_2$ then

$$E[c_{1k}] = \pi_1 - \pi_2 + \tau_1 - \tau_2$$

and

$$E[c_{2k}] = \pi_2 - \pi_1 + \tau_1 - \tau_2$$

If $\pi_1 = \pi_2$ these expectations are equal and consequently to test the null hypothesis we apply the two-sample t-test to the cross-over differences. That is, if $\pi_d = \pi_1 - \pi_2$ and $\hat{\pi}_d = \frac{1}{2}(\bar{c}_1. - \bar{c}_2.)$ then, on the null hypothesis,

$$T_\pi = \frac{\hat{\pi}_d}{(\hat{\sigma}_D^2 m/4)^{1/2}}$$

has Student's t-distribution on $(n_1 + n_2 - 2)$ d.f.

For our example data, $\hat{\pi}_d = \frac{1}{2}(-0\cdot1175 + 0\cdot3956) = 0\cdot1395$ and $T_\pi = 1\cdot176$ on 15 d.f. At the 5% level there is insufficient evidence $(P = 0\cdot26)$ to reject the null hypothesis of equal period effects.

What if $\lambda_1 \neq \lambda_2$?
If we reject the hypothesis that $\lambda_1 = \lambda_2$ then we cannot proceed to test $\tau_1 = \tau_2$ and $\pi_1 = \pi_2$ in the same way as done above. To see this we note that if $\lambda_d = \lambda_1 - \lambda_2 \neq 0$ then

$$E[\hat{\tau}_d] = E[\tfrac{1}{2}(\bar{d}_1. - \bar{d}_2.)] = \tau_d - \frac{\lambda_d}{2}$$

That is, $\hat{\tau}_d$ is no longer an unbiased estimator of τ_d if $\lambda_d \neq 0$.

By noting that

$$\hat{\lambda}_d = \bar{y}_{11\cdot} + \bar{y}_{12\cdot} - \bar{y}_{21\cdot} - \bar{y}_{22\cdot}$$

and

$$\hat{\tau}_d = \tfrac{1}{2}[\bar{y}_{11\cdot} - \bar{y}_{12\cdot} - \bar{y}_{21\cdot} + \bar{y}_{22\cdot}]$$

we see that an unbiased estimator of τ_d, given that $\lambda_d \neq 0$, is

$$\hat{\tau}_d | \lambda_d = \tfrac{1}{2}[\bar{y}_{11\cdot} - \bar{y}_{12\cdot} - \bar{y}_{21\cdot} + \bar{y}_{22\cdot}] + \tfrac{1}{2}[\bar{y}_{11\cdot} + \bar{y}_{12\cdot} - \bar{y}_{21\cdot} - \bar{y}_{22\cdot}]$$

$$= \bar{y}_{11\cdot} - \bar{y}_{21\cdot}.$$

That is, $\hat{\tau}_d | \lambda_d$ is the difference between the groups in terms of their first-period means. Also, $V[\hat{\tau}_d | \lambda_d] = m(\sigma_s^2 + \sigma^2)$, in our previous notation.

In other words, if $\lambda_d \neq 0$ then the estimator of τ_d is based on **between-subject** information and is the estimator we would have obtained if the trial has been designed as a parallel-group study. Whether or not this between-subjects estimator of τ_d will be sufficiently precise to detect a direct treatment difference of the size envisaged when the trial was planned will now be in doubt. At the planning stage, the size of the trial was probably determined on the assumption that the within-subjects estimator $\hat{\tau}_d$ was going to be used.

To test the null hypothesis that $\tau_d = 0$ given that $\lambda_d \neq 0$ we would still use a two-sample t-test, but would estimate $\sigma_s^2 + \sigma^2$ using only the first-period data. An example is given in Section 2.7.

A further problem of course is that if we reject the null hypothesis that $\lambda_d = 0$ we then have to decide if this is the result of differential carry-over effects, direct-by-period interaction or a difference between the two groups of subjects. We will take up this important point in Section 2.7, where we also mention some other suggestions of how to proceed if $\lambda_d \neq 0$.

2.4 Plotting subject differences and totals

It should be apparent from the results presented in the previous section that the test of the null hypothesis that $\lambda_d = 0$ is based on comparing the groups of subjects in terms of the subject totals. (Recall $\hat{\lambda}_d = \bar{t}_{1\cdot} - \bar{t}_{2\cdot}$.) The larger the difference between $\bar{t}_{1\cdot}$ and $\bar{t}_{2\cdot}$, the more evidence there is to reject the hypothesis that $\lambda_d = 0$.

Similarly, given $\lambda_d = 0$, the test of the null hypothesis that $\tau_d = 0$

is based on comparing the two groups in terms of the within-subject differences. (Recall $\hat{t}_d = \frac{1}{2}[\bar{d}_1. - \bar{d}_2.]$.) The larger the difference between $\bar{d}_1.$ and $\bar{d}_2.$, the more evidence there is to reject the hypothesis that $\tau_d = 0$.

We can visually portray what the data have to tell us about $\hat{\lambda}_d$ and $\hat{t}_d$ if we plot for each subject the difference d_{ik} against the total t_{ik} and use a different plotting symbol for each group. A separation of the groups along the horizontal (t_{ik}) axis would suggest that $\lambda_d \neq 0$, and (assuming $\lambda_d = 0$) a separation of the groups along the vertical (d_{ik}) axis would suggest that $\tau_d \neq 0$. This plot of differences against totals for the Example 2.1 data is given in Figure 2.3. To aid the comparison of the groups, we have also drawn the convex hull of each group. That is, we have joined up the outermost points of each group. One obvious feature of the plot is that subject 1 in group 2 stands out as having an unusually large difference, as already noted in the discussion of Figure 2.2. It will also be recalled that the SS for the group 2 differences was relatively large, and this is mainly the result of the unusually large difference for subject 1. If for medical

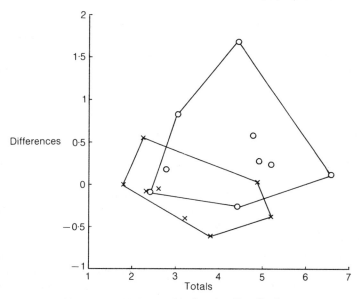

Figure 2.3. *Differences against totals plot for Patel's data.* × = *group 1;* ○ = *group 2.*

or other reasons it was decided that subject 1 in group 2 was no longer to be considered typical of the type of the subjects who should have been recruited into the trial, then it might be considered appropriate to remove subject 1 and reanalyse the data. We will not do this here, but will do it in the next section.

Comparing the groups in the horizontal direction there is quite clearly a good deal of overlap and hence there is no strong evidence to reject the hypothesis that $\lambda_d = 0$. We can therefore proceed to compare the groups in the vertical direction. The overlap this time is only slight and there is therefore some evidence to reject the hypothesis that $\tau_d = 0$.

The plot of the differences against the totals not only illustrates the features that would, hopefully, also be picked up by the t-tests, but it is a good way of getting an overall view of the whole data set. For example, the nature of the variability within and between the groups, in terms of the totals and differences, can easily be assessed. From this point of view this plot is one of the most useful and should be drawn as a matter of routine in any analysis of the 2 × 2 trial. Other plots have been suggested and some of these may prove useful additions to the differences against totals plot. For example, Huitson (1981), Hews (1981) and Barker *et al.* (1982) have suggested plotting for each subject, the period 2 observation against the period 1 observation and using a different plotting symbol for each group. Separation of the groups in various directions is then suggestive of differences between the period, direct treatment and carry-over effects.

2.5 The analysis of variance

Although we can test all the hypotheses of interest by using two-sample t-tests, it is important to note that we can also test these hypotheses using F-tests obtained from an analysis-of-variance table. The analysis-of-variance approach is also the most convenient one to follow for the higher-order designs that we will describe in later chapters.

The analysis-of-variance table for the 2 × 2 cross-over design has been a source of confusion in the past. Although Grizzle (1965) was the first to present the table, his results were only correct for the special case of $n_1 = n_2$. Grieve (1982) pointed out that Grizzle's later correction (Grizzle, 1974) did not clarify the situation, and went on to present the correct table. A correct table had earlier been given

Table 2.5 Analysis of variance of the full model

Source	d.f.	SS	EMS
Between-subjects: Carry-over	1	$\dfrac{2n_1 n_2}{(n_1+n_2)}(\bar{y}_{1\cdot\cdot} - \bar{y}_{2\cdot\cdot})^2$	$\dfrac{2n_1 n_2}{(n_1+n_2)}(\lambda_1 - \lambda_2)^2 + 2\sigma_s^2 + \sigma^2$
B-S residual	(n_1+n_2-2)	$\displaystyle\sum_{i=1}^{2}\sum_{k=1}^{n_i}\frac{y_{i\cdot k}^2}{2} - \sum_{i=1}^{2}\frac{y_{i\cdot\cdot}^2}{2n_i}$	$2\sigma_s^2 + \sigma^2$
Within-subjects: Direct Treatments (adjusted for Periods)	1	$\dfrac{n_1 n_2}{2(n_1+n_2)}(\bar{y}_{11\cdot} - \bar{y}_{12\cdot} - \bar{y}_{21\cdot} + \bar{y}_{22\cdot})^2$	$\dfrac{2n_1 n_2}{(n_1+n_2)}\left[(\tau_1-\tau_2) - \dfrac{(\lambda_1-\lambda_2)}{2}\right]^2 + \sigma^2$
Periods (adjusted for Treatments)	1	$\dfrac{n_1 n_2}{2(n_1+n_2)}(\bar{y}_{11\cdot} - \bar{y}_{12\cdot} + \bar{y}_{21\cdot} - \bar{y}_{22\cdot})^2$	$\dfrac{2n_1 n_2}{(n_1+n_2)}(\pi_1-\pi_2)^2 + \sigma^2$
W-S residual	(n_1+n_2-2)	$\displaystyle\sum_{i=1}^{2}\sum_{j=1}^{2}\sum_{k=1}^{n_i} y_{ijk}^2 - \sum_{i=1}^{2}\sum_{k=1}^{n_i}\frac{y_{i\cdot k}^2}{2} - \sum_{i=1}^{2}\sum_{j=1}^{2}\frac{y_{ij\cdot}^2}{n_i} + \sum_{i=1}^{2}\frac{y_{i\cdot\cdot}^2}{2n_i}$	σ^2
Total	$2(n_1+n_2)-1$	$\displaystyle\sum_{i=1}^{2}\sum_{j=1}^{2}\sum_{k=1}^{n_i} y_{ijk}^2 - \frac{y_{\cdots}^2}{2(n_1+n_2)}$	

by Hills and Armitage (1979) in an appendix to their paper. This is presented in Table 2.5.

The columns in Table 2.5 are for the source of variation (Source), degrees of freedom (d.f.), sums of squares (SS) and, for information only, the expected mean squares (EMS). It is clear for the EMS column that, as noted before, it is only sensible to test the hypothesis that $\tau_1 = \tau_2$ if it can first be assumed that $\lambda_1 = \lambda_2$.

It will be noted that the total corrected SS has been partitioned into a SS between subjects and a SS within subjects. The between-subjects SS is further partitioned into a SS for carry-over and a SS for residual. This residual we refer to as the between-subjects residual or B-S residual for short. The SS within-subjects is partioned into (a) a SS for direct treatments (adjusted for periods), (b) a SS for periods (adjusted for direct treatments), and (c) a SS for residual. This residual we refer to as the within-subjects residual or the W-S residual for short.

It will be noted that the 2 × 2 cross-over is a simple example of a split-plot design. The subjects form the main plots and the time points at which repeated measurements are taken are the subplots. It will be convenient to use the split-plot analysis of variance in the analyses of the more complicated designs to be described in the later chapters. However, the 2 × 2 cross-over is the only design in this book where it is necessary to further partition the between-subjects variability.

In the following $F_{1,v}$ denotes the F-distribution on 1 and v degrees of freedom.

The analysis-of-variance table for our example is given in Table 2.6.

Table 2.6 *Analysis of variance for Patel's data*

Source	d.f.	SS	MS	F
Between subjects:				
Carry-over	1	2·2212	2·2212	2·64
B-S residual	15	12·6415	0·8428	
Within-subjects:				
Direct Treatments	1	0·5574	0·5574	4·68
Periods	1	0·1637	0·1637	1·37
W-S residual	15	1·7882	0·1192	
Total	33	17·4102		

The table does not, of course, contain an EMS column, but a column of calculated mean squares (MS). Also given in the table is an F column which contains the calculated values of the F-ratios which we define below.

To test the null hypothesis that $\lambda_1 = \lambda_2$, we calculate the F-ratio

$$FC = \frac{\text{Carry-over MS}}{\text{B-S residual MS}}$$

$$= \frac{2 \cdot 2212}{0 \cdot 8428}$$

$$= 2 \cdot 64 \text{ on } (1, 15) \text{ d.f.}$$

On the null hypothesis, FC is an observed value from the $F_{1,(n_1 + n_2 - 2)}$ distribution. As before (of course), there is insufficient evidence $(P = 0 \cdot 13)$ to reject the null hypothesis. We can therefore proceed to test the null hypothesis that $\tau_1 = \tau_2$. We do this by calculating the F-ratio

$$FT = \frac{\text{Direct Treatments MS}}{\text{W-S residual MS}}$$

$$= \frac{0 \cdot 5574}{0 \cdot 1192}$$

$$= 4 \cdot 68 \text{ on } (1, 15) \text{ d.f.}$$

On the null hypothesis, FT is an observed value from the $F_{1,(n_1 + n_2 - 2)}$ distribution. As before, there is sufficient evidence $(P = 0 \cdot 05)$ to reject the null hypothesis at the 5% level.

To test the null hypothesis that $\pi_1 = \pi_2$ we calculate the F-ratio

$$FP = \frac{\text{Periods MS}}{\text{W-S residual MS}}$$

$$= \frac{0 \cdot 1637}{0 \cdot 1192}$$

$$= 1 \cdot 37 \text{ on } (1, 15) \text{ d.f.}$$

On the null hypothesis, FP is an observed value from the $F_{1,(n_1 + n_2 - 2)}$ distribution. At the 5% level there is insufficient evidence $(P = 0 \cdot 26)$ to reject the null hypothesis.

2.6   Analysing the residuals

Any analysis is incomplete if the assumptions which underlie it are not checked. Among the assumptions made above are that the repeated measurements on each subject are independent, normally distributed random variables with equal variances. These assumptions can be most easily checked by analysing the residuals. If $\hat{y}_{ijk}$ denotes the estimated value of the response based on the full model, then the residual r_{ijk} is defined as

$$r_{ijk} = y_{ijk} - \hat{y}_{ijk} = y_{ijk} - \bar{y}_{i\cdot k} - \bar{y}_{ij\cdot} + \bar{y}_{i\cdot\cdot}$$

The r_{ijk} are estimators of the e_{ijk} terms in the full model and, if the model is correct, should share similar properties. However, although the r_{ijk} are normally distributed with mean 0, they are not independent and do not have equal variances. Their variances and covariances are given below, where k is not equal to q:

$$V(r_{i1k}) = V(r_{i2k}) = \frac{(n_i - 1)}{2n_i}\sigma^2$$

$$\mathrm{Cov}\,[r_{i1k}, r_{i1q}] = \mathrm{Cov}\,[r_{i2k}, r_{i2q}] = -\,\mathrm{Cov}\,[r_{i1k}, r_{i2q}] = -\frac{\sigma^2}{2n_i}$$

$$\mathrm{Cov}\,[r_{i1k}, r_{i2k}] = -\frac{(n_i - 1)}{2n_i}\sigma^2$$

All other covariances are zero.

It can be seen that if n_1 and n_2 are large and approximately equal, the r_{ijk} are approximately independent with equal variances. Rather than use these raw residuals, however, it is more convenient to work with the following 'studentized' residuals:

$$t_{ijk} = \frac{r_{ijk}}{(\hat{V}(r_{ijk}))^{1/2}}$$

where $\hat{V}(r_{ijk})$ is the estimated value of $V(r_{ijk})$ obtained by replacing σ^2 by the W-S residual MS. Each t_{ijk} has mean 0 and variance 1. Although their joint distribution is complicated, little is lost in practice if the studentized residuals are treated as standard normal variables. The distribution of such residuals obtained from regression models is discussed by Cook and Weisberg (1982, pp. 18–20).

The values of t_{ijk} are given in Table 2.7, where it will be noted that only one residual is given for each subject because $r_{i\cdot k} = 0$. It

Table 2.7 *The fitted values and residuals for Patel's data*

Group 1 (AB)					*Group 2 (BA)*				
Subject	y_{ijk}	$\hat{y}_{ijk}$	r_{ijk}	t_{ijk}	*Subject*	y_{ijk}	$\hat{y}_{ijk}$	r_{ijk}	t_{ijk}
1	1·28	1·25	0·03	0·15	1	3·06	2·42	0·64	2·79
2	1·60	1·85	−0·25	−1·08	2	2·68	2·59	0·09	0·40
3	2·46	2·39	0·07	0·32	3	2·60	2·66	−0·06	−0·25
4	1·41	1·55	−0·14	−0·62	4	1·48	1·59	−0·11	−0·47
5	1·40	1·07	0·33	1·46	5	2·08	2·41	−0·33	−1·42
6	1·12	1·10	0·02	0·09	6	2·72	2·80	−0·08	−0·34
7	0·90	0·84	0·06	0·26	7	1·94	1·72	0·22	0·94
8	2·41	2·54	−0·13	−0·57	8	3·35	3·49	−0·14	−0·60
					9	1·16	1·40	−0·24	−1·05

can be seen that subject 1 in group 2 has an unusually large studentized residual of 2·79. If the model and assumptions are correct we should not expect to see 'large' studentized residuals. Lund (1975) has tabulated critical values for determining whether the largest studentized residual is significantly large (at the 10%, 5% and 1% levels). The response values corresponding to unusually large studentized residuals are called **outliers** or **discordant values**. The larger the residual, the more discordant is the corresponding response. If outliers are found in a set of data then their response values should be carefully examined. After such an examination it might be decided to remove the values and to reanalyse the depleted data set.

More often than not, plotting residuals in various ways can be most informative. One very useful plot is displayed in Figure 2.4. In this plot the t_{ijk} values are plotted against their corresponding $\hat{y}_{ijk}$ values. If the assumptions of the model are correct, this plot should have the appearance of a random scatter of points. Any strong pattern is indicative of a failure of the assumptions to hold. The pattern in Figure 2.4 is, apart from the outlier mentioned already, quite satisfactory. Whether or not the studentized residuals are normally distributed can also be determined by plotting the residuals against their corresponding expected normal order statistics (Cook and Weisberg, 1982, pp. 53–58). If the plotted points deviate markedly from linearity then this is indicative that the residuals are not normally distributed. The 'normal probability plot' for our data is given in Figure 2.5. The pattern of the points suggests that the residuals are quite consistent with having been sampled from a normal

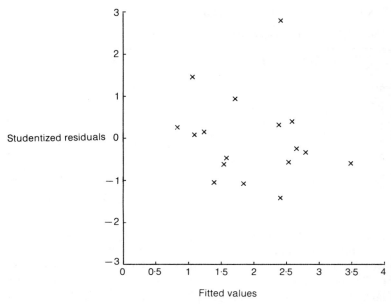

Figure 2.4 *Plot of t_{ijk} vs $\hat{y}_{ijk}$ for Patel's data.*

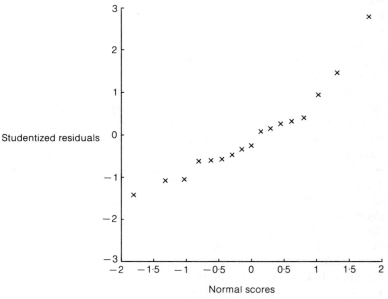

Figure 2.5 *Normal probability plot for Patel's data.*

Table 2.8 *Analysis of variance for Patel's data (subject 1 group 2 removed)*

Source	d.f.	SS	MS	F
Between subjects:				
Carry-over	1	2·0200	2·0200	2·24
B-S residual	14	12·6282	0·9020	
Within subjects:				
Direct Treatments	1	0·2485	0·2485	4·05
Periods	1	0·0276	0·0276	0·45
W-S residual	14	0·8602	0·0614	
Total	32	15·7846		

distribution. The null hypothesis that the residuals are normally distributed can also be checked using the test suggested by Shapiro and Wilk (1965). Applying this test here gives no evidence (at the 5% level) to reject the null hypothesis.

Let us suppose that subject 1 in group 2 is considered sufficiently unusual to be removed from the data set. The analysis of variance for the depleted data is given in Table 2.8. The group-by-period means, $\bar{y}_{11\cdot}, \bar{y}_{12\cdot}, \bar{y}_{21\cdot}$, and $\bar{y}_{22\cdot}$ are now 1·57, 1·69, 2·25 and 2·02, respectively. Removing this subject has reduced the difference between the means in the second group. The F-test for unequal carry-over effects is still not significant at the 10% level but now there is less evidence of a direct treatment difference. The value of FT is now 4·05 and P = 0·06.

The 95% confidence interval for the treatment difference is now $(-0·364, 0·012)$ and, of course, reflects the non-significant result from the F-test.

Although we have concentrated on the within-subject residuals r_{ijk}, we should also look at the between-subject residuals b_{ik}, where

$$b_{ik} = t_{ik} - \bar{t}_{i\cdot}.$$

Here b_{ik} is the residual for subject k in group i and t_{ik} and $\bar{t}_{i\cdot}$ are as defined in Section 2.3.

If the assumptions made about our model are correct, the b_{ik} should be i.i.d. with mean zero and variance

$$V[b_{ik}] = \frac{\sigma_T^2(n_i - 1)}{n_i}$$

where σ_T^2 was defined in Section 2.3.

Table 2.9 *Brown's (1980) data – improvement in dental hygiene*

	Group 1			Group 2	
Subject	Period 1	Period 2	Subject	Period 1	Period 2
1	0·83	1·83	1	1·67	0·33
2	1·00	2·17	2	2·50	0·50
3	0·67	1·67	3	1·00	−0·17
4	0·50	1·50	4	1·67	0·50
5	0·50	2·33	5	1·83	0·50
6	0·83	1·83	6	0·50	0·33
7	1·00	0·50	7	1·33	0·67
8	0·67	0·33	8	1·33	0·00
9	0·67	0·50	9	0·50	0·17
10	0·33	0·67	10	2·17	0·83
11	0·00	0·83	11	1·67	0·33
12	1·17	1·33	12	1·50	0·00
13	0·00	0·67	13	1·33	0·50
14	0·50	1·83	14	1·50	0·50
15	0·33	1·50	15	1·33	0·00
16	0·33	1·50	16	0·67	−0·17
17	0·50	1·17	17	1·67	0·50
18	1·00	1·67	18	2·50	0·67
19	0·00	1·33	19	1·83	0·00
20	0·50	1·50	20	0·83	0·67
21	−0·50	2·83	21	2·33	0·17
22	0·17	2·33	22	1·17	0·50
23	1·00	1·33	23	1·33	0·00
24	1·00	1·67	24	1·33	0·83
25	1.33	0·67	25	0·33	1·33
26	0·33	0·83	26	2.17	1·17
27	2·00	1·00	27	1·00	0·33
28	4·00	0·17	28	0·33	1·00
29	0·83	1·67	29	1·17	0·17
30	0·50	1·33	30	0·50	0·50
31	0·50	1·50			
32	0·50	1·67			
33	2·17	1·33			
34	0·67	1·17			

Reproduced from Brown, B.W. Jr. (1980) The crossover experiment for clinical trials. *Biometrics*, **36**, 69–79. With permission from the Biometric Society.

The studentized values of b_{ik} for Patel's data are, respectively, −0·54, 0·45, 1·34, −0·04, −0·84, −0·78, −1·20, 1·59, for group 1 and 0·13, 0·40, 0·52, −1·23, 0·11, 0·75, −1·01, 1·87, −1·53 for group 2. None of these is unusually large. Applying the Shapiro–Wilk test

Table 2.10 *Analysis of variance for Brown's data*

Source	d.f.	SS	MS	F
Within subjects:				
Carry-over	1	0·8626	0·8626	3·02
B-S residual	62	17·7364	0·2861	
Between subjects:				
Direct Treatments	1	18·9546	18·9546	39·96
Periods	1	0·9562	0·9562	2·02
W-S residual	62	29·4070	0·4743	
Total	127	67·4607		

confirms that there is no reason to reject the null hypothesis that the b_{ik} are normally distributed. In conclusion then, we have no reason to doubt our model as far as the subject totals are concerned.

We will return to these data again in Section 2.9 when the use of baseline measurements is considered.

Before leaving the topic of residuals, it is interesting to take another look at the well-known data set given by Brown (1980). These data are given in Table 2.9 and their analysis of variance is given in Table 2.10. Using this latter table, and following Grizzle's advice of using a 10% significance level, it will be found that the null hypothesis of equal carry-over effects is rejected (FC = 3·02, P = 0·09). The studentized residuals reveal, however, that subject 28 in group 1 has a studentized residual of 4·61. This is clearly an outlier and should be investigated further, but as is often the case with published data, it is not possible to do this here. If subject 28 is removed, however, and the data reanalysed, the null hypothesis of equal carry-over effects is now no longer rejected (FC = 2·19, P = 0·14). The decision to include subject 28 is therefore crucial to the subsequent analysis.

2.7 Follow-up analysis when carry-over effects are significantly different

The interpretation of the data in Example 2.1 was straightforward because there was no evidence to suggest that the carry-over effects were different. It was then possible to calculate an estimate and a confidence interval for the direct treatment difference $(\tau_1 - \tau_2)$. However, when the null hypothesis of equal carry-over effects is rejected the interpretation is much more difficult.

The main reason for the difficulty is that, in most cases, there is no unique explanation of why the null hypothesis was rejected. This stems from the inherent problem, mentioned earlier in Section 2.3, that the carry-over effects are aliased with the direct-by-period interaction and the group effects. To see this more clearly, consider writing the fixed effects in the full model as given below:

	Period 1	Period 2
Group 1	$\mu + \pi_1 + \tau_1 + (\tau\pi)_{11}$	$\mu + \pi_2 + \tau_2 + (\tau\pi)_{22}$
Group 2	$\mu + \pi_1 + \tau_2 + (\tau\pi)_{21}$	$\mu + \pi_2 + \tau_1 + (\tau\pi)_{12}$

Here $(\tau\pi)_{ij}$ is the interaction parameter associated with treatment i and period j.

If the usual constraints $\pi_1 + \pi_2 = 0$ and $\tau_1 + \tau_2 = 0$ are applied to the parameters, and we set $\pi_1 = -\pi$ and $\tau_1 = -\tau$, the model can be written as:

	Period 1	Period 2
Group 1	$\mu - \pi - \tau + (\tau\pi)_{11}$	$\mu + \pi + \tau + (\tau\pi)_{22}$
Group 2	$\mu - \pi + \tau + (\tau\pi)_{21}$	$\mu + \pi - \tau + (\tau\pi)_{12}$

If the usual constraints

$$(\tau\pi)_{11} + (\tau\pi)_{12} = 0$$
$$(\tau\pi)_{21} + (\tau\pi)_{22} = 0$$
$$(\tau\pi)_{11} + (\tau\pi)_{21} = 0$$
$$(\tau\pi)_{12} + (\tau\pi)_{22} = 0$$

are applied to the interaction parameters, and we set $(\tau\pi)_{11} = (\tau\pi)$, the model becomes:

	Period 1	Period 2
Group 1	$\mu - \pi - \tau + (\tau\pi)$	$\mu + \pi + \tau + (\tau\pi)$
Group 2	$\mu - \pi + \tau - (\tau\pi)$	$\mu + \pi - \tau - (\tau\pi)$

Using these constraints therefore reveals the aliasing of the interaction and the group effects. If, however, we use the less familiar constraints

$$(\tau\pi)_{11} = 0$$
$$(\tau\pi)_{21} = 0$$
$$(\tau\pi)_{12} + (\tau\pi)_{22} = 0$$

and set $(\tau\pi)_{22} = -(\tau\pi)$, the model becomes:

	Period 1	Period 2
Group 1	$\mu - \pi - \tau$	$\mu + \pi + \tau - (\tau\pi)$
Group 2	$\mu - \pi + \tau$	$\mu + \pi - \tau + (\tau\pi)$

That is, the interaction effects are now associated with the carry-over effects. See Cox (1984) for further, related discussion.

The constraints applied do not affect the numerical values obtained for the sums of squares in an analysis of variance or the estimates of any treatment contrasts. Therefore, whichever constraints are applied, the same numerical values will be obtained: it is their interpretation which will differ. For example, the analysis presented by Barker *et al.* (1982) is in terms of a model which includes parameters for the groups, rather than for the interaction or carry-over effects. The formulae for the sums of squares in their analysis of variance table are as given in Table 2.5 above, but they refer to the carry-over SS as the Groups (interaction) SS and their expression for EMS for Treatments is

$$\frac{2n_1 n_2}{(n_1 + n_2)}(\tau_1 - \tau_2)^2 + \sigma^2$$

A danger, therefore, of including group parameters is that it may appear that the null hypothesis $\tau_1 = \tau_2$ can be tested even if carry-over effects are present. This is not the case, of course, as Barker *et al.* point out, but such a parameterization might mislead the unwary. A difference between the groups implies that we cannot test for treatments.

If the null hypothesis of equal carry-over effects is rejected, there are, as suggested above, a number of possible causes, and additional information must be used to decide between them. The main point to note, however, is that once the null hypothesis of equal carry-over effects is rejected we have evidence of a treatment difference. Because of the intrinsic aliasing the problem left to sort out is that of deciding on a meaningful estimate and a meaningful interpretation of the difference between the treatments. The solution to this problem cannot be obtained from the results of the trial alone: additional background information on the nature of the treatments and periods must be used.

Some reasons why the null hypothesis $\lambda_1 = \lambda_2$ may be rejected are listed below:

1. There is a true carry-over effect. That is, the physical effects of the first treatment are still present when the subject enters the second treatment period. Using a 'wash-out' period between the two treatment periods should lessen the chances of a significant carry-over effect.
2. There is a psychological carry-over effect. Here the attitudes of the subjects as they enter the second treatment period depend on their experiences in the first treatment period. For example, if one of the treatments is a placebo and the other an active agent which relieves pain, the subjects who received the placebo may have suffered discomfort in the first period and feel unhappy about entering the second period. Such feelings might then affect their rating of the active agent.
3. There is a direct-by-period interaction. This literally means that the difference between the two direct treatments depends on the period in which they were administered. This might happen if the size of the difference between the treatments depends on the level of the response, e.g. the higher the response, the larger the treatment difference. If there is a period effect such that the response is higher (lower) in period 2 than in period 1, then the treatment difference observed in period 2 will be higher (lower) than in period 1. As an example, suppose that the level of response depended on whether the outdoor temperature was low or high. If all the responses in period 1 happened to coincide with a warm spell and those in period 2 with a cold one, there is likely to be a significant interaction effect.
4. The two groups of subjects differ significantly. This might happen if the randomization resulted in an unfortunate allocation of subjects to groups. This can sometimes be detected if additional measurements on each subject, such as age, sex, weight, etc., are recorded on entry to the trial.

Koch (1987) has also noted that the parameter associated with an interaction between the direct treatment effects in period 2 and the carry-over effects of the treatments in period 1 is also aliased with the carry-over difference and direct-by-period interaction. This new interaction could manifest itself in a way that would give the impression that the null hypothesis is being rejected because of reason

2 above. See Koch (1987) for further details and discussion.

Having found a significant difference in the carry-over effects (i.e. a direct-by-period interaction, etc.) the next step is to decide which of the above four possibilities (or combination of them) is most likely. The choice will depend on the particular features of the trial and so it is difficult to give detailed advice. However, Hills and Armitage (1979) have considered this matter and suggest that the presence of an interaction or different carry-over effects can sometimes be detected by looking at a plot of the four means $\bar{y}_{11\cdot}, \bar{y}_{12\cdot}, \bar{y}_{21\cdot}$ and $\bar{y}_{22\cdot}$. This groups-by-periods plot was described in Section 2.2, where it will be recalled that these four means were labelled as 1A, 1B, 2B and 2A, respectively. However, unlike Hills and Armitage, we join 1A with 2A and 2B with 1B. Some typical plots which might be obtained are given in Figure 2.6 (a), (b), (c) and (d). In all of these plots there is a period effect so that the means in period 2 are higher.

The parallel lines in plot (a) indicate that the direct treatment difference is the same in both periods, i.e. there is no direct-by-period interaction. Real data, however, will contain random variation and so exactly parallel lines will not be seen, even if there is no interaction. The significance test for parallelism is the t-test (or F-test) for carry-over effects as used earlier. If this is not significant, then the lines are parallel except for random perturbations. If the test is significant, the shape of the plot will indicate the nature of the non-parallelism. Then, of course, the plot will look like (b), (c) or (d).

These plots suggest either a true direct-by-period interaction or different carry-over effects. Plot (b) may be interpreted as suggesting that A has a large effect in period 1 which is carried over into period 2. Alternatively, the response may be such that it cannot exceed some natural limit. The difference is smaller in period 2 therefore, because A has reached this limit. Plot (c) may be interpreted as suggesting that there is a true direct-by-period interaction if the response is such that a large treatment difference is obtained if the response is high. Another explanation is that B has a carry-over effect which pushes up A in period 2. However, this is unlikely as B does not have a large effect in period 1. Plot (d) indicates a strong direct-by-period interaction as the treatment order is reversed. This could be explained by A having a very large carry-over effect, but it is more likely to be the result of a true interaction effect.

If it is decided that there is a significant direct-by-period interaction, it is sometimes possible to remove it by analysing transformed values of the response, e.g. analysing $\log(y)$ or $y^{1/2}$ instead of y. Of

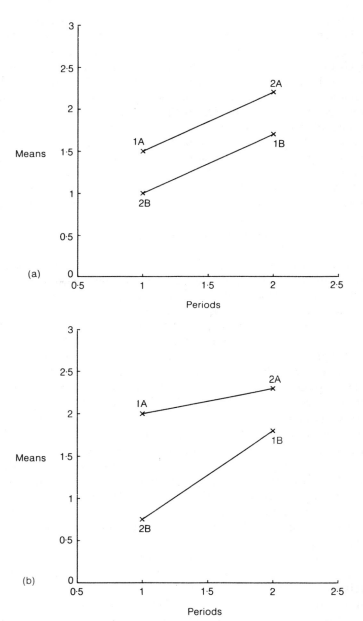

Figure 2.6 *Some typical groups-by-periods plots.*

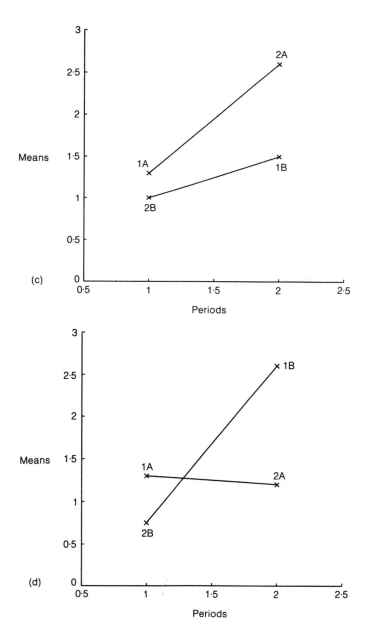

Table 2.11 *Grizzle's (1965) data – difference between pre- and post-treatment haemoglobin*

	Group 1 (AB)			Group 2 (BA)	
Subject	Period 1	Period 2	Subject	Period 1	Period 2
1	0·2	1·0	1	1·3	0·9
2	0·0	−0·7	2	−2·3	1·0
3	−0·8	0·2	3	0·0	0·6
4	0·6	1·1	4	−0·8	−0·3
5	0·3	0·4	5	−0·4	−1·0
6	1·5	1·2	6	−2·9	1·7
			7	−1·9	−0·3
			8	−2·9	0·9

Reproduced from Grizzle, J.E. (1965) The two-period change-over design and its use in clinical trials. *Biometrics*, **21**, 467–80. With permission from the Biometric Society.

course, the assumptions we made earlier about our model must now apply to the transformed data. If such a transformation cannot be found, or it is not convenient to present results on a transformed scale, then in the presence of a significant interaction we must decide whether: the treatment difference obtained in period 1 is to be used as our estimate of the true treatment difference; we should use the difference obtained in period 2; present both differences; take an average over the two periods; or abandon the trial.

If the significant interaction is the result of a difference between the carry-over effects, then one solution is to use only the data from the first period. These data are free of carry-over effects and might provide an unbiased estimator of the direct treatment difference.

Table 2.12 *Analysis of variance for Grizzle's data*

Source	d.f.	SS	MS	F
Within subjects:				
Carry-over	1	4·5733	4·5733	4·57
B-S residual	12	12·0067	1·0001	
Between subjects:				
Direct Treatments	1	3·5630	3·5630	2·86
Periods	1	6·2430	6·2430	5·01
W-S residual	12	14·9442	1·2453	
Total	27	42·9100		

However the situation is complicated by the use of the first period data **only following a significant interaction test**. We return to this point in Section 2.13. Also the variance of this estimator, as we said in Section 2.3, includes a component due to the between-subject variability and consequently may be too imprecise to be useful.

In both the Patel and the Brown data sets, which we have used as our examples so far, there was no convincing evidence to suggest that the carry-over effects were significantly different. (Although the groups-by-periods plot for Patel's data did suggest that there might be a significant interaction.) A set of data which when analysed does provide evidence of unequal carry-over effects is that given by Grizzle (1965). These data are given in Table 2.11 and their analysis of variance is given in Table 2.12. The test for equal carry-over effects gives $FC = 4.57$ on $(1, 12)$ d.f. There is evidence $(P = 0.05)$, therefore, to reject the null hypothesis of equal carry-over effects. Consequently, it is necessary to consider these data further.

The studentized residual for subject 6 in group 2 is 1.98 which, although on the large side, is probably not large enough to warrant removing that subject from the data set. Apart from this, the plot

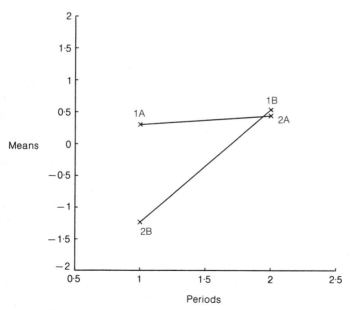

Figure 2.7 *Groups-by-periods plot for Grizzle's data.*

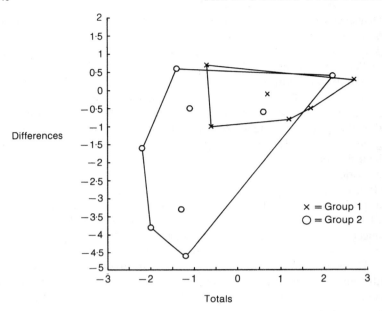

Figure 2.8 *Differences-vs-totals plot for Grizzle's data.*

of the residuals reveals nothing odd. The plot of the means, given in Figure 2.7, suggests that there is a strong direct-by-period interaction: the estimate of the treatment difference $\tau_1 - \tau_2$ in period 1 is large and positive whereas in period 2 it is small and negative. Such a dramatic change cannot be explained sensibly without more information concerning the conduct of the trial and of the nature of the treatments. However, for the purposes of illustration, these data will be considered further.

The plot of the differences vs the totals, as described in Section 2.4, is given in Figure 2.8.

It is apparent from Figure 2.8 that the variability of the differences is much larger in group 2. If the model is correct, the variance should be the same in both groups. Clearly, there is some evidence that the model is not correct. We reconsider the fitted model at the end of this section.

It would appear from the pattern of the means in Figure 2.7 that an explanation in terms of unequal carry-over effects seems reasonable: treatment A has a strong effect and a large carry-over into period 2, whereas B is relatively ineffective. A large direct treatment difference is observed in period 1, therefore, but not in period 2.

As mentioned earlier, an estimate of the direct treatment difference can be obtained by using the data from period 1, i.e.

$$\hat{\tau}_1 - \hat{\tau}_2 = \bar{y}_{11\cdot} - \bar{y}_{21\cdot} = 1\cdot5375$$

The pooled estimate of $\sigma_s^2 + \sigma^2$ obtained from the period 1 data in each group is $1\cdot5666$ on 12 d.f.

A 95% confidence interval for $(\tau_1 - \tau_2)$ is given by

$$1\cdot5375 \pm 2\cdot179 \times \left(\frac{14}{48} 1\cdot5666 \right)^{1/2}$$

That is, $1\cdot5375 \pm 2\cdot179 \times 0\cdot6760 = (0\cdot06, 3\cdot01)$.

Some authors suggest using the data from both periods even when there is a significant direct-by-period interaction. Poloniecki and Daniel (1981), for example, suggest that the relative sizes of the estimated direct treatment difference and the interaction, obtained using both periods, should be compared. They argue that a statistically significant interaction effect may, in fact, be clinically unimportant and draw attention away from a real treatment difference. Conversely, a large interaction may be statistically insignificant and get overlooked. Expressed in terms of our earlier notation, they make the point that if $|(\tau\pi)| \geqslant |\tau|$, then this would imply that one treatment is better in one period but not in the other. If this condition on $(\tau\pi)$ does not hold then, of course, a treatment preference may be deduced even though, perhaps, the exact size of the treatment difference is in doubt. See also Poloniecki and Pearce (1983) and the subsequent comments of Grieve (1985).

Willan and Pater (1986a) also take issue with the advice given by Grizzle (1965) that the data in the second period should not be used if the hypothesis of equal carry-over effects ($H_\lambda: \lambda_1 = \lambda_2$) is rejected. In order to present their findings we recall that $\hat{\tau}_d = \frac{1}{2}[\bar{y}_{11\cdot} - \bar{y}_{12\cdot} - \bar{y}_{21\cdot} + \bar{y}_{22\cdot}]$ is the estimator of τ_d obtained from using the data in both periods and that $\hat{\tau}_d | \lambda_d = \bar{y}_{11\cdot} - \bar{y}_{21\cdot}$ is the estimator of τ_d obtained using only the data from period 1. Also, as done in Section 2.5, let FT denote the F-ratio used to test the null hypothesis of equal treatment effects ($H_\tau: \tau_1 = \tau_2$) and let FT1 denote the corresponding F-ratio obtained from the analysis of variance of the first-period data.

Willan and Pater show that, even though $\hat{\tau}_d$ is biased ($E[\hat{\tau}_d] = \tau_d - \lambda_d/2$), using FT will provide a more powerful test of H_τ than that provided by FT1, if and only if

$$\frac{\lambda_d}{\tau_d} < 2 - [2(1 - \rho)]^{1/2}$$

where $\rho = \sigma_s^2/(\sigma_s^2 + \sigma^2)$ is the correlation between the two repeated measurements on a subject, and it is assumed, for convenience, that $n_1 = n_2$. The strategy they propose using in practice is to use $F_{max} = \max(FT, FT1)$ as the test-statistic to test H_τ.

They also compared $\hat{\tau}_d$ and $\hat{\tau}_d | \lambda_d$ in terms of their mean squared error (MSE). The MSE of $\hat{\tau}_d$ is smaller than that of $\hat{\tau}_d | \lambda_d$, if and only if

$$\frac{\lambda_d^2}{4} < \frac{(1 + \rho)}{(1 - \rho)} \frac{\sigma^2}{n}$$

where $n = n_1 = n_2$.

Grizzle, it will be recalled, suggested that H_λ should be tested at the 10% two-sided level. If H_λ is rejected, Grizzle recommends that only the first-period data should be used. The disadvantage of this approach is, as Brown (1980) pointed out, that the test of H_λ lacks power as it is based on between-subject comparisons. Willan and Pater have also determined the power of rejecting H_λ for situations in which the analysis of the first-period data would be more powerful for testing H_τ than the analysis which uses the data from both periods. They concluded that in many circumstances in which the analysis of the first-period data provides a more powerful test of H_τ and a more precise estimate of τ_d, the Grizzle procedure is unlikely to result in its use.

In conclusion then, Willan and Pater have demonstrated that, even though $\hat{\tau}_d$ is a biased estimator, in many cases the bias is more than compensated for by the reduction in variance brought about by using the data from both periods.

In a follow-up paper, Willan (1988) calculated the nominal significance levels to specify when using the F_{max} statistic. These results, like those of Willan and Pater, are based on the assumption that no direct treatment difference in the first period implies no carry-over difference in the second period. Willan also considered the power associated with F_{max} and the precision of the resulting estimator of τ_d. Overall, he showed that the strategy of using F_{max} works quite well.

Grieve (1987a) pointed out that the Grizzle approach to testing H_τ is equivalent to a Behrens–Fisher problem, Behrens (1929); Fisher (1941), if the direct-by-period interaction is significant. This is because $\hat{\tau}_d$ can be expressed as the sum of two uncorrelated statistics which have unequal variances. Grieve compared three well-known approximations which have been suggested in the literature for solving the Behrens–Fisher problem but did not recommend any one in particular. The choice between them depends on one's favourite approach to inference: frequency, fiducial or Bayesian. One advantage of this approach is that even though the estimate of τ_d is obtained from the first-period data only, the estimate of the variance of $\hat{\tau}_d$ is obtained using the data from both periods. Yet another approach is to use a full Bayesian analysis and we do this in Section 2.12, where we describe the work of Grieve (1985).

We return now to take up the point mentioned earlier that the model used for Grizzle's data was incorrect. The estimated value of ρ for these data is $\hat{\rho} = -0.11$, which Grizzle suggests is evidence that the correlation among the repeated measurements is not large enough to have warranted using a cross-over trial. The basic problem with Grizzle's data is not this, however. Rather, it is that his data are differences between pre- and post-treatment responses and so any subject effects have been 'differenced out'. This feature is also present in Brown's data which were considered in Section 2.6. The estimated value of ρ is -0.21 when the outlier is removed. Brown's data were also obtained by differencing the raw data.

2.8 Nonparametric analysis

If the data from a cross-over trial are such that it would be unreasonable to assume that they are normally distributed, then the usual t-tests, as described in Section 2.3, can be replaced by Wilcoxon rank-sum tests, or equivalently by Mann–Whitney U-tests. As with normal data these nonparametric tests are based on subject totals and differences.

A nonparametric test would be required, for example, if the data could not be transformed to satisfy the usual assumptions or the observed response was categorical with more than four or five categories. The analysis of binary data and categorical data with a small number of categories is described in Chapter 3.

The nonparametric analysis for the 2×2 cross-over was first

Table 2.13 *Data from mouthwash trial*

Subject	Group 1 (AB) Period 1	Period 2
1	0·796	0·709
2	0·411	0·339
3	0·385	0·596
4	0·333	0·333
5	0·550	0·550
6	0·217	0·800
7	0·086	0·569
8	0·250	0·589
9	0·062	0·458
10	0·429	1·339
11	0·036	0·143
12	0·036	0·661
13	0·200	0·275
14	0·065	0·226
15	0·177	0·435
16	0·121	0·224
17	0·250	1·271
18	0·180	0·460

Subject	Group 2 (BA) Period 1	Period 2
1	0·062	0·000
2	0·143	0·000
3	0·453	0·344
4	0·235	0·059
5	0·792	0·937
6	0·852	0·024
7	1·200	0·033
8	0·080	0·000
9	0·241	0·019
10	0·271	0·687
11	0·304	0·000
12	0·341	0·136
13	0·462	0·000
14	0·421	0·395
15	0·187	0·167
16	0·792	0·917

described by Koch (1972) and later illustrated by Cornell (1980) in the context of evaluating bioavailability data. To illustrate the nonparametric tests we will use the data described in Example 2.2 and presented in Table 2.13. When analysed under the usual assumptions of normality, equal variance, etc., the residuals from the fitted model indicate that not all these assumptions hold. Transforming the data (using the log and square-root transformations) was not totally successful and so a nonparametric analysis is used.

Example 2.2

In this 2×2 trial an oral mouthwash (treatment A) was compared with a placebo mouthwash (treatment B). The trial was double-blind and lasted fifteen weeks. This period was divided into two six-week treatment periods and a three-week wash-out period. One variable of interest was the average plaque score. This was obtained for each subject by allocating a score of 0, 1, 2 or 3 to each tooth and averaging over all teeth present in the mouth. The scores of 0, 1, 2 and 3 for each tooth corresponded, respectively, to (0) no plaque, (1) a film of plaque visible only by disclosing, (2) a moderate accumulation of deposit visible to the naked eye and (3) an abundance of soft matter.

Of the 41 subjects who entered the trial, only 38 completed it. The reasons for the withdrawals were unrelated to the treatments. Of these 38, complete records were obtained for only 34. The reasons for the missing data were again unrelated to the treatments. The complete records are given in Table 2.13.

The analysis proceeds in exactly the same way as described in Section 2.3, except that the significance test we use is the Wilcoxon rank-sum test rather than the t-test.

The subject totals, period differences and cross-over differences are given in Table 2.14, along with their corresponding ranks. The ranking is done in terms of the total number of subjects, not separately for each group.

Testing $\lambda_1 = \lambda_2$

Although it has not happend with our subject totals, it is possible that some of them will be the same, i.e. there may be ties in the data. If this happens we assign to the tied observations the average of the

Table 2.14 *Subject totals and differences and their ranks*

Group 1 (AB)

Subject	Total	Rank	Period difference	Rank	Cross-over difference	Rank
1	1·505	30	0·087	25·0	0·087	31·0
2	0·750	20	0·072	23·0	0·072	30·0
3	0·981	26	−0·211	11·0	−0·211	15·0
4	0·666	18	0·000	18·5	0·000	28·5
5	1·100	28	0·000	18·5	0·000	28·5
6	1·017	27	−0·583	4·0	−0·583	6·0
7	0·655	17	−0·483	5·0	−0·483	7·0
8	0·839	23	−0·339	8·0	−0·339	10·0
9	0·520	14	−0·396	7·0	−0·396	9·0
10	1·768	34	−0·910	2·0	−0·910	3·0
11	0·179	4	−0·107	15·0	−0·107	21·0
12	0·697	19	−0·625	3·0	−0·625	5·0
13	0·475	12	−0·075	17·0	−0·075	24·0
14	0·291	6	−0·161	12·0	−0·161	18·0
15	0·552	15	−0·318	9·0	−0·318	11·0
16	0·345	9	−0·103	16·0	−0·103	22·0
17	1·521	31	−1·021	1·0	−1·021	2·0
18	0·640	16	−0·280	10·0	−0·280	13·0

Group 2 (BA)

Subject	Total	Rank	Period difference	Rank	Cross-over difference	Rank
1	0·062	1	0·062	22·0	−0·062	25·0
2	0·143	3	0·143	27·0	−0·143	19·0
3	0·797	21	0·109	26·0	−0·109	20·0
4	0·294	7	0·176	28·0	−0·176	17·0
5	1·729	33	−0·145	13·0	0·145	33·0
6	0·876	24	0·828	33·0	−0·828	4·0
7	1·233	29	1·167	34·0	−1·167	1·0
8	0·080	2	0·080	24·0	−0·080	23·0
9	0·260	5	0·222	30·0	−0·222	14·0
10	0·958	25	−0·416	6·0	0·416	34·0
11	0·304	8	0·304	31·0	−0·304	12·0
12	0·477	13	0·205	29·0	−0·205	16·0
13	0·462	11	0·462	32·0	−0·462	8·0
14	0·816	22	0·026	21·0	−0·026	26·0
15	0·354	10	0·020	20·0	−0·020	27·0
16	1·709	32	−0·125	14·0	0·125	32·0

ranks they would have got if they had been slightly different from each other. This can be seen in the columns of Table 2.14 which refer to the period and cross-over differences. There are, for example, two period differences which take the value 0·000. They have both been assigned the average of the ranks 18 and 19, i.e. a rank of 18·5. Let R_i = the sum of the ranks of group $i, i = 1, 2$. Under the null hypothesis that $\lambda_1 = \lambda_2$,

$$E[R_1] = n_1(n_1 + n_2 + 1)/2$$
$$E[R_2] = n_2(n_1 + n_2 + 1)/2$$

and

$$V[R_1] = V[R_2] = n_1 n_2(n_1 + n_2 + 1 - T)/12$$

where T is a correction for ties.

If there are no ties then $T = 0$. If there are v tied sets, with t_s ties in each set, then

$$T = \frac{\sum_{s=1}^{v} t_s(t_s^2 - 1)}{[(n_1 + n_2)(n_1 + n_2 - 1)]}$$

For our subject totals

$$E[R_1] = 315$$
$$E[R_2] = 280$$
$$T = 0$$

and

$$V[R_1] = V[R_2] = 840$$

An asymptotic test of the null hypothesis can be based on either R_1 or R_2. For R_1 we calculate

$$z = \frac{R_1 - E[R_1]}{(V[R_1])^{1/2}}$$

and compare it with the standard normal distribution.

The two-sided hypothesis would be rejected at the 5% significance level if $|z| \geqslant 1·96$. A similar test can be based on R_2. For our data $R_1 = 349$ and

$$z = \frac{349 - 315}{(840)^{1/2}} = 1·17$$

Therefore, there is insufficient evidence (P = 0·24) to reject the null hypothesis.

Testing $\tau_1 = \tau_2$, *given that* $\lambda_1 = \lambda_2$
The period differences and their ranks are given in Table 2.14. Letting R_1 now refer to the sum of the ranks of the period differences for group 1, our test statistic is

$$z = \frac{205 - 315}{(840)^{1/2}} = -3\cdot79$$

There is very strong evidence (P = 0·0002) of a direct treatment difference.
In the above test, $R_1 = 205$ and $E[R_1]$ and $V[R_1]$ are as before. In fact, as there are ties in the period differences, $V[R_1]$ should have been adjusted by using the value of T as defined above. However, as $T = 0\cdot00535$ here, we did not bother to include it in the test statistic, as it would have made little difference to the result.

Testing $\pi_1 = \pi_2$, *given that* $\lambda_1 = \lambda_2$
Using the ranks of the cross-over differences, we obtain $R_1 = 284$ and the test statistic is $-1\cdot07$. There is no evidence (P = 0·28) therefore to suggest a period difference.

The exact version of the Wilcoxon rank-sum test
If $n_1 + n_2$ is small (less than 12 according to Gibbons, 1985, p. 166) then the asymptotic test should be replaced by its exact version. To conduct this test we need the null distribution of the rank-sum statistic. The upper tail of this distribution has been tabulated by, for example, Hollander and Wolfe (1973, Table A.5). This table is in terms of m and n, where n is the size of the smaller group and m is the size of the larger. The table covers the following values of m and n: $m = 3, 4, \ldots, 10$ and $n = 1, 2, \ldots, m$ and $m = 11, 12, \ldots, 20$ and $n = 1, 2, 3$ and 4.
As we require $n = 16$ and $m = 18$ the tables are of no use. Indeed, for these group sizes, the asymptotic test was quite suitable. To provide an illustration of the exact test we will use the data from the subjects in the first half of each group. The resulting table obtained from these data is given as Table 2.15. We must emphasize that we are using this smaller set of data for the purposes of illustration only, and do not recommend basing inferences on fewer than the observed number of subjects!
To test each of our null hypotheses we compare the value of the

Table 2.15 *Subject totals and differences and their ranks (first-half data)*

Group 1 (AB)

Subject	Total	Rank	Period difference	Rank	Cross-over difference	Rank
1	1·505	16	0·087	12·0	0·087	16·0
2	0·750	8	0·072	10·0	0·072	15·0
3	0·981	12	−0·211	5·0	−0·211	7·0
4	0·666	7	0·000	7·5	0·000	13.5
5	1·100	14	0·000	7·5	0·000	13·5
6	1·017	13	−0·583	1·0	−0·583	3·0
7	0·655	6	−0·483	2·0	−0·483	4·0
8	0·839	10	−0·339	4·0	−0·339	6·0
9	0·520	5	−0·396	3·0	−0·396	5·0

Group 2 (BA)

Subject	Total	Rank	Period difference	Rank	Cross-over difference	Rank
1	0·062	1	0·062	9·0	−0·062	12·0
2	0·143	3	0·143	14·0	−0·143	9·0
3	0·797	9	0·109	13·0	−0·109	10·0
4	0·294	4	0·176	15·0	−0·176	8·0
5	1·729	17	−0·145	6·0	0·145	17·0
6	0·876	11	0·828	16·0	−0·828	2·0
7	1·233	15	1·167	17·0	−1·167	1·0
8	0·080	2	0·080	11·0	−0·080	11·0

rank-sum statistic for the group with the smaller number of subjects with the appropriate lower- and upper-tail values of the null distribution. As the distribution is discrete, we may not be able to achieve exactly the significance level we would like. For example, for $n = 8$ and $m = 9$ the closest we can get to a probability of 0·025 in each tail is to use the values of 51 and 93 obtained from Table A.5 of Hollander and Wolfe. These values correspond to a probability of 0·023 in each tail. If our observed statistic is 51 or smaller or is 93 or larger, we would reject the null hypothesis at the 4·6% significance level.

The observed rank-sum for testing $\lambda_1 = \lambda_2$ is 62, and so we have no reason to reject the null hypothesis. For testing $\tau_1 = \tau_2$ the rank-sum is 101, and so there is evidence of a direct treatment difference. For testing $\pi_1 = \pi_2$ the rank-sum is 70, and there is, therefore, no evidence of a period difference.

Point estimate of $\delta = \tau_2 - \tau_1$
Let us label the period differences in group 1 as $X_i, i = 1, 2, \ldots, m$ and the period differences in group 2 as $Y_j, j = 1, 2, \ldots, n$, where n is the size of the smaller group.
Before we can calculate the point estimate we must first form the $m \times n$ differences $Y_j - X_i$, for $i = 1, 2, \ldots, m$ and $j = 1, 2, \ldots, n$. The point estimate $\hat{\delta}$ is then half the value of the median of these differences.
To obtain the median we first order the differences from smallest to largest. If $m \times n$ is odd and equals $2p + 1$, say, then the median is the $(p + 1)$th ordered difference. If $m \times n$ is even and equals $2p$, say, then the median is the average of the pth and $(p + 1)$th ordered differences.
For the smaller of our example data sets, $m = 9$ and $n = 8$. Therefore, $m \times n = 72$ and the median is the average of the 36th and 37th ordered differences.
The ordered differences for the smaller data set are:

-0.232 -0.217 -0.145 -0.145 -0.025 -0.010 -0.007 0.008 0.022
0.037 0.056 0.062 0.062 0.066 0.071 0.080 0.080 0.089 0.104 0.109
0.109 0.143 0.143 0.176 0.176 0.194 0.251 0.273 0.291 0.320 0.338
0.354 0.387 0.401 0.419 0.438 0.448 0.458 0.476 0.482 0.505 0.515
0.539 0.545 0.563 0.572 0.592 0.626 0.645 0.659 0.663 0.692 0.726
0.741 0.756 0.759 0.828 0.828 1.039 1.080 1.095 1.167 1.167 1.167
1.224 1.311 1.378 1.411 1.506 1.563 1.650 1.750

The point estimate is $\hat{\delta} = (0.438 + 0.448)/4 = 0.221$.
Using the larger data set, the point estimate is $\hat{\delta} = 0.207$.

Confidence interval for $\delta = \tau_2 - \tau_1$
To obtain a symmetric two-sided confidence interval for δ, with confidence coefficient $1 - \alpha$, we first obtain an integer C_α using Table A.5 of Hollander and Wolfe (1973). To obtain this integer for our particular values of m, n and α we first obtain the value $w(\alpha/2, m, n)$ from the table. This value is such that, on the null hypothesis,

$P[W \geqslant w(\alpha/2, m, n)] = \alpha/2$, where W is the rank-sum statistic. The value of C_α is then obtained by noting that $[n(2m + n + 1)/2] - C_\alpha + 1 = w(\alpha/2, m, n)$.

On the null hypothesis, the integer C_α is, in fact, such that

$$P\left[\left(\frac{n(n + 1)}{2} + C_\alpha \right) \leqslant W \leqslant \left(\frac{n(2m + n + 1)}{2} - C_\alpha \right) \right] = 1 - \alpha$$

We then order the differences $Y_j - X_i$ as done in the previous subsection.

The $(1 - \alpha)$ confidence interval is then $(\frac{1}{2}\delta_L, \frac{1}{2}\delta_U)$, where δ_L is the C_αth ordered difference and δ_U is the $(mn + 1 - C_\alpha)$th ordered difference.

For our smaller data set $w(0.023, 9, 8) = 93$ and hence $C_\alpha = 16$. The confidence interval is then obtained as half the values of the 16th and 57th ordered differences. That is, a 95.4% confidence interval for δ is $(0.040, 0.414)$.

For large m and n, the integer C_α may, according to Hollander and Wolfe, be approximated by

$$C_\alpha = \frac{mn}{2} - z_{\alpha/2} \left[\frac{mn(m + n + 1)}{12} \right]^{1/2}$$

where $z_{\alpha/2}$ is the upper $(1 - \alpha/2)$ point of the standard normal distribution.

For our larger data set, and taking $z_{0.025} = 1.96$, we get $C_\alpha = 87$. That is, the 95% confidence interval is obtained by taking δ_L as the 87th ordered difference and δ_U as the 202nd ordered difference. The resulting 95% confidence interval for δ is $(0.102, 0.343)$.

We also note that for the smaller data set the asymptotic approximation gives 16, as we obtained from the exact formula.

Testing for equality of dispersion
For the above Wilcoxon rank-sum tests to be valid the data in each group must have the same variability. As our groups of subjects are (or should be) a random division of those available for the trial, this assumption will usually hold for cross-over data. However, if we are worried about this we can apply a nonparametric test to compare the variabilities of the groups. A test which does not assume that the medians of the two groups are the same is given by Moses (1963), and described in Hollander and Wolfe (1973, pp. 92–9).

2.9 The use of baseline measurements

It will be recalled that the test for the presence of a direct-by-period interaction (or different carry-over effects) uses the subject totals from which the subject differences have not been eliminated. Hence this test will generally be less powerful than that for a direct treatment difference. Although in the presence of a direct-by-period interaction we can still get an estimate of the treatment difference from the first-period data, this again uses between-subject comparisons. One way to increase the power of these tests is to use baseline measurements taken during the run-in and wash-out periods. Sometimes, for ethical reasons, for example, a wash-out period is not possible and only the first of the baseline measurements is taken. The analysis in this case is straightforward since the first baseline can be treated as a genuine covariate (see Section 2.10). We shall concentrate here on the case where both baseline measurements are available and the appropriate analysis is not so obvious.

To illustrate the analysis we return to Example 2.1 and the data given in Table 2.1. We will present a simple analysis based on the use of within-subject information only.

We have four periods and two sequence groups, hence a total of six within-subject degrees of freedom from which to estimate effects. Three of these correspond to the period effects. The remaining three correspond to the group-by-period interaction and contain information on the direct treatment effects, carry-over effects and direct-by-period interaction. There are two possible carry-over effects, a difference in treatment carry-over at the time of the second baseline measurement (first-order carry-over) and a difference in treatment carry-over at the time of the second treatment measurement (second-order carry-over). This second carry-over is aliased with the direct-by-period interaction. The way in which we partition the three degrees of freedom of the group-by-period interaction depends on the order in which we examine these various effects. In order to illustrate this we first define a linear model for the expectations of the observations. Let $[x_{i1k}, y_{i1k}, x_{i2k}, y_{i2k}]$ represent the four observations, in order of collection, from the kth subject in the ith group, that is the baseline and treatment measurements are represented by x_{ijk} and y_{ijk} respectively. We can write the expectations of these as in Table 2.16.

The parameter μ represents an overall mean, π_j the jth period

Table 2.16 *Expectations of the responses in each group*

Group 1 (AB)	Group 2 (AB)
$E(x_{11k}) = \mu - \gamma + \pi_1$	$E(x_{21k}) = \mu + \gamma + \pi_1$
$E(y_{11k}) = \mu - \gamma + \pi_2 - \tau$	$E(y_{21k}) = \mu + \gamma + \pi_2 + \tau$
$E(x_{12k}) = \mu - \gamma + \pi_3 - \theta$	$E(x_{22k}) = \mu + \gamma + \pi_3 + \theta$
$E(y_{12k}) = \mu - \gamma + \pi_4 + \tau - \lambda$	$E(y_{22k}) = \mu + \gamma + \pi_4 - \tau + \lambda$

effect ($\pi_1 + \pi_2 + \pi_3 + \pi_4 = 0$), and γ the group effect. Given correct randomization there is no real reason to expect a group effect, and the inclusion of γ from this point of view is rather artificial. However, its role in the model is rather to ensure that the least squares estimators of the other effects will all be within-subject contrasts. The remaining three parameters, τ, θ and λ represent, respectively, direct treatment and first- and second-order carry-over effects. (It should be noted that $-2\tau = \tau_d$ as defined in Section 2.3.) In more general terms, θ represents any difference between groups of the second baseline means and λ any direct-by-period interaction, whether due to carry-over differences or not. There are many ways in which effects can arise which are aliased with these two parameters. Our aim is to produce appropriate ways of isolating the two degrees of freedom which will include any such effects, should they exist. Some authors, for example Willan and Pater (1986b), set $\pi_1 = \pi_2$ and $\pi_3 = \pi_4$. Unless the treatment periods are very short compared with the wash-out period there seems little justification for this.

We now need to consider the assumptions to be made about the covariance structure of the four observations from each subject. This has really been unnecessary previously when we had only two observations from each subject. Conventional split-plot analyses of variance are based on the so-called **uniform** covariance structure in which the variances of the observations taken on a subject are constant and the covariances between pairs of observations on the same subject are constant. Observations from different subjects are independent. In other words the pattern of the dispersion matrix of the four repeated observations on each subject is:

$$\sigma^2 \begin{bmatrix} 1 & \rho & \rho & \rho \\ \rho & 1 & \rho & \rho \\ \rho & \rho & 1 & \rho \\ \rho & \rho & \rho & 1 \end{bmatrix}$$

This is the structure generated by a model which includes a random subject effect with variance $\sigma^2\rho$, and an error term with variance $\sigma^2(1 - \rho)$. In spite of the conventional adoption of this structure, we have found it to be too restrictive for general application in the 2 × 2 trial with baseline measurements (Kenward and Jones, 1987b, Section 3). For this reason the analyses in this section have been constructed in such a way that they are valid under any covariance structure. However, although we make no requirements about the covariance structure we shall still use ordinary least squares (OLS) estimates of the parameters defined in Table 2.16. Strictly, these are only optimal under the uniform structure (and some other less practically important structures) but they have the great advantage of simplicity and it is unlikely in practice that they will be much less efficient than the alternatives. In Chapter 7 we consider in more detail the implications of departures from uniformity and we describe there how generalized least squares estimators can be constructed for this problem.

We want to make inferences about the effects represented by τ, θ and λ and we shall always allow for possible period effects, i.e. the parameters π_j will always be retained in any model. We shall get different least squares estimators of τ, θ and λ, depending on the assumptions made about the others, but in all cases the estimators will take the form $\hat{c}_1 - \hat{c}_2$ where $\hat{c}_i$ is a contrast among the four means from group i, that is,

$$\hat{c}_i = w_1 \bar{x}_{i1\cdot} + w_2 \bar{y}_{i1\cdot} + w_3 \bar{x}_{i2\cdot} + w_4 \bar{y}_{i2\cdot}$$

where

$$\sum_{i=1}^{4} w_i = 0, \qquad \bar{x}_{ij\cdot} = \frac{1}{n_i} \sum_{k=1}^{n_i} x_{ijk}$$

and similarly for $\bar{y}_{ij\cdot}$. This means that any of the estimators can be defined using the set (w_1, w_2, w_3, w_4).

In the following we test hypotheses using t-tests. If a nonparametric analysis of the data is thought to be appropriate, then these t-tests should be replaced by Wilcoxon rank-sum tests.

If the linear model is fitted with all parameters present, then the estimators of the three effects of interest are defined by the following contrasts:

$$\tau \,|\, \theta, \lambda \colon \tfrac{1}{2}(1, -1, 0, 0)$$
$$\theta \,|\, \tau, \lambda \colon \tfrac{1}{2}(1, 0, -1, 0)$$

and

$$\lambda \mid \tau, \theta: \tfrac{1}{2}(2, -1, 0, -1)$$

where the notation $\psi_1 \mid \psi_2, \psi_3$ indicates the contrast for ψ_1, given that ψ_2 and ψ_3 are in the model. It is assumed that the other parameters (μ, γ and π_j, $j = 1, 2, 3$) are always included. We can interpret these estimators as follows. By including both θ and λ in the model we are in effect saying that the second pair of measurements cannot be used to compare the direct treatments. Hence the estimator of τ is based on the first treatment and baseline difference. This is standard practice, see for example Hills and Armitage (1979), although sometimes the first baseline is used as a covariate to improve on the precision of the estimator based on the simple difference. Since the estimators are optimal under our full model, whatever the covariance structure, the question arises as to the origin of this extra precision. By using the baseline as a covariate we have implicitly changed the model slightly. We return to this in Chapter 7 when the use of generalized least squares is considered.

The simple baseline differences, $x_{i1k} - x_{i2k}$, are used to estimate θ. This has also been suggested by Wallenstein (1979), Patel (1983) and Hills and Armitage (1979).

Finally, the difference between the average of the two treatment measurements and the first baseline measurement, $\bar{y}_{i..} - \bar{x}_{i1.}$, is used in the estimator of the direct-by-period interaction, λ. The average alone, $\bar{y}_{i..}$, is used in a 2×2 trial without baseline measurements, and here we use the first baseline measurement to remove the between-subject variation from the comparison based on this average.

In general, of course, we would not want to use the estimator of τ based on the first two measurements only, unless there was evidence that there was a carry-over effect or direct-by-period interaction. This points to the use of a sequential procedure which we discuss shortly. For this sequential procedure we need OLS estimators under forms of the model in which some parameters are set to zero. The estimator of λ under the assumption that $\theta = 0$ is defined by

$$\lambda \mid \tau: \tfrac{1}{2}(1, -1, 1, -1)$$

In this case we use the standard estimator of the direct-by-period interaction from a 2×2 trial without baselines, but replace the treatment measurements, y_{ijk}, by the (treatment – baseline) differences,

$y_{ijk} - x_{ijk}$. The only remaining model of interest is the one in which both θ and λ are zero. We then get the estimator of τ defined by

$$\tau: \tfrac{1}{4}(0, -1, 0, 1)$$

This does not involve the baseline measurements at all, and is the same estimator as we would use in a 2×2 trial without baseline measurements. In the absence of a carry-over effect or direct-by-period interaction this defines, under the uniform covariance structure, the optimal (i.e. least squares) estimator of τ. Hence an appropriate estimator of τ does not necessarily use baseline measure-

Table 2.17 *Contrasts for effects of interest*

Subject	$\theta\mid\tau,\lambda$	$\lambda\mid\tau$	τ
	Group 1 (AB)		
1	−0·0750	−0·1400	0·0125
2	−0·2600	−0·2650	0·1525
3	0·0400	−0·2150	−0·0075
4	−0·0650	−0·2050	0·1000
5	0·2300	−0·0450	−0·1375
6	−0·0800	−0·1200	0·0200
7	−0·0600	−0·1800	0·0000
8	−0·1050	−0·8050	0·0950
Mean	−0·0469	−0·2469	0·0294
Variance	0·0193	0·0055	0·0078

Subject	$\theta\mid\tau,\lambda$	$\lambda\mid\tau$	τ
	Group 2 (BA)		
2	0·1400	−0·1200	−0·1450
3	0·4350	0·1550	−0·0700
4	−0·1050	−0·0850	−0·0450
5	−0·0255	−0·2550	0·0650
6	−0·0800	−0·6300	−0·0600
7	0·0850	−0·7200	−0·2075
8	−0·2100	−0·6700	−0·0300
9	−0·0250	−0·2200	0·0225
Mean	−0·0019	−0·3181	−0·0588
Variance	0·0490	0·1019	0·0075

ments, as some authors have implied, for example, Willan and Pater (1986b, p. 284).

In order to produce a simple and robust analysis we confine ourselves to the comparison between groups of the contrasts defined above. For each effect, a particular contrast is calculated from each subject and the mean of this contrast is compared between groups using standard two-sample procedures, typically t-tests or corresponding confidence intervals. In this way it is not necessary to make any assumptions about the covariance structure, apart from the fact that the contrast has the same variance in each group. The values of the contrasts for $\theta|\tau, \lambda, \lambda|\tau$ and τ are given in Table 2.17.

It is only possible to use the measurement from the second treatment period in the estimation of the direct treatment effect if we are confident that there is no carry-over effect or direct-by-period interaction. We therefore begin by examining these effects, starting with the comparability of the groups at the time of the second baseline measurement, i.e. with θ. There are two reasons for starting with this effect. First, it is only logical to examine the direct-by-period interaction (λ) if the subjects are still comparable at the time of the start of the second treatment period, i.e. if $\theta = 0$. Second, the test with lowest power is likely to be the test for direct-by-period interaction and so it is desirable to increase this as much as possible. We get a more powerful test for λ if we can first assume that $\theta = 0$. It could also be argued that the comparability of groups at the end of the second wash-out period, that would be implied by $\theta = 0$, could also be taken to imply that a carry-over effect in the second treatment period would be unlikely. Hence one could perhaps regard this single test as a sufficient check on the validity of the direct treatment comparison. However, the absence of first-order carry-over could not be taken to imply the absence of a more general form of direct-by-period interaction, and this would need to be checked using the test associated with λ.

We therefore estimate θ using the contrast defined by $\frac{1}{2}(1, 0, -1, 0)$, i.e. we use the differences $\frac{1}{2}(x_{i1k} - x_{i2k})$ for each subject. We now apply this to the data from the asthma trial. Using Table 2.1 we have

$$\hat{\theta} = \tfrac{1}{2}(\bar{x}_{11.} - \bar{x}_{12.} - \bar{x}_{21.} + \bar{x}_{22.})$$

$$= -0.045.$$

The pooled variance of $\frac{1}{2}(x_{i1k} - x_{i2k})$ is 0.035 on 14 degrees of freedom,

hence the standard error of θ is 0·093. We could now test the null
hypothesis $\theta = 0$ using a two-sample t-test. A confidence interval is
more informative, for example the 90% interval for θ is ($-0·209$,
0·119). The effect is far from statistical significance, even at the 10%
level.

We next examine the direct-by-period interaction using the
contrast defined by $\frac{1}{2}(1, -1, 1, -1)$. From this we get $\hat{\lambda} = 0·071$ with
a standard error of 0·140. A 90% confidence interval is given by
($-0·175, 0·317$). As with θ, the effect is far from statistical significance.
Note that the confidence interval for λ is somewhat longer than that
for θ. However, in comparison to the estimate of λ we would have
used if we had not first assumed that $\theta = 0$, we have gained in
precision: the standard error for the estimate corresponding to
$\frac{1}{2}(2, -1, 0, -1)$ is 0·201. If we had no baseline measurements at all, we
would have had to estimate λ using the subject totals $y_{i\cdot k} = y_{i1k} + y_{i2k}$.
The corresponding standard error is 0·336, more than twice that of
$\hat{\lambda}$, indicating the importance of using within-subject comparisons.

In the absence of the two effects corresponding to θ and λ we use
the estimator for the direct treatment effect τ defined by $\frac{1}{4}(0, -1, 0, 1)$.
For the example we get $\hat{\tau} = 0·088$, with a standard error of 0·044.
When testing assumptions, as above, it is sensible to use a less extreme
level of significance than when testing the principal effect of interest.
In the confidence intervals for θ and λ, tests were made implicitly at
the 10% level. We reduce this to 5% for τ, for which we get a 95%
confidence interval of (0·011, 0·165). One end of this interval is close
to zero, hence the direct treatment effect is on the borderline of
statistical significance at the 5% level. The positive sign of $\hat{\tau}$ indicates
that treatment B is associated with the higher average FEV_1 levels.

The simple procedure therefore consists of three two-sample
comparisons, based on the three contrasts defined by $\frac{1}{2}(1, 0, -1, 0)$,
$\frac{1}{2}(1, -1, 1, -1)$ and $\frac{1}{4}(0, -1, 0, 1)$. These are orthogonal and hence
the contrasts comprise a complete decomposition of the three degrees
of freedom of the group-by-period interaction, although the usual
analysis-of-variance decomposition into independent sums of squares
is not appropriate under a general covariance structure.

If the observations have a distribution which is very non-normal
the two-sample t-tests can be replaced, as noted earlier, by appropriate nonparametric tests: the analysis is still based on the same three
contrasts.

If it is believed that either θ or λ is not zero, the treatment effect could be estimated using only the first two observations, i.e. using the contrast $\frac{1}{2}(1, -1, 0, 0)$. In the example the resulting estimate of τ is 0·101, with a standard error of 0·094, about twice the standard error of $\hat{\tau}$ obtained using both the treatment observations from each subject.

2.10 The use of covariates

It often happens in clinical trials that additional information is available about each subject, for example age, weight or disease state. These additional data are usually called **covariates** and they can be put to two important uses. It may be that we wish to know if a treatment effect is related to the values taken by a covariate. Or, if a covariate does not seem to be related to any treatment effect, it may be that it is still related to a subject's response and then the possibility exists that some of the between-subject variation can be accounted for by the covariate values. In this way the between-subject residual variance might be reduced. We can only use a covariate for this purpose if it is first established that the covariate is indeed unrelated to the treatment effect. In the 2×2 cross-over this second use of the covariate is relevant only for the investigation of the direct-by-period interaction because other comparisons are based on within-subject differences from which between-subject variation is eliminated. In this section we shall outline the ways in which covariates are used. The computation required by the analyses is standard, although more involved than that described previously, and can be done by most statistical computer packages. For further details of the computation involved we refer to Armitage and Berry (1987, Chapters 8 and 9).

A covariate may be categorical, like sex, or continuous, like weight. We shall begin by looking at the use of the former. The introduction of a categorical covariate is equivalent to introducing a further factor into the trial and we simply need to generalize the analysis of variance, as given in Table 2.5. Quite often the trial is run at a number of different treatment centres. The variable which identifies the centre is then a categorical covariate. Suppose, for example, that we have a single additional factor A (e.g. centre) with a levels. If the trial has a total of n subjects, the corresponding analysis of variance has the skeleton form given in Table 2.18.

An association between the covariate and the direct treatment

Table 2.18 *Skeleton analysis of variance for a 2 × 2 cross-over trial with an additional categorical covariate*

Source	d.f.
Between subjects:	
A main effect	$a - 1$
Direct treatment × Period interaction	1
A × Direct treatment × Period interaction	$a - 1$
Between-subjects residual	$n - 2a$
Within subjects:	
Period main effect	1
Direct treatment main effect	1
A × Period interaction	$a - 1$
A × Direct treatment interaction	$a - 1$
Within-subjects residual	$n - 2a$
Total	$2n - 1$

effect is indicated by a large *A*-by-direct treatment interaction. In the presence of such an interaction it is necessary to examine the treatment effect at each of the levels of *A*. This does not preclude the possibility of there being a clear overall treatment effect, but any such conclusion will depend on the differences in direction of the treatment effect among the levels of *A* and on the relative sizes of the treatment main effect and *A*-by-direct treatment interaction. It is possible to examine in a similar way the interaction between *A* and the direct-by-period interaction. The *A*-by-period interaction is included in the analysis-of-variance table for completeness but is unlikely to be of great interest. The generalization of this procedure to more covariate factors should be clear at this point. Should there be no interaction between *A* and direct treatments then the incorporation of *A* into the analysis with the aim of reducing the between-subject error amounts to its use as a blocking factor. Its effectiveness will then depend on the size of the *A* main effect mean square relative to the between-subjects residual mean square. If it was known before the trial that *A* was to be used in this way then subjects should be randomized within each level of *A* and it would then be essential that *A* be included in the analysis.

Suppose that we now have a continuous covariate. We take as an example a 2 × 2 trial from an investigation of the relationship between plasma oestradiol levels in women and visuo-spatial ability.

The study was carried out by Dr Robert Woodfield at King's College Hospital, London. Populations of women were chosen to reflect the widest possible range of plasma oestradiol concentration and our example is taken from one such population: women undergoing in-vitro fertilization (IVF). These were evaluated in the proliferative phase and at the end of ovarian hyperstimulation. These two conditions, corresponding to low and high oestradiol concentrations respectively, define the two 'treatments' in the trial. By selecting the times of the first test period it was possible to determine which condition a subject would have first. Hence it was possible to

Table 2.19 *Log (EFT) and IQ values*

	Group 1 (AB)		
Subject	Covariate (IQ)	Period 1	Period 2
1	98·8	4·399	3·779
2	75·0	4·748	4·524
3	92·5	4·202	3·185
4	82·5	4·487	4·154
5	100.0	4·614	3·724
6	117·5	2·376	1·297
7	90·0	4·123	3·656
8	103·8	3·463	2·452
9	106·3	3·123	1·258
10	108·8	3·455	3·089
11	106·3	4·132	2·734
12	103·8	3·539	2·742

	Group 2 (BA)		
Subject	Covariate (IQ)	Period 1	Period 2
1	117·5	3·166	3·625
2	118·8	3·714	3·273
3	88·8	3·209	2·667
4	112·5	2·692	3·175
5	91·3	4·406	4·638
6	87·5	4·890	4·971
7	101·3	3·470	2·141
8	101·3	3·732	4·008
9	101·3	4·644	4·307
10	107·5	3·792	3·646
11	103·8	3·605	2·452

randomize the allocation to the two sequence groups. After allowing for exclusions there were respectively 12 and 11 women in the two groups (low-to-high and high-to-low). Visuo-spatial ability was assessed using several tests. We use the results from one, the embedded figures test (EFT). This response is the time taken to complete a task, and therefore lower values correspond to a higher measured ability. The distribution of these times is highly skewed and following the investigator's approach we use a log transformation. The log-transformed EFT scores are given in Table 2.19 along with an IQ score for each subject. It is known that EFT score and IQ are strongly associated and we therefore introduce as our covariate the IQ score obtained at the time of the first-period test. The IQ score is obtained from a series of tests and is considered to be quite stable to changes in the conditions being compared. As well as accounting for some of the between-subject variation in log (EFT)

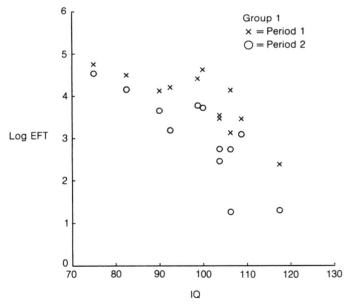

Figure 2.9 *Scatter plots of log (EFT) time against IQ for each group/period category.*

scores the inclusion of the IQ as a covariate allows us to investigate a possible association between IQ and the effect of condition on EFT score, should such an effect be found to exist.

We start by plotting the data. A scatter plot of log(EFT) times against IQ is given for each group in Figure 2.9. In these plots a different symbol is used for each period. As expected, there is a strong negative association between IQ and log(EFT) time, although this is much more apparent in group 1, and the relationship appears to be roughly linear. If the slope of this relationship were not the same for the two conditions (the 'treatments') this would indicate a relationship between IQ and the condition effect. However, it is difficult to detect this from the plots in the presence of possible period effects and, given the strong association, it is difficult to judge whether there is an overall effect associated with the conditions. As before, we get a clearer picture by looking separately at the subject totals and differences.

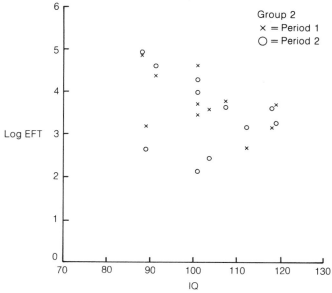

Figure 2.9 *Continued*

We first look at the subject totals. The plots of these are given in Figure 2.10 for each of the two groups. The strong negative trend is clear from this. As before, we use the subject totals to investigate the direct-by-period interaction, in this case the condition-by-period interaction, and a difference in the trend between the two groups would indicate that there is a condition-by-period interaction that changes with IQ, that is, a condition-by-period-by-IQ interaction. If the trend lines have the same slope in each group but are at different heights, this indicates the presence of a condition-by-period interaction that is independent of IQ. In keeping with conventional analysis of covariance we are assuming that relationships with covariates are linear. This need not be true of course, although it appears to be a reasonable assumption in this case, and the arguments used here can be extended to allow for nonlinear relationships. We test formally for these effects using the analysis of covariance of the

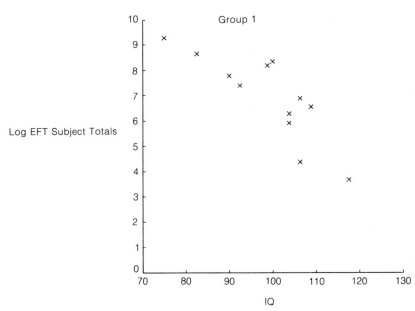

Figure 2.10 *Scatter plots of the subject totals of log (EFT) time against IQ for each group.*

Table 2.20 *Analysis of covariance of the subject totals*

Source	d.f.	SS	MS	F
Covariate (IQ)	1	21·030	21·030	14·68
Groups (Condition × Period)	1	2·982	2·982	2·08
Group × Covariate (Condition × Period × IQ)	1	2·463	2·463	1·72
Residual	19	27·214	1·432	

totals. We have here the simplest example of such an analysis, with one factor (Groups) with two levels and one covariate (IQ). The analysis of covariance table is presented in Table 2.20.

The large F-ratio for IQ confirms the strong association observed in the plots. The remaining effects are negligible. Although there is

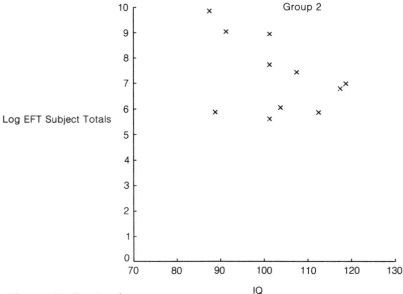

Figure 2.10 *Continued*

no evidence of an interaction with IQ this does not mean that the inclusion of the covariate has served no purpose. Its use has led to a reduction in the residual mean square from 2·52 to the observed value of 1·43. It can be seen from this how the use of a suitably chosen covariate is one method for increasing the sensitivity of the test for direct-by-period interaction.

We now consider the analysis of the within-subject differences. First we plot the differences in log(EFT) times against IQ for each of the two groups (Figure 2.11). The first thing to note is the preponderance of negative values, particularly in the first group. The period 2 − period 1 differences are being used in the analysis and this therefore suggests a large period effect with the second period scores being the lower. This is in fact expected from the nature of the test, for which there is likely to be a marked learning effect. There is a hint of a slope in the scatter plot for group 1 but not for group 2, which suggests at most a small interaction between IQ and the difference between the conditions. The analysis-of-covariance table for the differences is given in Table 2.21. Note the inclusion of the correction factor as a row in the table: in this analysis this corresponds to the period main effect and, as expected, the effect is very large. There are no effects associated with IQ but there is a large condition effect. Ignoring the covariate, the mean difference (low − high) in log(EFT) times between the conditions is 0·619 with a standard error of 0·229. This indicates a larger EFT time, that is lower ability, under the low oestradiol condition.

Table 2.21 *Analysis of covariance of the within-subject differences*

Source	d.f.	SS	MS	F
Correction factor	1	6·775	6·775	24·11
(Period main effect)				
Covariate	1	0·072	0·072	0·26
(IQ × Period)				
Groups	1	2·434	2·434	8·65
(Condition main effect)				
Group × Covariate	1	0·654	0·654	2·32
(Condition × IQ)				
Residual	19	5·344	0·281	

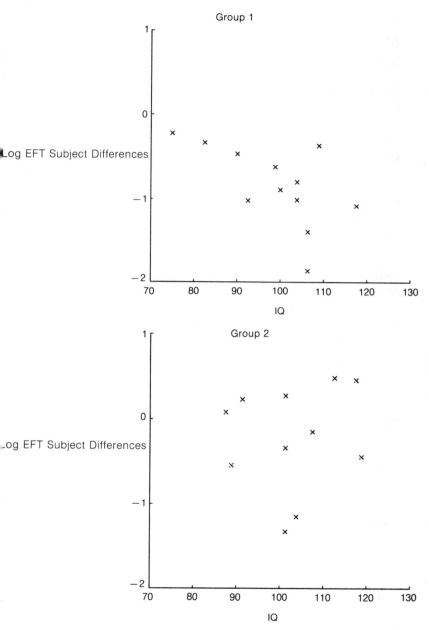

Figure 2.11 *Scatter plots of within-subjects log (EFT) differences against IQ for each group.*

2.11 Missing values

In this section we consider the analysis of data from the 2×2 trial in which some pairs of observations are incomplete. We assume that the reason why the observations are missing is unconnected either with the treatments or with the subjects' response. If this is not the case then the analysis is very much more difficult (see Gould, 1980, for example, in the context of parallel group trials). Suppose that in group i we have n_i subjects with complete pairs of observations (y_{i1k}, y_{i2k}), and m_{ij} subjects with a single observation z_{ijk} in the jth period ($j = 1, 2; i = 1, 2$). In the following we consider three methods of analysis. The first is the simplest: analyse only the complete pairs. Since the remaining data contain only between-subject information, the effect of discarding these observations is likely to be greater for the test of direct-by-period interaction. This test is already of low power so any further loss of sensitivity is undesirable, and arguably all the data should be used, if possible, unless only a small proportion of the subjects have missing values.

The second method of analysis was suggested by Patel (1985) and makes use of the simplification that occurs when observations are missing from the second period only, that is when $m_{12} = m_{22} = 0$. By using an unconditional dispersion matrix for the pairs (y_{i1k}, y_{i2k}),

$$V\left\{ \begin{bmatrix} y_{i1k} \\ y_{i2k} \end{bmatrix} \right\} = \Sigma = \begin{bmatrix} \sigma_{11} & \sigma_{12} \\ \sigma_{21} & \sigma_{22} \end{bmatrix}$$

and by using unconstrained cell means

$$E[y_{ijk}] = E[z_{ijk}] = \mu_{ij}$$

it is possible, with a suitable reparameterization, to partition the likelihood of the data into two components

$$l(\mathbf{y}_1, \mathbf{z}_1; \mu_{11}, \mu_{21}, \sigma_{11}) \times l(\mathbf{y}_2 | \mathbf{y}_1; \mu_{12}^*, \mu_{22}^*, \beta, \sigma_{2\cdot1})$$

where

$$\mathbf{y}_1 = (y_{111}, y_{112}, \ldots, y_{21n_2})^{\mathrm{T}}$$
$$\mathbf{z}_1 = (z_{111}, z_{112}, \ldots, z_{21m_{21}})^{\mathrm{T}}$$
$$\mathbf{y}_2 = (y_{121}, y_{122}, \ldots, y_{22n_2})^{\mathrm{T}}$$

and

$$\mu_{i2}^* = \mu_{i2} - \beta\mu_{i1}$$
$$\beta = \sigma_{12}/\sigma_{11}$$
$$\sigma_{2\cdot1} = \sigma_{22} - \beta\sigma_{12}$$

Since none of the newly defined parameters occurs in both components of the likelihood, the two components can be maximized separately. From standard results, we get from the first component

$$\hat{\mu}_{i1} = (n_i + m_{i1})^{-1}(y_{i1\cdot} + z_{i1\cdot})$$
$$= p_i \bar{y}_{i1\cdot} + (1 - p_i)\bar{z}_{i1\cdot}, \qquad i = 1, 2$$

where

$$p_i = \frac{n_i}{n_i + m_{i1}}$$

and

$$\hat{\sigma}_{11} = s_{11} = \frac{1}{n_1 + n_2 + m_{11} + m_{21} - 2}$$
$$\times \sum_{i=1}^{2} \left[\sum_{k=1}^{n_1} (y_{i1k} - \hat{\mu}_{i1})^2 + \sum_{k=1}^{m_{i1}} (z_{i1k} - \hat{\mu}_{i1})^2 \right]$$

and from the second component

$$\hat{\beta} = s_{12}^{(y)}/s_{11}^{(y)}$$
$$\mu_{i2}^* = \bar{y}_{i2\cdot} - \hat{\beta}\bar{y}_{i1\cdot}$$

and

$$\hat{\sigma}_{2\cdot1} = s_{22}^{(y)} - \hat{\beta}s_{12}^{(y)}$$

where

$$s_{jj'}^{(y)} = \frac{1}{n_1 + n_2 - 2} \sum_{i=1}^{2} \sum_{k=1}^{n_i} (y_{ijk} - \bar{y}_{ij\cdot})(y_{ij'k} - \bar{y}_{ij'\cdot})$$

are the sample variances and covariance from the complete pairs. Note that following conventional practice, the divisor in the maximum likelihood estimators of the dispersion parameters has been modified to make the estimators unbiased. From these estimators we can recover the estimators of the original parameters:

$$\hat{\mu}_{i2} = \mu_{i2}^* + \hat{\beta}\hat{\mu}_{i1}$$
$$= \bar{y}_{i2\cdot} - \hat{\beta}(1 - p_i)(\bar{y}_{i1\cdot} - \bar{z}_{i1\cdot}), \qquad i = 1, 2$$

and

$$\hat{\sigma}_{12} = \hat{\beta}\hat{\sigma}_{11}$$
$$\hat{\sigma}_{22} = \hat{\sigma}_{21} + \hat{\beta}^2\hat{\sigma}_{11}$$

Also the variances and covariances of $\hat{\mu}_{i1}$ and $\hat{\mu}_{i2}$ are:

$$V[\hat{\mu}_{i1}] = \frac{p_i}{n_i}\sigma_{11}$$

$$V[\hat{\mu}_{i2}] = \frac{1}{n_i}\left[\left(\frac{n_1 + n_2 - 3 - p_i}{n_1 + n_2 - 4}\right)\sigma_{22} - (1 - p_i)\left(\frac{n_1 + n_2 - 3}{n_1 + n_2 - 4}\right)\frac{\sigma_{12}^2}{\sigma_{11}}\right]$$

and

$$\text{Cov}\,[\hat{\mu}_{i1}, \hat{\mu}_{i2}] = \frac{p_i\sigma_{12}}{n_i}$$

These can be estimated by substituting the estimates given above for the unknown parameters.

The analysis is then based on the standard contrasts among the $\hat{\mu}_{ij}$. We have the direct-by-period interaction:

$$\hat{\lambda} = \tfrac{1}{2}[\hat{\mu}_{11} + \hat{\mu}_{12} - \hat{\mu}_{21} - \hat{\mu}_{22}]$$

and direct treatment effect:

$$\hat{\tau} = \tfrac{1}{4}[\hat{\mu}_{11} - \hat{\mu}_{12} - \hat{\mu}_{21} + \hat{\mu}_{22}]$$

The standard errors of these are obtained from the estimated variances and covariances of the $\hat{\mu}_{ij}$ and conventional statistics, e.g. $\hat{\lambda}/[\text{s.e.}(\hat{\lambda})]$, are used to construct the usual tests. Patel (1985) suggests using the t-distribution with degrees of freedom based on the number of completed pairs, i.e. $(n_1 + n_2 - 2)$, as an approximation to the null distribution of these statistics. He shows in a simulation study that this approximation is adequate in small trials, except possibly when the proportion of incomplete pairs is large, say greater than 40%. However, trials with so many missing values would arguably be of dubious value.

The third method of analysis to be described has a more *ad hoc* nature, but can be used when observations are missing from both periods. Simply, estimates are obtained separately from the complete and incomplete data and then combined using the estimated inverse variances as weights. For example, for the direct-by-period interaction we have from the complete pairs:

$$\hat{\lambda}_C = \tfrac{1}{2}[\bar{y}_{11\cdot} + \bar{y}_{12\cdot} - \bar{y}_{21\cdot} - \bar{y}_{22\cdot}]$$

and from the incomplete pairs:

$$\hat{\lambda}_I = \tfrac{1}{2}[\bar{z}_{11\cdot} + \bar{z}_{12\cdot} - \bar{z}_{21\cdot} - \bar{z}_{22\cdot}]$$

Assuming that the variance is the same in both periods we can write

$$\Sigma = \begin{bmatrix} \sigma^2 + \sigma_s^2 & \sigma_s^2 \\ \sigma_s^2 & \sigma^2 + \sigma_s^2 \end{bmatrix}$$

and then

$$V[\hat{\lambda}_C] = \frac{1}{2}\left(\frac{1}{n_1} + \frac{1}{n_2}\right)(2\sigma_s^2 + \sigma^2)$$

$$= K_C(2\sigma_s^2 + \sigma^2)$$

and

$$V[\hat{\lambda}_I] = \frac{1}{4}\left(\frac{1}{m_{11}} + \frac{1}{m_{12}} + \frac{1}{m_{21}} + \frac{1}{m_{22}}\right)(\sigma_s^2 + \sigma^2)$$

$$= K_I(\sigma_s^2 + \sigma^2)$$

Combining the two estimates $\hat{\lambda}_C$ and $\hat{\lambda}_I$ we get

$$\hat{\lambda} = \frac{K_C^{-1}(2\sigma_s^2 + \sigma^2)^{-1}\hat{\lambda}_C + K_I^{-1}(\sigma_s^2 + \sigma^2)^{-1}\hat{\lambda}_I}{K_C^{-1}(2\sigma_s^2 + \sigma^2)^{-1} + K_I^{-1}(\sigma_s^2 + \sigma^2)^{-1}}$$

$$= \frac{K_I\hat{\lambda}_C + (1 + \rho^2)K_C\hat{\lambda}_I}{K_I + (1 + \rho^2)K_C}$$

where

$$\rho^2 = \frac{\sigma_s^2}{\sigma^2 + \sigma_s^2}$$

The variance of $\hat{\lambda}$ is approximately

$$V[\hat{\lambda}] = \sigma^2 \frac{K_C K_I \rho^2 (1 + \rho^2)}{K_C(1 + \rho^2) + K_I \rho^2}$$

There are a number of ways of estimating the dispersion parameters. For example, the sum $(\sigma^2 + \sigma_s^2)$ could be obtained from the pooled variances of combined sets $(\mathbf{y}_1, \mathbf{z}_1)$ and $(\mathbf{y}_2, \mathbf{z}_2)$ and the correlation ρ from the complete pairs.

An approximation to the d.f. of the combined estimator can be obtained using the results given by Satterthwaite (1946). An example of using these results in a different context is given in Section 4.9.

Finally, in addition to the methods described above, we should note that a Bayesian analysis of the 2×2 trial with missing data in the second period has been described by Racine *et al.* (1986) in reply to the discussion of their paper. An example of using this method has been given by Grieve (1987b).

2.12   A Bayesian analysis of the 2 × 2 trial

Here we describe the Bayesian analysis of the 2 × 2 trial as presented by Grieve (1985, 1986). A Bayesian analysis of the 2 × 2 trial as used in bioequivalence testing, and for equal group sizes, was given earlier by Selwyn, Dempster and Hall (1981). Other related references are Dunsmore (1981a) and Fluehler et al. (1983). An excellent review (with discussion) of the use of Bayesian methods in the pharmaceutical industry has been given by Racine et al. (1986).

The model we shall assume is for the two-period design without baselines and is as given in Section 2.3, with the addition of the constraints $T = \tau_1 = -\tau_2$ and $R = \lambda_1 = -\lambda_2$. In other words, the difference between the carry-over effects is $\lambda_1 - \lambda_2 = 2R$ and the difference between the direct treatment effects is $\tau_1 - \tau_2 = 2T$. It will be recalled that $\hat{T} = (\bar{y}_{11.} - \bar{y}_{12.} - \bar{y}_{21.} + \bar{y}_{22.})/4$ and $\hat{R} = (\bar{y}_{11.} + \bar{y}_{12.} - \bar{y}_{21.} - \bar{y}_{22.})/2$. Also we will define $\sigma_A^2 = 2\sigma_s^2 + \sigma^2$ and note that $m = (n_1 + n_2)/n_1 n_2$.

The joint (uninformative) prior distribution for our model parameters is assumed to be proportional to $(\sigma_A^2 \times \sigma^2)^{-1}$. The following posterior distributions are then obtained, where $\mathbf{y}$ denotes the observed data:

$$p(T, R \,|\, \mathbf{y}) \propto \left(\frac{Q_1 Q_2}{\text{SSE SSP}} \right)^{-(n_1 + n_2 - 1)/2} \tag{2.1}$$

$$p(R \,|\, \mathbf{y}) \propto \left(\frac{Q_2}{\text{SSP}} \right)^{-(n_1 + n_2 - 1)/2} \tag{2.2}$$

$$p(T \,|\, R, \mathbf{y}) \propto \left(\frac{Q_1}{\text{SSE}} \right)^{-(n_1 + n_2 - 1)/2} \tag{2.3}$$

Here,

SSE = Within-subjects residual SS

SSP = Between-subjects residual SS

$$Q_1 = \frac{8(T - R/2 - \hat{T})^2}{m} + \text{SSE}$$

and

$$Q_2 = \frac{2(R - \hat{R})^2}{m} + \text{SSP}$$

In fact, from the above it can be seen that

$$p(R \mid \mathbf{y}) = t\left[\hat{R}, \frac{m \, \text{SSP}}{2(n_1 + n_2 - 2)}, n_1 + n_2 - 2 \right] \qquad (2.4)$$

where $t[a, b, c]$ denotes a shifted and scaled t-distribution with c d.f., location parameter a and scale parameter $b^{1/2}$. The variance of $t[a, b, c]$ is $bc/(c - 2)$.

The marginal distribution of $T, p(T \mid \mathbf{y})$, does not have a convenient form and must be obtained by numerically integrating out R from the joint posterior distribution for T and R given in equation (2.1). However, Grieve (1985) has shown that, to a very good approximation,

$$p(T \mid \mathbf{y}) = t\left[\hat{T} + \frac{\hat{R}}{2}, \frac{mb_0}{8b_1}, b_1 \right] \qquad (2.5)$$

where

$$b_1 = \frac{(\text{SSE} + \text{SSP})^2 (n_1 + n_2 - 6)}{(\text{SSE})^2 + (\text{SSP})^2} + 4$$

and

$$b_0 = \frac{(b_1 - 2)(\text{SSE} + \text{SSP})}{(n_1 + n_2 - 4)}$$

Also,

$$p(T \mid R, \mathbf{y}) = t\left[\hat{T} + \frac{R}{2}, \frac{m \, \text{SSE}}{8(n_1 + n_2 - 2)}, n_1 + n_2 - 2 \right] \qquad (2.6)$$

Grieve has also considered the effect of including the extra constraint $\sigma_A^2 > \sigma^2$ in the prior information and concludes that it makes very little difference.

To provide an illustration of the Bayesian approach we give in Figure 2.12 the posterior distributions obtained for Patel's data with the outlier removed. For these data $n_1 = n_2 = 8$ and the analysis of variance was given in Table 2.8.

The posterior distribution, $p(R \mid \mathbf{y})$, has mean -0.5025 and variance 0.1315 on 14 d.f. Although the posterior distribution is suggestive of

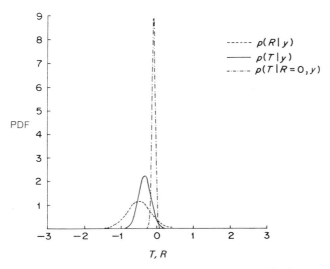

Figure 2.12 *The posterior distributions for Patel's data.*

a difference in carry-over effects, the 90% credible (confidence) interval for R is $(-1·14, 0·14)$ and does therefore support the null hypothesis that $R = 0$.

If we assume that $R = 0$, then the appropriate posterior distribution for T is $p(T|R = 0, \mathbf{y})$. The difference between $p(T|R = 0, \mathbf{y})$ and $p(T|\mathbf{y})$ is quite dramatic, however, and it is important to make a sensible choice between them. The distribution $p(T|R = 0, \mathbf{y})$ has mean $-0·0881$ and variance $0·0022$ on 14 d.f. The 95% credible interval for T is $(-0·1715, 0·0048)$, i.e. the 95% credible interval for $\tau_1 - \tau_2$ is $(-0·343, 0·010)$. If we assume that $R \neq 0$, the posterior we would use is $p(T|\mathbf{y})$ which has mean $-0·3394$ and variance $(mb_0/8b_1) = 0·0351$ on $b_1 = 15·36$ d.f., where $b_0 = 15·01$. The 95% credible interval for $\tau_1 - \tau_2$ is then $(-1·473, 0·116)$.

Further examples of a Bayesian analysis are given by Grieve (1985, 1987b, 1989) and in Racine *et al.* (1986). The Bayesian analysis of Brown's data, which we analysed in Section 2.7 is given in Grieve (1989), among others.

In the analysis so far, we have assumed an uninformative prior for the parameters. Naturally, in the Bayesian approach it is appealing to make use of informative prior information which may be subjective or may have been obtained in earlier trials. Selwyn et al. (1981) show how an informative prior distribution on R can be included in the analysis. Although this is a step forward, it does seem to us that if prior information on R is available there must be prior information on T also and this should be used.

Grieve (1985) and Racine et al. (1986) have also considered the approach of Selwyn et al. (1981) and conclude that it is likely to be difficult to put into practice: they prefer an approach which uses a Bayes factor to assess the significance of the carry-over effect. (See also the remarks of Spiegelhalter in the discussion of Racine et al., 1986).

In order to explain the Bayes factor approach, we let M_1 denote the model (as defined in Section 2.3) which includes the carry-over parameters and let M_0 denote the model with the carry-over parameters omitted.

The prior odds on no carry-over difference is then defined as $P = P(M_0)/P(M_1)$, where $P(M_i)$ denotes the prior probability of model M_i, $i = 0, 1$. The posterior probabilities for the two models are then

$$p(M_0|\mathbf{y}) = \frac{PB_{01}}{1 + PB_{01}}$$

and

$$p(M_1|\mathbf{y}) = \frac{1}{1 + PB_{01}}$$

where B_{01} is the Bayes factor obtained from

$$B_{01} = \left(\frac{p(M_0|\mathbf{y})}{p(M_1|\mathbf{y})}\right) \bigg/ \left(\frac{P(M_0)}{P(M_1)}\right) = \frac{p(\mathbf{y}|M_0)}{p(\mathbf{y}|M_1)}$$

Inference on T is then based on the mixture posterior form:

$$p_{\mathbf{M}}(T|\mathbf{y}) = \frac{PB_{01}}{1 + PB_{01}} p(T|\mathbf{y}, M_0) + \frac{1}{1 + PB_{01}} p(T|\mathbf{y}, M_1)$$

where $p(T|\mathbf{y}, M_0)$ is given by (2.6) with $R = 0$ and $p(T|\mathbf{y}, M_1)$ is obtained by either integrating out R from (2.1) or by using the approximation (2.5).

For the 2 × 2 trial

$$B_{01} = \left(\frac{3}{2m}\right)^{1/2} \left(1 + \frac{FC}{n_1 + n_2 - 2}\right)^{-(n_1 + n_2)/2}$$

where FC is as defined in Section 2.5.

The sensitivity of the conclusions to the prior belief of a carry-over difference can then be obtained by displaying summaries of $p_M(T|y)$ as a function of $P(M_1) = 1/(1 + P)$. Examples of doing this are given in Grieve (1985, 1989) and Racine *et al.* (1986).

2.13   A critical review of the 2 × 2 trial

The 2 × 2 trial has been the source of much debate and some confusion in the past and we finish our examination of the trial with a discussion of those issues over which there has been some disagreement. If we limit ourselves for the moment to the purely statistical properties of the 2 × 2 trial, then we would have to conclude that it is a design to be avoided. It suffers from two 'classic' faults. First, potentially important effects are aliased (sequence group, carry-over and direct-by-period interaction). Unless we make assumptions about two of these we are not entitled to draw conclusions about any of them. Second, it is a split-plot design with a large expected main-plot component to the error in which (the same) potentially important effects occur in the main-plot stratum. This strict and rather formal criticism of the design, however, has not precluded its use in practice; indeed, its widespread use indicates at least a moderately successful record. Its adoption generally rests on a further assumption. We can remove both objections to the design at a stroke if we can assume that all three aliased effects are negligible in size compared with the direct treatment effect, the primary effect of interest in the trial (strictly, a simple group effect would not bias the usual treatment comparison, but this is anyway of least concern given proper randomization).

Given this assumption, the use of the design, and the appropriate treatment comparison from the within-subject differences, are unobjectionable. Further, the design is clearly superior to the corresponding parallel-group design with the same numbers of subjects in terms of precision, power and realistic costs. These comparisons are based on very straightforward calculations; we refer to Chassan (1970) and Brown (1980) for details.

Unsurprisingly, the contention lies with the additional assumption. It has been argued that it should first be tested using the data at hand. In Grizzle's (1965) procedure the assumption is tested at the 10% level of significance using between-subject totals. If it is significant, the first-period data alone are used to estimate the treatment effect. First we note that there is implicit in this process the assumption that there can be no group effect or direct-by-period interaction, an assumption that several authors have made but few have recognized explicitly. Even given this assumption, however, there are very serious objections to the approach. It now appears to be widely accepted that the power of the preliminary test is quite inadequate in realistically sized trials; see for example Brown (1980), Poloniecki and Daniel (1981), Armitage and Hills (1982), Willan and Pater (1986a), Kenward and Jones (1987b) and Clayton and Hills (1987). We have seen in Sections 2.9 and 2.10 how this power can be improved through the use of baseline measurements or covariates. Hence it is possible in some circumstances to have a reasonable chance of detecting a carry-over difference or a direct-by-period interaction.

However, as Freeman (1988) has shown, the problem with Grizzle's procedure does not just lie in the lack of power of the preliminary test. The problem lies more in the automatic use of the first-period data to provide a treatment comparison in the event of discovering a significant interaction. (We leave aside, for the moment, the objection that this implies an interpretation of the interaction effect that will not necessarily be appropriate in all cases.) The argument for using the first-period comparison has typically been that it provides an unbiased estimate of the treatment difference. This is true, in the sense intended, only if it were always used. The problem lies in its use conditional on discovering a significant carry-over effect. Since the test statistics for the carry-over and direct treatment are correlated, the test statistic for the direct treatment will not then be unbiased. Moreover, because of Type II errors, failure to reject the null hypothesis of equal carry-over effects will not necessarily imply an unbiased estimator from the within-subject differences either. Freeman explores the consequences of these points by examining the behaviour of the overall Grizzle procedure. He shows that the actual significance levels for the direct treatment comparison can be much too large unless carry-over is very small, and also that confidence intervals for the direct treatment difference can be misleading. Most importantly, this undesirable behaviour gets worse as the number of subjects increases. Freeman concludes that Grizzle's procedure should not be used in any circumstances.

Freeman's criticism of the Grizzle procedure is a cogent one and raises the spectre of a long history of misleading 2 × 2 cross-over trials. We would conjecture, however, that the situation in which Freeman's results are critical is rather limited, and in practice they are relevant only when Grizzle's procedure is adopted as a substitute for using prior knowledge about the absence of a carry-over difference. Commonly the 2 × 2 trial is only used when the occurrence of carry-over is thought to be unlikely, and there may be much past experience or medical knowledge on which to base such a judgement. In the absence of a carry-over difference even the Grizzle procedure deviates only mildly from its nominal properties. In practice the argument is also complicated by the collection of several measurements from each subject, which may run into tens or even hundreds. The analysis of one particular type of measurement will not be considered in isolation and this has implications for the accumulation of evidence on particular effects. At the moment this generally appears to be done in an informal manner, and many questions remain open about the appropriate way to approach the joint analysis of multiple measurements from the 2 × 2 cross-over trial.

From Freeman's results it appears that Grizzle's procedure is at its worst when a carry-over difference is present even in the absence of a difference between the direct treatment effects. This point has been discussed by several authors. Freeman takes the extreme view that the direct and carry-over effects are at most only slightly related, whereas Willan and Pater (1986a) and Willan (1988) take a more moderate view and consider several types of relationship, including high and low dependence. At the moment it is only possible to conjecture about such relationships, but we would tend to endorse Willan and Pater's view, and note that although one can conceive of good examples of a carry-over difference occurring in the absence of a direct treatment difference, there are many more instances that one can conceive of where the carry-over and the direct effects are associated. This relationship between direct and carry-over effects has implications for the two approaches (already discussed in Sections 2.7 and 2.12) which claim to circumvent, at least to some extent, the problems of carry-over.

Grizzle's procedure can be misleading because the two stages are considered separately, and the consequences of the preliminary test are not incorporated into the process. If the 2 × 2 trial is to be seriously considered in situations in which there may be carry-over, then clearly any analysis must consider the overall procedure used. This is Willan and Pater's (1986a) approach, which is developed further in Willan (1988). As they point out, however, the justification for their analysis rests firmly on the assumption that a carry-over effect must be accompanied by a direct treatment effect. Although they acknowledge that there will be situations in which this is not true, it is interesting that it is just this relationship that Freeman rejects.

The Bayesian analysis discussed in Section 2.12 also provides an informative overall view when non-informative priors are used, in the sense that the two-dimensional posterior distribution makes quite clear the statistical dependence of the information of carry-over and direct treatment effects. This does not solve the problem of carry-over, however, it rather provides a useful viewpoint. A move towards a solution requires the use of an informative prior and here the Bayesian analysis runs into problems (see for example the discussion of Racine et al., 1986). While technically it is simple to introduce an informative prior for the carry-over effect, there are logical objections. The use of such a prior presupposes that knowledge exists about the likelihood of a carry-over effect occurring yet, at the same time there is no prior knowledge about the direct effect. Again we are led to the question of the relationship between the carry-over and the direct treatment effects. Clearly on many occasions, we will have prior information on both, and then we have the problem of combining this information. Also, if the prior information indicates that the probability of a carry-over effect is not negligible, this information should have been used in the choice of design, either by changing the length of the wash-out period (if this was appropriate, or indeed practical) or by abandoning the 2 × 2 design altogether in favour of a parallel-group design or higher-order cross-over. Both of these objections to the use of an informative prior disappear if the prior simply states that the probability of a carry-over is negligible. But this is precisely what generally occurs in practice when the analysis does not present a problem, regardless of one's viewpoint of statistical inference.

Finally, we add that neither the Willan and Pater, nor the Bayesian approaches, addresses the problem caused by the aliasing of the group, carry-over and direct-by-period interaction effects. These are not 'identical' in this design, as Freeman (1988) asserts, but could in principle occur in any combination and represent quite different effects, as explained by Koch (1987). The approaches to this question that are described in Section 2.7 are admittedly very informal, but this is perhaps inevitable.

This brings us to our final point, one that has not always been made as clear as it could be in discussions of the 2 × 2 trial. There are a variety of purposes behind the use of such a trial and before arguing the case of a particular analysis it is desirable to state clearly just what the trial is meant to achieve in the first place and to consider the context of the trial. Is it one of many on the same treatments? Have there been many preceding trials? Are many measurements being taken from each subject?, and so on. There has in the past been much emphasis on hypothesis testing, but it has been argued that the main purpose behind a 2 × 2 trial, given its common use in the early phases of drug development, is estimation (Clayton and Hills, 1987). The perspective described in Racine et al. (1986) is also a useful one, that of accumulating evidence on the behaviour of particular treatments. Clearly, there is much further scope for critical appraisal of the 2 × 2 trial along these lines. While the trial continues in common use, and there is no sign yet of its impending disappearance, then it is inevitable, and desirable, that it remains the subject of critical attention.

CHAPTER 3

The analysis of binary and categorical data

3.1 Introduction

In this chapter we consider the analysis of binary and categorical data from cross-over trials. We shall be concentrating on the 2×2 trial, hence much of the material forms a natural progression from Chapter 2. However, we shall also be laying the groundwork for analyses with higher-order designs and so to a certain extent we shall be looking ahead to later chapters.

A **categorical** observation can only take a fixed, usually small, number of values, which typically correspond to some form of classification. Examples are colour, e.g. blue/red/green/other, or change in condition, e.g. worse/same/better. The latter of these two examples is **ordered**, that is, we can rank the different categories. In clinical trials categorical observations are often generated by the answers to questionnaires and are very commonly ordered. A **binary** response is a special case of a categorical observation which can take only two values, traditionally labelled 0 and 1; examples are no/yes, failure/success and no effect/effect. In keeping with standard practice we shall refer to the responses '0' and '1' as failure and success respectively. We shall be considering the following examples.

Example 3.1

This example consists of safety data from a trial on the disease cerebrovascular deficiency in which a placebo (A) and an active drug (B) were compared. A 2×2 design was used at each of two centres, with 33 and 67 subjects respectively at each centre. The response measured was binary and was defined according to whether an electrocardiogram was considered by a cardiologist to be normal (1) or abnormal (0). In such a trial each subject supplies a pair of observations $(0, 0), (0, 1), (1, 0)$ or $(1, 1)$ where (a, b) indicates a response a in period 1 and b in period 2. We can therefore summarize the data from one 2×2 trial in the form of a 2×4 contingency table:

Group	$(0, 0)$	$(0, 1)$	$(1, 0)$	$(1, 1)$	Total
1(AB)	n_{11}	n_{12}	n_{13}	n_{14}	$n_{1.}$
2(BA)	n_{21}	n_{22}	n_{23}	n_{24}	$n_{2.}$
Total	$n_{.1}$	$n_{.2}$	$n_{.3}$	$n_{.4}$	$n_{..}$

In the table, the entry n_{11} for example is the number of subjects in sequence group 1 who gave a $(0, 0)$ response. The other entries in the body of the table are defined in a similar way and the sizes of the two groups are given by the marginal totals $n_{1.}$ and $n_{2.}$. The tables of data for the two centres are given in Table 3.1.

Example 3.2

This is also a 2×2 trial, but with a three-category outcome. The condition being treated is primary dysmenorrhea and the categories

Table 3.1 *Example 3.1: Data from a two-centre 2×2 trial on cerebrovascular deficiency. Outcomes 0 and 1 correspond to abnormal and normal electrocardiogram readings*

Centre 1

Group	$(0, 0)$	$(0, 1)$	$(1, 0)$	$(1, 1)$	Total
1(AB)	6	2	1	7	16
2(BA)	4	2	3	8	17
Total	10	4	4	15	33

Centre 2

Group	$(0, 0)$	$(0, 1)$	$(1, 0)$	$(1, 1)$	Total
1(AB)	6	0	6	22	34
2(BA)	9	4	2	18	33
Total	15	4	8	40	67

Table 3.2 *Example 3.2: Data from a 2×2 trial on a treatment for primary dysmenorrhea. Treatments: A (placebo), B (high dose analgesic)*

Group	Outcome									Total
	(1,1)	(1,2)	(1,3)	(2,1)	(2,2)	(2,3)	(3,1)	(3,2)	(3,3)	
1(AB)	2	3	6	1	2	2	0	0	0	16
2(BA)	3	2	0	1	1	1	6	0	0	14
Total	5	5	6	2	3	3	6	0	0	30

are amounts of relief obtained: 1 (none or minimal), 2 (moderate) and 3 (complete). Note that these are ordered. The treatments are a placebo (A) and a high dose analgesic (B). There are nine possible outcomes $(1, 1), (1, 2), \ldots, (3, 3)$ from the two periods and the numbers responding in each category in each sequence group are given in Table 3.2.

In the next section we discuss the analysis of binary data from 2×2 trials using simple contingency table procedures. Although these techniques are now fairly well established, and arguably quite adequate for a typical 2×2 trial, we need to generalize them in several ways to accommodate both higher-order designs and discrete data with more than two categories. We shall base these generalizations on a **log-linear model**, an approach which is not yet well established in the analysis of categorical cross-over data but which is very common in other areas of statistics. To introduce the model we first apply it to the 2×2 trial with binary data and in Section 3.3 we show how all the tests described in Section 3.2 can be derived through the model, together with some additional tests. Having established the principles behind this approach we then show how binary data from higher-order designs can be analysed (Section 3.4) and how the generalization to categorical data can be made (Section 3.5). The approach is based on a particular model for correlated categorical observations. There is no naturally 'obvious' model to use in this situation (unlike, for example, those based on the multivariate normal distribution for continuous data) and there are other possibilities that could be considered. In Section 3.6 we discuss briefly some alternative approaches to the problem.

3.2 Contingency table analyses for 2×2 trials

In this section we describe several tests for binary data from 2×2 trials. These are largely well established and are particularly simple to use, being based on the 2×4 contingency table which can be used to describe the results. To illustrate these tests we use the trial at the second centre from Example 3.1. These tests are based on standard contingency table methods, and those readers not already familiar with these are referred to Everitt (1977) and Armitage and Berry (1987, Chapters 4 and 12). The emphasis in this section is on hypothesis testing; this is a consequence of using contingency table methods and of avoiding explicit statistical models. Some comments on estimation will be made when appropriate, but a full treatment will have to wait until the next section.

The first three tests we consider are for a direct treatment effect in the absence of a direct-by-period interaction. The first two of these use results only from those subjects who show a preference, that is, who have a $(0, 1)$ or $(1, 0)$ outcome.

3.2.1 McNemar's test

In the absence of a period effect and under the null hypothesis of no direct treatment effect then, given that a subject has shown a preference, the choice is equally likely to have been for either treatment. There is a total of $n_P = n_{.2} + n_{.3}$ subjects who show a preference and out of these $n_A = n_{13} + n_{22}$ show a preference for A. Hence, under the null hypothesis, n_A has a binomial distribution with probability $\frac{1}{2}$ and index n_P. We write

$$n_A \sim B(\tfrac{1}{2}, n_P)$$

To obtain the probability of a result as extreme as this under the null hypothesis we sum the appropriate binomial probabilities. This gives, for a one-sided test, for $n_A/n_P > \frac{1}{2}$,

$$P = \sum_{r=n_A}^{n_P} \binom{n_P}{r} (\tfrac{1}{2})^r (\tfrac{1}{2})^{n_P - r}$$

$$= (\tfrac{1}{2})^{n_P} \sum_{r=n_A}^{n_P} \binom{n_P}{r}$$

For $n_A/n_P < \frac{1}{2}$, n_A is replaced by $n_B = n_P - n_A$ in this expression. For a two-sided test, P is doubled. This is known as McNemar's test (McNemar, 1947) and is just an example of the well-known sign test. We can also construct an approximate two-sided version of the test which is easier to calculate. Under the null hypothesis, $V(n_A) = n_P/4$ and hence the ratio

$$\frac{(n_A - \frac{1}{2}n_P)^2}{V(n_A)} = \frac{(n_A - n_B)^2}{n_P}$$

has an asymptotic χ_1^2 distribution.

Example 3.1 (cont.)

In this example $n_A = 10$ and $n_B = 2$ giving $n_P = 12$. We then have $P = 0 \cdot 019$ and doubling this for a two-sided test we get a probability of $0 \cdot 038$. For the approximate version we compare

$$\frac{(10 - 2)^2}{12} = 5 \cdot 33$$

with the χ_1^2 distribution to get a two-sided probability of $0 \cdot 021$. This is rather more extreme than the exact probability above.

3.2.2   The Mainland–Gart test

The main problem with McNemar's test is the assumption that there is no period effect. Strictly, when this assumption does not hold, the test is invalid. In practice the consequences are only serious when $n_{12} + n_{13}$ and $n_{22} + n_{23}$ differ substantially, for only then will the period effect favour one of the two treatments (Nam, 1971; Prescott, 1979, 1981). However, since the reason for counterbalancing the treatments on the two sequences is to allow for a possible period effect, an analysis that assumes this effect is negligible seems particularly inappropriate. In this absence of convincing evidence that there is no period effect we suggest that the following test is to be preferred to McNemar's; in particular we do not draw conclusions about the example from the tests above. To derive this alternative test we apply the following argument. We can associate with each entry in the 2 × 4 table a probability, ρ_{ij}, and obtain the following table:

Group	(0, 0)	(0, 1)	(1, 0)	(1, 1)	Total
1(AB)	ρ_{11}	ρ_{12}	ρ_{13}	ρ_{14}	1
2(BA)	ρ_{21}	ρ_{22}	ρ_{23}	ρ_{24}	1
Total	$\rho_{\cdot 1}$	$\rho_{\cdot 2}$	$\rho_{\cdot 3}$	$\rho_{\cdot 4}$	2

The odds in favour of a $(1, 0)$ response in group 1 as opposed to a $(0, 1)$ response is the ratio of probabilities ρ_{13}/ρ_{12}. If there were no direct-by-period interaction or direct treatment effect we ought to get the same odds in group 2, i.e. $\rho_{23}/\rho_{22} = \rho_{13}/\rho_{12}$. If these two odds were not equal this would indicate that there was a direct treatment effect. A natural way to express this effect is as the ratio of the odds

$$\psi_\tau = \frac{\rho_{23}/\rho_{22}}{\rho_{13}/\rho_{12}} = \frac{\rho_{12}\rho_{23}}{\rho_{13}\rho_{22}}$$

This is just the odds-ratio in the 2×2 contingency table with probabilities proportional to

ρ_{12}	ρ_{13}
ρ_{22}	ρ_{23}

and the absence of a direct treatment effect corresponds to no association in this table. This points to a test for direct treatment effect in terms of the 2×2 contingency table

n_{12}	n_{13}	m_1
n_{22}	n_{23}	m_2
$n_{\cdot 2}$	$n_{\cdot 3}$	$m_{\cdot}$

where $m_1 = n_{12} + n_{13}$ and $m_2 = n_{22} + n_{23}$. To test for this association we can apply the standard tests for a 2×2 contingency table to this table, where evidence of association indicates a direct treatment effect. Mainland (1963, pp. 236–8) derived this test using a heuristic argument based on the randomization of subjects to groups, while Gart (1969) gave a rigorous derivation in which he conditioned on subject effects in a linear logistic model for each individual observation in each period. This derivation is described in more detail at the end of Section 3.3.

The literature on testing in 2×2 contingency tables is very large; see for example Bishop, Fienberg and Holland (1975, Section 2.2) and Everitt (1977, Chapter 2). Yates (1984) provides a thorough discussion of some of the more controversial aspects of the problem. Refer to these for details of the procedures discussed below.

3.2.3   Fisher's exact test

Two main approaches to test construction are used. The first, leading to Fisher's exact test, uses a conditional argument. The second is based on an asymptotic approximation using the χ_1^2 distribution and is sometimes called the unconditional approach.

Fisher's exact test is constructed as follows (Everitt, 1977, Section 2.4). Conditional on the observed margins we can write down the probability of obtaining any particular arrangement of the table entries. The one-sided significance probability is obtained by adding the probabilities of those tables which show as much or more association than the observed table, where the association in a table is measured by the odds-ratio. The necessary arithmetic can be done relatively simply on a computer. In order to obtain a two-sided test the usual method is to double the value of P. It can happen that P is greater than one-half and then doubling the value will not produce a meaningful probability. In this situation we have an observed table that lies at the mode of the distribution of possible tables and arguably the most sensible two-sided probability for this case is one: certainly there is no evidence of association in the table.

Example 3.1 (cont.)

In the example we have the 2×2 table

0	6	6
4	2	6
4	8	12

We first note that only 12 out of the 67 subjects have actually made a preference, so in this analysis the results from less than one-fifth of the subjects are used. The associated odds-ratio is $(0 \times 2)/(4 \times 6) = 0$. Only 2 out of the 12 subjects showing a preference gave this for treatment B and the estimated odds-ratio is zero. It can be seen that if any cell in the 2×2 table is zero the sample odds-ratio will either be zero or not defined, and this is most likely to occur if one or both of the groups are very small. This is simply a reflection of the fact that we have little information if there are few subjects in one group. Note that in practice there are better ways of estimating this odds-ratio (see for example, Plackett 1981, Section 4.4). In the next section we use the method of maximum likelihood. For the exact test the probabilities are added from the tables with the same margins and odds-ratios no larger than that observed. In our example we have only the observed table, which has probability $P = 0.030$. Doubling this we get a two-sided pobability of 0.06. There is some evidence of a direct treatment effect, but this is not strong. The fact that this evidence is not stronger in a probabilistic sense, in spite of the extreme table observed, is a consequence of the small number of subjects showing a preference. This is a common problem with the analysis of binary data from the 2×2 cross-over trial. Direct information about the treatment effect comes from the subjects who make a preference. Yet we cannot say when the trial is planned what proportion of the total will fall into this category and so it is not uncommon for there to be too little information available to make a sufficiently sensitive treatment comparison.

3.2.4 Unconditional tests

As an alternative to the conditional exact test the following statistics can be compared with the χ_1^2 distribution:

1. The standard χ^2 statistic:

$$X^2 = \frac{(n_{12}n_{23} - n_{22}n_{13})^2 m.}{n_{.2}n_{.3}m_1 m_2}$$

2. The standard χ^2 statistic with Yates's correction:

$$X_C^2 = \frac{(|n_{12}n_{23} - n_{22}n_{13}| - \frac{1}{2}m.)^2 m.}{n_{.2}n_{.3}m_1 m_2}$$

3. The likelihood ratio statistic:

$$X_{LR}^2 = 2 \sum_{i=1}^{2} \sum_{j=2}^{3} n_{ij} \log(n_{ij}m_./n_{.j}m_i)$$

The two tests 1 and 3 are examples of unconditional tests and will generally give very similar results to each other. As asymptotic approximations to the Fisher's exact test, however, they may be poor in small samples and the corrected test, 2, is intended as an improvement on this approximation. In small samples it may well differ somewhat from the other two. In a sense neither the unconditional nor the conditional approach is the 'better', and the choice between them depends on an appreciation of the difference in the questions that they answer, and unfortunately this is just the point on which there is disagreement. This is not the place to enter the argument and we refer to Yates (1984) for further discussion. In large samples there is very little difference between the results from the two approaches. The same distinction between the conditional and unconditional approaches applies to all the tests that follow and so we present both types of test even where this means, for the exact tests, introducing some slightly awkward computation. In small tables, such as the examples here, we would normally prefer to use the conditional exact test.

Example 3.1 (cont.)

As a comparison with the exact test we now apply the alternatives to the example. We have $X^2 = 6.00$ (P = 0.014), $X_C^2 = 3.38$ (P = 0.066) and $X_{LR}^2 = 7.64$ (P = 0.006). The two unconditional tests produce more extreme results than the exact test, which is well approximated by the corrected test.

As a final point on these tests, it should be remembered that the comparison made is conditional on a preference occurring, and a full description of the results, particularly with respect to the prediction of the effects of using one treatment rather than the other in the population as a whole, must take into account the number likely to make a preference. Even if the one treatment were always preferred to the other, when a preference were made, this would be of little help if a preference were only made very rarely.

3.2.5   *Prescott's test*

The Mainland–Gart test has the advantage that it does not depend
on the randomization of subjects to groups, at least under Gart's
logistic model. This advantage is obtained at a price, however: the
test does not make use of any additional information that randomization provides and this is reflected in the exclusion from the analysis
of the data from subjects who show no preference. Prescott (1981)
introduced a test for a direct treatment difference which does depend
on the randomization for its validity but which can, at the same
time, exploit the extra information from the randomization. Given
randomization one would then expect Prescott's test to be more
sensitive than the Mainland–Gart test and this is confirmed by the
limited studies that have been done. Effectively the test is based on
the same odds-ratio as the Mainland–Gart test and the additional
subjects provide information on the distribution of the observed
odds-ratio. This means that there is a limit to the increase in
sensitivity that Prescott's test can provide, and in particular it does
not really solve the problem of few subjects making a preference, for
these subjects still provide the direct information on the treatment
comparison.

The test makes use of all the data from the trial although the
responses from the subjects who show no preference are combined.
The relevant contingency table is then the 2 × 3 table:

Group	$(0, 1)$	$(0, 0)$ *and* $(1, 1)$	$(1, 0)$	*Total*
1(AB)	n_{12}	$n_{11} + n_{14}$	n_{13}	$n_{1.}$
2(BA)	n_{22}	$n_{21} + n_{24}$	n_{23}	$n_{2.}$
Total	$n_{.2}$	$n_{.1} + n_{.4}$	$n_{.3}$	$n_{..}$

Formally, Prescott's test is the test for linear trend in this table. This
may be less familiar than the usual test for association in the table;
its importance in practice is usually with ordered categorical data,
see for example Armitage and Berry (1987, Section 12.2) or Everitt
(1977, Section 3.6). The test for association in this table, which is on
two degrees of freedom, would provide a legitimate test for direct
treatments in the absence of direct-by-period interaction and in fact
can be used in this way, as for example Farewell (1985) suggests.

However, this test can be decomposed into two components, each on one degree of freedom, one of which corresponds to Prescott's test and the other, which does not correspond to a simple treatment effect, will be discussed later. Given random allocation of subjects to groups one would not expect this second component to contribute anything to the association in the table and Prescott's test is constructed under this assumption. Thus Prescott's test extracts the single degree of freedom in the test for association that might be expected to show a treatment difference if one exists, and in this lies its advantage over the simple test for association on two degrees of freedom.

Prescott gives an informative derivation of the test which shows up its analogies with the t-test for direct treatments that was discussed in Chapter 2 for continuous data. As in the t-test, a comparison is made between groups of the differences in mean response from the two periods. In terms of the original binary observations y_{ijk} we have the mean difference for group 1

$$\bar{d}_1 = \frac{1}{n_{1.}} \sum_{k=1}^{n_{1.}} (y_{i2k} - y_{i1k}) = \frac{n_{12} - n_{13}}{n_{1.}}$$

and similarly for group 2. In the absence of a direct treatment difference (and direct-by-period interaction) $E(\bar{d}_1 - \bar{d}_2) = 0$, which is the analogous result to that in Chapter 2. At this point, however, we must depart from the previous development as the theory based on the normal distribution is no longer appropriate. Instead the distribution of the mean difference is derived from the distribution of the 2×3 contingency table conditional on the observed margins and the resulting test is another example of a conditional exact test. The computation involved is somewhat greater than for Fisher's exact test and methods for constructing efficient algorithms for this purpose are discussed in the appendix to this chapter.

There are also unconditional tests which correspond to the three tests X^2, X_C^2 and X_{LR}^2 for the 2×2 table. We only present the first two of these here as the likelihood ratio test is less convenient to calculate than these two and belongs more properly in the next section. These statistics have asymptotic χ_1^2 distributions under the null hypothesis, and for small samples the corrected test should provide the better approximation to the exact test. They are calculated as follows:

$$X^2(P) = [(n_{12} - n_{13})n.. - (n._2 - n._3)n_1.]^2/V$$
$$X_C^2(P) = [|(n_{12} - n_{13})n.. - (n._2 - n._3)n_1.| - \tfrac{1}{2}n..]^2/V$$

where

$$V = n_1.n_2.[(n._2 + n._3)n.. - (n._2 - n._3)^2]/n..$$

$X^2(P)$ is a special case of the statistic defined in Armitage and Berry (1987, equation (12.1)).

Example 3.1 (cont.)

We now apply these to the example. The 2×3 table of preference data is

0	28	6	34
4	27	2	33
4	55	8	67

The one-sided probability from the exact test is 0·020 and doubling this we get the significance probability of 0·04. This is similar to the probability from the Mainland–Gart test (0·06). From the two approximate tests we get $X^2(P) = 5·36$ (P $= 0·021$) and $X_C^2(P) = 4.10$ (P $= 0·043$).

Before moving on to tests for other effects we remark that each of the three tests for a direct treatment effect (McNemar, Mainland–Gart, Prescott) has a corresponding test for period effect which is obtained by interchanging n_{22} and n_{23} in the appropriate table.

3.2.6 Tests for direct-by-period interaction

All the tests so far discussed in this section have depended for their validity on the absence of a direct-by-period interaction in any of its possible forms. In testing for this interaction we are in a similar position to that for continuous data: there exists a test for the interaction but it cannot distinguish between the different causes or origins of the interaction; we cannot expect the test to be very sensitive so other relevant information is likely to be equally, or more, important when assessing the existence of such an interaction.

The test for interaction uses the non-preference observations, i.e. those for categories $(0,0)$ and $(1,1)$, and is usually justified by analogy with the 'difference in mean response' used with continuous data to test for the interaction. With binary data the equivalent effect can be expressed as an odds-ratio. In the absence of an interaction and whether or not there are period or treatment differences, the odds in favour of a $(1,1)$ response as opposed to a $(0,0)$ response should be the same in both groups. That is to say, the odds-ratio

$$\psi_\lambda = \frac{\rho_{11}\rho_{24}}{\rho_{14}\rho_{21}}$$

should be equal to one. The test for this is the test for association in the corresponding 2 × 2 table

n_{11}	n_{14}
n_{21}	n_{24}

This test for interaction was proposed by Altham (1971, Section 8) and Hills and Armitage (1979).

Example 3.1. (cont.)

For the example the appropriate 2 × 2 table is

6	22	28
9	18	27
15	40	55

for which we have the odds-ratio $(6 \times 18)/(9 \times 22) = 0.55$. The one-sided probability from the exact test is 0.246 with corresponding two-sided probability equal to 0.49. There is no evidence from this test of an interaction.

In a later paper Armitage and Hills (1982) proposed a second test for the direct-by-period interaction. This has the same form as Prescott's test but is based on the 2 × 3 table in which the preferences have been combined:

Group	$(0,0)$	$(0,1)$ and $(1,0)$	$(1,1)$	Total
1(AB)	n_{11}	$n_{12}+n_{13}$	n_{14}	$n_{1\cdot}$
2(BA)	n_{21}	$n_{22}+n_{23}$	n_{24}	$n_{2\cdot}$
Total	$n_{\cdot 1}$	$n_{\cdot 2}+n_{\cdot 3}$	$n_{\cdot 4}$	$n_{\cdot\cdot}$

However, we do not recommend the use of this test, for reasons we give in the next section.

3.2.7   Cox and Plackett's test

In the introduction to Prescott's test, mention was made of a second component of the association between rows and columns in the 2×3 contingency table. We now consider the interpretation of this component and tests for its significance. The component makes a comparison, between the two groups, of the difference in within-subject dependence. Recall that we are assuming that the two observations from a particular subject need not be independent, and here we test to see if the degree of this dependence is the same in each group. We call this comparison the **group-by-dependence** interaction. The random allocation of subjects to groups ought to ensure that this effect is negligible and thus in Prescott's test we could assume that this component contributed nothing to the association in the table. However, even if a trial has been randomized it is still possible, especially with small numbers of subjects, that through bad luck the two groups are rather different. Such a difference can affect the results in many ways; one manifestation might be the presence of a significant group-by-dependence interaction. Hence the detection of such an interaction does suggest some differences between the groups which should be followed up.

Strictly, if the only difference between the groups is the existence of this interaction then we can still isolate a valid comparison between the treatments. But, by questioning the comparability of the groups, one questions the foundations of the trial and, even though it may not be possible to identify statistically a reason for doubting the validity of the treatment comparison, a further examination of the other factors involved in the trial, the conduct and so on, may suggest caution in interpreting the results. Thus, while a group-by-dependence interaction may not be very interesting in itself, or necessarily undermine the validity of the treatment comparison, it may be taken to suggest that a second look be given to the trial as a whole, and in particular to the composition of the two subject groups. In our own experience, however, we have not yet detected such an interaction with genuine data.

The test that Cox and Plackett (1980) suggested for this interaction is the test for second-order association in the $2 \times 2 \times 2$ table

1st level		2nd level	
n_{11}	n_{13}	n_{21}	n_{23}
n_{12}	n_{14}	n_{22}	n_{24}

For details of such a test see Everitt (1977, Section 4.6). Cox and Plackett (1980) described this as a test for stability of the experimental conditions. Unfortunately neither the conditional nor unconditional tests are very easy to construct. We obtain the former using the enumeration discussed in the appendix to this chapter, while the latter is most easily obtained through the likelihood ratio procedures discussed in the next section. Here we just quote the results from the example.

Example 3.1 (cont.)

The appropriate $2 \times 2 \times 2$ table is

6	6	9	2
0	22	4	18

For this table the exact one-sided probability is 0·536, which corresponds to a modal table in the distribution, and the likelihood ratio test leads to a probability of 0·230. There is no evidence of a group-by-dependence interaction.

3.2.8   Analysis using the first period only

If the analysis is to be based on the data from the first period only, whether because of a detected or suspected direct-by-period interaction, or for some other reason, we construct the test for a direct treatment difference as follows. The appropriate test is a standard comparison of proportions and can be constructed using a 2×2 contingency table. The odds in favour of a subject in group 1 getting a success in the first period is $(\rho_{13} + \rho_{14})/(\rho_{11} + \rho_{12})$. In the absence of a treatment difference one would expect the same odds in group 2, or, equivalently, the odds-ratio

$$\psi_{\text{FPT}} = \frac{(\rho_{11} + \rho_{12})(\rho_{23} + \rho_{24})}{(\rho_{13} + \rho_{14})(\rho_{21} + \rho_{22})}$$

would be equal to one. We therefore use the test for association in the 2×2 table

$n_{11} + n_{12}$	$n_{13} + n_{14}$	$n_{1\cdot}$
$n_{21} + n_{22}$	$n_{23} + n_{24}$	$n_{2\cdot}$
$n_{\cdot 1} + n_{\cdot 2}$	$n_{\cdot 3} + n_{\cdot 4}$	$n_{\cdot\cdot}$

It is important to recognize, however, that the odds-ratio in this table is not related in a simple way to the Mainland–Gart odds-ratio,

$$\psi = \frac{\rho_{12}\rho_{23}}{\rho_{13}\rho_{22}}$$

which was used earlier to measure the direct treatment difference, unless the observations from a subject are independent. The main reason for this is that the interpretation of the Mainland–Gart odds-ratio is in terms of probabilities of the joint outcomes from a subject, not the marginal probabilities. This distinction should become clearer in the next section. However, in the absence of any effects associated with treatments, both odds-ratios will be equal to one. They differ in the way in which they measure the treatment effect when it is not negligible.

In this section we have described the basic contingency table tests that can be applied to binary data from the 2×2 cross-over. Naturally most of the various issues discussed in Chapter 2, particularly concerning the role of the direct-by-period interaction and the relevance of a carry-over effect (see Sections 2.7 and 2.13 in particular), are equally relevant here but should not need reiteration.

For example Altham (1971, Section 8) and Dunsmore (1981b) discuss Bayesian analyses for the binary 2 × 2 trial and presumably a binary version of the Willan and Pater (1986a) procedure described in Section 2.7 could be constructed. To incorporate baselines and covariates we need to introduce models for binary data for more complex designs, and we return to this type of problem in Section 3.4.

3.3 A model for the binary 2 × 2 cross-over

The tests just described are probably adequate for most analyses of binary data from 2 × 2 cross-over trials. However, they do not immediately point to appropriate analyses either for binary data from more complex trials or for categorical data. To develop such analyses we need to establish the principles behind the tests already described and this is most conveniently done using a formal statistical model. We first consider the problem of binary data and then show how the same principles can be applied to construct models for observations with more than two categories. Essentially we are choosing a particular model for correlated binary observations. Unlike the analogous case with correlated continuous data, where the multivariate normal distribution is typically used, there is no obviously 'natural' approach to use. With multivariate binary data it is not possible to have simultaneously simple representations, in terms of the effects of interest, of the joint, marginal and conditional distributions of the observations.

Broadly, models have tended to fall into one of two classes. Either the **marginal** probabilities are modelled directly, in which case the joint distribution, and in particular the second-order moments, are complicated functions of the parameters, or the **conditional and joint** probabilities are modelled, leading to awkward expressions for the marginal probabilities. For a general discussion of such models see Ware *et al.* (1988) and the references given there.

The approach to be described is based on that of Kenward and Jones (1987a) and Jones and Kenward (1987) and falls into the second class. We have chosen it because it generalizes in a natural way the majority of tests for the 2 × 2 trial and because it has several practical advantages. The model is a formalization of the representation of effects in terms of **logarithms of odds-ratios**, or **logits**, and falls into the very general class of log-linear models. Such models are in widespread use in many areas of statistics and consequently there exists a large literature on the subject; see for example McCullagh and Nelder (1983) and Bishop, Fienberg and Holland (1975) and the references given there. There also exists a wide range of suitable computer software: examples are GLIM (Numerical Algorithms Group, Oxford, UK), Genstat (Rothamsted Experimental Station, Harpenden, UK) and FREQ (Haberman, 1979). We shall also see that this approach allows us to construct appropriate models for binary and categorical data directly from the corresponding linear models for continuous data, which are generally easy to formulate.

3.3.1 A model for bivariate binary data

We begin by describing the model for the 2×2 trial. This allows us to illustrate the principles behind the use of the model in the simplest case. In Section 3.4 and 3.5 we then apply these same principles to obtain models for more complex designs and for categorical data. In Section 3.6 we discuss briefly other approaches that have been suggested for modelling binary data from the 2×2 trial.

We assume that each row of the 2×4 table of counts $[n_{ij}]$ is an independent observation from a multinomial distribution with probabilities $[\rho_{i1}, \rho_{i2}, \rho_{i3}, \rho_{i4}]$ and index $n_{i\cdot}$, $i = 1, 2$. Hence the construction of the model amounts to a representation of the probabilities $[\rho_{ij}]$ in terms of the effects of interest. We base these representations on a bivariate logistic model (Cox, 1970, Section 7.6; McCullagh and Nelder, 1983, Section 6.5.2). For a pair of correlated binary random variables Y_1 and Y_2 this takes the general form

$$P(Y_1 = y_1, Y_2 = y_2) = \exp(\beta_0 + \beta_1 y_1 + \beta_2 y_2 + \beta_{12} y_1 y_2) \qquad (3.1)$$

where, for this expression only, we code the binary responses as $+1$ and -1. The parameter β_0 is a normalizing term, chosen so that the probabilities sum to one over the four outcomes, and consequently can be written as a function of the other three parameters. The parameter β_{12} determines the statistical dependence of the two observations and this is expressed in terms of a difference in the conditional logits (or log odds-ratios):

$$4\beta_{12} = \ln\left[\frac{P(Y_1 = 1 \mid Y_2 = 1)}{P(Y_1 = -1 \mid Y_2 = 1)} \right] - \ln\left[\frac{P(Y_1 = 1 \mid Y_2 = -1)}{P(Y_1 = -1 \mid Y_2 = -1)} \right]$$

$$= \text{logit}\,[P(Y_1 = 1 \mid Y_2 = 1)] - \text{logit}\,[P(Y_1 = 1 \mid Y_2 = -1)] \qquad (3.2)$$

This difference will be positive or negative according to the sign of the correlation between the observations and zero only if they are independent. The remaining two parameters can be described as 'design' terms, and their interpretation is again through logits of conditional probabilities. We have the basic expression

$$\text{logit}\,[P(Y_a = 1\,|\,Y_b = y_b)] = 2(\beta_a + y_b \beta_{12})$$

where (a, b) takes the value $(1, 2)$ or $(2, 1)$. A comparison within a subject takes the form

$$2(\beta_1 - \beta_2) = \text{logit}\,[P(Y_1 = 1\,|\,Y_2 = r)] - \text{logit}\,[P(Y_2 = 1\,|\,Y_1 = r)]$$

$$(3.3)$$

and for a comparison between two groups, with the same dependence parameter β_{12}, we have the general form

$$2(\beta_{a(1)} - \beta_{a(2)}) = \text{logit}\,[P(Y_{a(1)} = 1\,|\,Y_{b(1)} = r)]$$

$$- \text{logit}\,P(Y_{a(2)} = 1\,|\,Y_{b(2)} = r)] \qquad (3.4)$$

where the subscript (1) or (2) indicates the group and, as before, (a, b) represents a permutation of the two periods. There is an expression like (3.1) for each group, hence there is a total of six independent parameters. The effects such as period and direct treatment will be defined using linear combinations of the β_i parameters from the two groups.

Construction of the model for the 2 × 2 trial

Rather than simply presenting the model, and showing how the parameters are interpreted, we first demonstrate its construction from a linear model for continuous data from a 2 × 2 trial. This construction can be generalized in a simple and obvious way for more complex designs and represents one of the advantages of this form of modelling. It is important, however, that the construction of the model is not confused with the subsequent interpretation. The former is merely a procedure for arriving at the correct parameterization whereas the latter explains how the parameters relate to trial effects. Let Y_{ijk} represent the response from the kth subject in the jth period of the ith group. There are three steps in the construction of the model:

1. It is first assumed that the pair of observations from a subject are

independent. For each group and period, standard linear models for the expectations of continuous observations from the 2×2 trial are used to represent the logits of the success probabilities. That is,

$$\text{logit}\,[P(Y_{11k} = 1)] = \ln \left[\frac{P(Y_{11k} = 1)}{1 - P(Y_{11k} = 1)} \right] = \alpha + \pi_1 + \tau_1$$

$$\text{logit}\,[P(Y_{12k} = 1)] = \alpha + \pi_2 + \tau_2 + \lambda_1$$

$$\text{logit}\,[P(Y_{21k} = 1)] = \alpha + \pi_1 + \tau_2$$

and

$$\text{logit}\,[P(Y_{22k} = 1)] = \alpha + \pi_2 + \tau_1 + \lambda_2$$

where π_j, τ_j and λ_j are the effects associated with period, direct treatment and carry-over j respectively.

2. The joint probabilities under independence are obtained by taking the product of probabilities defined above. For example, for group 1,

$$P(Y_{11k} = 0, Y_{12k} = 0) = \exp(\xi)$$

$$P(Y_{11k} = 0, Y_{12k} = 1) = \exp(\xi + \alpha + \pi_2 + \tau_2 + \lambda_1)$$

$$P(Y_{11k} = 1, Y_{12k} = 0) = \exp(\xi + \alpha + \pi_1 + \tau_1)$$

and

$$P(Y_{11k} = 1, Y_{12k} = 1) = \exp(\xi + 2\alpha + \pi_1 + \pi_2 + \tau_1 + \tau_2 + \lambda_1)$$

where ξ is a normalizing term. This determines the appropriate parameterization of the 'design' terms in (3.1)

3. In the final step the dependency parameters, the β_{12}, are introduced. Denoting the parameter from the ith group by $\beta_{12(i)}$, we introduce one parameter, σ, which determines the 'average' dependence, $(\sigma \propto \beta_{12(1)} + \beta_{12(2)})$ and a second, ϕ, which determines the difference in dependence or group-by-dependence interaction $(\phi \propto \beta_{12(1)} - \beta_{12(2)})$.

The resulting model is conveniently expressed in terms of the log probabilities $L_{ij} = \ln \rho_{ij}$. Avoiding over-parameterization by setting $\pi = -\pi_1 = \pi_2$, $\tau = -\tau_1 = \tau_2$ and $\lambda = -\lambda_1 = \lambda_2$, we have

Outcome	Group 1	Group 2
$(0,0)$	$L_{11} = \mu_1 + \sigma + \phi$	$L_{21} = \mu_2 + \sigma - \phi$
$(0,1)$	$L_{12} = \mu_1 + \alpha + \pi + \tau - \lambda - \sigma - \phi$	$L_{22} = \mu_2 + \alpha + \pi - \tau + \lambda - \sigma + \phi$
$(1,0)$	$L_{13} = \mu_1 + \alpha - \pi - \tau - \sigma - \phi$	$L_{23} = \mu_2 + \alpha - \pi + \tau - \sigma + \phi$
$(1,1)$	$L_{14} = \mu_1 + 2\alpha - \lambda + \sigma + \phi$	$L_{24} = \mu_2 + 2\alpha + \lambda + \sigma - \phi$

$$(3.5)$$

The two parameters μ_1 and μ_2 are normalizing terms.

Interpretation of the parameters
The model defined in (3.1) is an example of a log-linear model, and the parameters are interpreted through the logits defined earlier. It must be remembered, however, that not all the terms in the model are orthogonal, hence the interpretation of some will depend on which others are set to zero. This is particularly important with respect to the direct treatment effect, τ.

1. α: This is a constant from which the other effects are defined as deviations. It has no direct interpretation in the presence of the other effects unless the observations are independent.
2. σ, ϕ: These determine the within-subject dependence structure and are respectively proportional to the sum and difference between the two groups of the expression (3.2).
3. π: This represents the difference in period effects. It can be expressed in terms of the logits (3.3) from each group, from which we can get the odds-ratio from the Mainland–Gart test for a period effect,

$$\pi = \tfrac{1}{4}\ln\left(\frac{\rho_{12}\rho_{22}}{\rho_{13}\rho_{23}}\right)$$
$$= \tfrac{1}{4}(L_{12} - L_{13} + L_{22} - L_{23})$$

4. λ: This was chosen to represent a difference in carry-over effects but, because of the aliasing described in Section 2.7, the tests that are based on it correspond to tests for any type of direct-by-period interaction. We have

$$\lambda = \tfrac{1}{2}\ln\left(\frac{\rho_{11}\rho_{24}}{\rho_{14}\rho_{21}}\right)$$
$$= \tfrac{1}{2}(L_{11} - L_{14} - L_{21} + L_{24})$$

To construct all the tests in Section 3.2 we need to introduce one additional parameter which is closely related to λ. We denote it by λ^* and it can be taken to represent a non-specific form of direct-by-period interaction, although it can only be given this interpretation when τ is also in the model. A parameter can be defined by its corresponding column in the design matrix $\mathbf{A}$ in the expression

$$\mathbf{L} = \mathbf{A}\gamma$$

where $\mathbf{L} = [L_{11}, \ldots, L_{24}]^T$ and $\gamma = [\mu_1, \mu_2, \alpha, \pi, \tau, \lambda, \sigma, \phi]^T$. For example, the column corresponding to λ is

$$\mathbf{a}_\lambda = [0, -1, 0, -1, 0, 1, 0, 1]^T$$

The corresponding column for λ^* is

$$\mathbf{a}_\lambda^* = [\tfrac{1}{2}, 0, 0, -\tfrac{1}{2}, -\tfrac{1}{2}, 0, 0, \tfrac{1}{2}]^T$$

In the full model, or in the model without ϕ, the two parameters are aliased, that is, whichever we include in the model we obtain the same estimate. The same is not true, however, if τ is dropped from the model.

5. τ: This represents the comparison of the direct treatment effects in the absence of a direct-by-period interaction. It can be expressed in terms of the logits (3.4) through which we can obtain the odds-ratio from the Mainland–Gart test:

$$\tfrac{1}{4} \ln \left(\frac{\rho_{12}\rho_{23}}{\rho_{13}\rho_{22}} \right) = \tau$$

It was mentioned in Section 3.2 that the odds ratio from the direct treatment comparison using the first period corresponds to the Mainland–Gart odds-ratio, $\exp(4\tau)$, only when the two observations from a single individual are independent. We can now show this explicitly. With the full model we have

$$\frac{(\rho_{11} + \rho_{12})(\rho_{23} + \rho_{24})}{(\rho_{13} + \rho_{14})(\rho_{21} + \rho_{22})} = e^{2\tau} \frac{(1 + e^{\alpha + \pi + \tau - \lambda - 2\phi})(1 + e^{\alpha + \pi - \tau + \lambda + \sigma - 2\phi})}{(1 + e^{\alpha + \pi + \tau - \lambda + \sigma + 2\phi})(1 + e^{\alpha + \pi - \tau + \lambda + 2\phi})}$$

The observations are independent when $\sigma = \phi = 0$ and, when this is true, the ratio reduces to $\exp(2\tau)$, the square root of the Mainland–Gart odds-ratio. In general, however, we should not expect equivalence between the odds-ratios. The effects in the current model are defined in terms of joint and conditional probabilities and their interpretation does not carry over to the marginal probabilities.

This does not mean that marginal probabilities calculated from the fitted model cannot be used to aid interpretation of the results, however, and we shall make use of this in later sections.

3.3.2   Hypothesis tests

We now consider the construction from the model of the tests described above in Section 3.2, together with some additional tests. Each is a test for the significance of a particular parameter in the model. We denote this parameter in general by ψ; in practice it will be one of τ, λ or λ^*, and ϕ. At the same time it will be assumed that a selection of the remaining parameters, possibly none, are zero. We denote the remaining nonzero parameters by $\eta_1, \eta_2, \ldots, \eta_s, s \leqslant 5$, and we shall write $\boldsymbol{\eta} = [\eta_1, \eta_2, \ldots, \eta_s]^T$. For each test $\boldsymbol{\eta}$ will consist of α, σ and π together with at most two from τ, λ or λ^*, and ϕ. We use the notation $[\psi | \eta_1, \ldots, \eta_s]$ to represent a test of the null hypothesis $\psi = 0$.

Conditional exact tests
We consider two types of test statistic based on the model: conditional exact and likelihood ratio tests. The construction of the conditional exact tests follows the general procedure described in Cox (1970, Section 4.2). These tests are based on the conditional distribution of the sufficient statistic for ψ given the observed value of the sufficient statistic for the nuisance parameters $\eta_1, \ldots, \eta_s$. One requirement for this is the existence of the relevant sufficient statistics and it can be shown that this holds for the tests described below. We denote the set of joint sufficient statistics for $\boldsymbol{\eta} = [\eta_1, \eta_2, \ldots, \eta_s]^T$ by $[t_{\eta_1}, t_{\eta_2}, \ldots, t_{\eta_s}]$ and write $\mathbf{t}_\eta = [t_{\eta_1}, \ldots, t_{\eta_s}]^T$. In fact we have

$$t_{\eta_k} = \mathbf{a}_{\eta_k}^T \mathbf{n}$$

where $\mathbf{a}_{\eta_k}$ is the column of $\mathbf{A}$ which corresponds to the parameter η_k and $\mathbf{n} = [n_{11}, n_{12}, \ldots, n_{24}]^T$. Similarly, the sufficient statistic for ψ is $t_\psi = \mathbf{a}_\psi^T \mathbf{n}$. Inferences about ψ are then made using the conditional distribution of t_ψ given the observed value of $\mathbf{t}_\eta$. By definition this distribution is free of the nuisance parameters $\boldsymbol{\eta}$.

The construction of the distribution, which is discrete, is a matter of enumeration. In general this requires lengthy computation but a great simplification occurs from the presence in $\boldsymbol{\eta}$ of the three parameters α, σ and π. Conditional on t_α, t_σ and t_π, the distribution of the original data $\mathbf{n}$ is that of a 2×4 contingency table conditional on the observed margins $[n_{1.}, n_{2.}]$ and $[n_{.1}, n_{.2}, n_{.3}, n_{.4}]$. As a consequence the probability for the hypothesis test $\psi = 0$ versus $\psi > 0$ is obtained by summing the conditional probabilities (which are known) from those 2×4 tables with the observed margins, which also produce the same sufficient statistics as those observed for the remaining nuisance parameters and for which the sufficient statistic for ψ is greater than or equal to t_ψ. The probability for the other one-sided alternative $\psi < 0$ is obtained from a similar summation from those tables for which the sufficient statistic for ψ is less than or equal to t_ψ. The probability for the two-sided alternative is obtained by doubling the smaller of the two one-sided probabilities. As we saw in the previous section, the summation can often be simplified further to give a simple sum of probabilities from a 2×2 or 2×3 table. We describe some of the computational procedures involved in the appendix to this chapter.

Likelihood ratio tests
The construction of the likelihood ratio tests is completely standard, and the resulting statistics are normally similar in value to the other unconditional tests described in Section 3.2. If we denote the maximized likelihood for the data **n** and the model with parameters $\boldsymbol{\eta}$ by $L(\mathbf{n}; \hat{\boldsymbol{\eta}})$, we have the likelihood ratio statistic for the hypothesis $\psi = 0$ versus $\psi \neq 0$, in the presence of $\boldsymbol{\eta}$, given by

$$\Lambda(\mathbf{n}; \psi \mid \boldsymbol{\eta}) = -2[\ln L(\mathbf{n}; \hat{\boldsymbol{\eta}}) - \ln L(\mathbf{n}; \hat{\psi}, \hat{\boldsymbol{\eta}})]$$

Under the null hypothesis $\psi = 0$, and given that the model corresponding to $\boldsymbol{\eta}$ is adequate, $\Lambda(\mathbf{n}; \psi \mid \boldsymbol{\eta})$ has an asymptotic χ_1^2 distribution. Any computer package with facilities for log-linear models should allow the calculation of the appropriate statistics. Although the observed counts have a product multinomial distribution, the correct likelihood ratio tests can be obtained if, for each model fitted, it is assumed that the data consist of eight independent Poisson observations with expectations $\{\rho_{ij}\}$ and no constraints on μ_1 and μ_2. This relationship between the multinomial and Poisson distributions is an important feature of certain log-linear models; see for example Bishop, Fienberg and Holland (1975, Chapter 13) and McCullagh and Nelder (1983, Section 6.4). Alternatively, given the presence of α, σ and π among the nuisance parameters $\eta_1, \dots, \eta_s$, it can be assumed that the set $[n_{11}, n_{12}, n_{13}, n_{14}]$ comprises four independent binomial observations $n_{1j} \sim B(\rho_j^*, n_{.j})$ where the ρ_j^* are defined as follows:

j	Outcome	logit(ρ_j^*)
1	(0, 0)	$\mu_* + 2\phi$
2	(0, 1)	$\mu_* + 2\tau - 2\lambda - 2\phi$
3	(1, 0)	$\mu_* - 2\tau - 2\phi$
4	(1, 1)	$\mu_* + 2\phi - 2\lambda$

where $\mu_* = \mu_1 - \mu_2$. Note the absence of α, σ and π from these expressions.

In terms of the model parameters the tests are constructed as follows. We omit McNemar's test from this list because, for the reasons given in Section 3.2, we do not consider it wholly suitable for cross-over trials.

1. The Mainland–Gart test

$$[\tau | \alpha, \sigma, \pi, \lambda^*, \phi]$$

We remark here on the presence of both λ^* and ϕ in the model. It is shown at the end of this section how the Mainland–Gart test can be derived through an alternative approach that does not depend on the same dependence structure in each group, hence the presence of ϕ. Strictly the test is not valid, however, in the presence of a direct-by-period interaction and so λ^* is redundant. A parameter is being included in the model which is assumed to be equal to zero. This does not invalidate the test but one would expect this to reduce its sensitivity and this is consistent with the expected superiority of Prescott's test, at least in terms of the current model. From the example (the second centre data from Example 3.1) we obtain

$$\Lambda(\mathbf{n}; \tau | \alpha, \pi, \sigma, \lambda^*, \phi) = 7\cdot64 \qquad (P = 0\cdot006)$$

a rather more extreme result than the probability (0·06) obtained from Fisher's exact test in Section 3.2. Generally in small samples the conditional exact tests will, on average, be more conservative than the likelihood ratio tests.

2. Prescott's test

$$[\tau | \alpha, \sigma, \pi]$$

Here the redundant parameter λ^* is dropped and, since for this test it is assumed that the groups are properly randomized, it is also assumed that $\phi = 0$. In this case, we have for the example,

$$\Lambda(\mathbf{n}; \tau \,|\, \alpha, \pi, \sigma) = 5 \cdot 85 \qquad (P = 0 \cdot 016)$$

slightly more extreme than the exact test.

3. The direct-by-period interaction
The first test, defined by the test for association in the 2×2 table of non-preference data, corresponds to

$$[\lambda \,|\, \alpha, \sigma, \pi, \tau, \phi]$$

From the example we get the likelihood ratio statistic equal to $0 \cdot 987$ $(P = 0.320)$.

Given properly randomized groups we might consider the alternative test with ϕ set to zero. We then get a second test for the interaction:

$$[\lambda \,|\, \alpha, \sigma, \pi, \tau]$$

In the example this produces similar results to the previous test, the two-sided probability from the exact test is $0 \cdot 398$, and from the likelihood ratio test we get $P = 0 \cdot 247$. It is difficult to conceive of a realistic situation in which these two tests would differ much. The former does have the practical advantage of greater simplicity, however. The other test for direct-by-period interaction mentioned in Section 3.2 (proposed by Armitage and Hills, 1982) corresponds to

$$[\lambda^* \,|\, \alpha, \sigma, \pi]$$

The omission of the treatment parameter τ from the model when testing for a direct-by-period interaction is inconsistent with the marginality relations involved and the use of this test is therefore hard to justify.

4. The group-by-dependence interaction
Cox and Plackett's test is defined by

$$[\phi \,|\, \alpha, \sigma, \pi, \tau, \lambda]$$

From the example we get the likelihood ratio statistic of $1 \cdot 44$ $(P = 0 \cdot 230)$. Such a test could also be constructed in the absence of the direct-by-period interaction, giving a second test,

$$[\phi \,|\, \alpha, \sigma, \pi, \tau]$$

This is the test for nonlinearity in the 2 × 3 table used in Prescott's test and corresponds to the second degree of freedom for association in the table. Farewell (1985) mentions this test, referring to it as G'_1, but he does not make it clear to which hypothesis it refers. For the example the exact one-sided probability is 0·44 and the likelihood ratio statistic is 1·79 (P = 0·181).

3.3.3 Estimation of the model parameters

The method of maximum likelihood provides an obvious way of getting estimates of the parameters in the model. The details are standard and we refer to McCullagh and Nelder (1983, Chapter 5) or Bishop, Fienberg and Holland (1975, Chapters 3 and 5). Most computer packages that produce the likelihood ratio tests will also produce the associated maximum likelihood estimates, together with their corresponding asymptotic standard errors.

Example 3.1 (cont.)

The series of tests given earlier indicate, for the example, the presence of a direct treatment difference but provide no evidence of either direct-by-period or group-by-dependence interactions. It is sensible therefore to estimate the parameters from the model containing $\{\alpha, \sigma, \pi, \tau\}$. We get the maximum likelihood estimates:

Parameter	α	σ	π	τ
MLE	0·490	0·883	− 0·365	− 0·814
s.e.	0·151	0·215	0·318	0·389

Note in particular the large size of the estimate of σ relative to its standard error. We could test the significance of this term either through the asymptotic distribution of the ratio of the estimate to its standard error, or through a likelihood ratio test. The two procedures are asymptotically equivalent. Either way we would get in this case an overwhelmingly significant result, which together with the sign of the estimate, indicates a strong positive dependence between the two observations from a subject.

The estimate of τ is negative, indicating that the odds are in favour of the treatment as opposed to the placebo. We can write the estimate odds-ratio as

$$\hat{\psi}_\tau = \exp(4\hat{\tau}) = e^{-3 \cdot 256} = 0 \cdot 0385$$

This gives us the odds-ratio with respect to a preference having been made, or equivalently, the odds-ratio comparing the direct treatments in one period conditional on the same response in the other period. This provides a legitimate treatment comparison but to interpret this in terms of clinical practice we need additional information on the likelihood of a preference being made. For example, we might also wish to know the simple probabilities of a success under each treatment for a randomly chosen individual. This involves both the estimated direct treatment effect and the probability of a preference and can be obtained using predictions from the fitted model. This can be done in several ways. One approach, which has analogues in other areas of log-linear modelling and which is particularly useful with more complex designs, is to predict each outcome from the fitted model and then sum these to obtain the marginal probabilities. As an illustration we apply the procedure to the example. From the fitted model we obtain the table of estimated or predicted probabilities $\{\hat{\rho}_{ij}\}$:

Group	(0, 0)	(0, 1)	(1, 0)	(1, 1)
1(AB)	0·2145	0·0184	0·1949	0·5721
2(BA)	0·2355	0·1022	0·0416	0·6227

The marginal probability of a success under treatment A can then be obtained from the combination

$$P_A = \tfrac{1}{2}(\hat{\rho}_{13} + \hat{\rho}_{14} + \hat{\rho}_{22} + \hat{\rho}_{24}) = 0 \cdot 746$$

and under treatment B from

$$P_B = \tfrac{1}{2}(\hat{\rho}_{12} + \hat{\rho}_{14} + \hat{\rho}_{23} + \hat{\rho}_{24}) = 0.627$$

There are other ways of obtaining estimates of the marginal probabilities, and these effectively correspond to different forms of averaging, but the former approach is convenient and is easily generalized for other designs. In a similar way, other functions of the probabilities can be calculated to aid interpretation and presentation of the results. These represent ways of examining the implications of the inferences drawn from the earlier tests and model selection. A different approach would be to attempt to draw inferences directly from these functions of the probabilities, and this leads to some of the alternative methods described in Section 3.6.

3.3.4 Fixed subject effects

The modelling approach used in this section can be modified to include **fixed** subject effects. Although this is not of great use in the 2 × 2 trial, it does provide an alternative derivation of the Mainland–Gart test, and more importantly, illustrates a technique that can usefully be applied with higher-order designs. We assume that conditional on the subject effect δ_{ik} the two observations from the (i, k)th subject are independent with probabilities p_{ijk}, where

$$\text{logit}\,(p_{ijk}) = \text{logit}\,[P(Y_{ijk}|\delta_{ik})] = \delta_{ik} + \omega_{ij}$$

where ω_{ij} denotes the effects from period j of group i. In the present notation we can write for ω_{ij}:

i/j	1	2
1	$\omega_{11} = -\pi - \tau$	$\omega_{12} = \pi + \tau - \lambda$
2	$\omega_{21} = -\pi + \tau$	$\omega_{22} = \pi - \tau + \lambda$

The subject effects $\{\delta_{ik}\}$ can be regarded as nuisance parameters which we want to eliminate and this can be done by conditioning on the observed subject totals $\{y_{i\cdot k}\}$. To see how this works we consider the conditional probability

$$P(Y_{i1k} = r\,|\,y_{i\cdot k} = t)$$

If t is equal to 0 or 2, corresponding to the outcomes $(0, 0)$ and $(1, 1)$, then this probability is just 0 or 1. Hence, conditional on the subject totals, information about the effects of interest is contained only in the preferences $(0, 1)$ and $(1, 0)$, and we discard the non-preference observations. This is analogous to the use only of the within-subject differences with continuous data. We have

$$P(Y_{i1k} = 1 | y_{i \cdot k} = 1) = \frac{p_{i1k}(1 - p_{i2k})}{p_{i1k}(1 - p_{i2k}) + (1 - p_{i1k})p_{i2k}}$$

$$= \frac{e^{\omega_{i1} - \omega_{i2}}}{1 + e^{\omega_{i1} - \omega_{i2}}}$$

which does not depend on the subject effect δ_{ik}. We can then summarize the relevant data and their distribution in the form of two independent binomial observations,

$$n_{i2} \sim B(p_i, n_{i2} + n_{i3}), \qquad i = 1, 2$$

where

$$p_1 = \frac{e^{-2\pi - 2\tau + \lambda}}{1 + e^{-2\pi - 2\tau + \lambda}}$$

and

$$p_2 = \frac{e^{-2\pi + 2\tau - \lambda}}{1 + e^{-2\pi + 2\tau - \lambda}}$$

In order to test the null hypothesis $\tau = 0$ it must first be assumed that $\lambda = 0$. The appropriate test is then for the equality of the two binomial proportions and this is the test for association in the Mainland–Gart 2 × 2 contingency table.

To show the relationship between the model used earlier in this section and the fixed-effects model we first write down an expression for the probabilities of the joint outcomes (r, s) conditional on the subject effects, where r and s take the values 0 or 1. The outcomes in the two periods from a subject are conditionally independent so we get these probabilities simply from the appropriate products of p_{ijk} and $1 - p_{ijk}$, i.e.

$$P_i(r, s | \delta_{ik}) = P(y_{i1k} = r, y_{i2k} = s | \delta_{ik})$$

$$= \frac{\exp \left[(r + s)\delta_{ik} + r\omega_{i1} + s\omega_{i2} \right]}{[1 + \exp(\delta_{ik} + \omega_{i1})][1 + \exp(\delta_{ik} + \omega_{i2})]}$$

Next we need to introduce a probability distribution for the $\{\delta_{ik}\}$, say $f(\delta)$. We then get the **unconditional** probabilities of the joint outcomes:

$$P_i(r, s) = \int P_i(r, s | \delta) f(\delta) d\delta$$

To relate Gart's model to ours we need a distribution $f(\delta)$ such that

$$P_i(r, s) = \frac{\exp\left[r(\alpha + \omega_{i1}) + s(\alpha + \omega_{i2}) + rs\sigma\right]}{1 + e^{\alpha}(\exp\omega_{i1} + \exp\omega_{i2}) + \exp(2\alpha + \omega_{i1} + \omega_{i2} + \sigma)}$$

We have assumed that the distribution $f(\delta)$ is the same in each group so the resulting probabilities would not be expected to involve ϕ. To introduce this parameter we would need to let the distribution differ between groups. Finally, whatever distribution is used, provided that it is the same in each group, and in the absence of a direct-by-period interaction, we have under the null hypothesis $H_{0:}\ \tau = 0$,

$$\omega_{1j} = \omega_{2j}, \qquad j = 1, 2$$

which implies that

$$P_1(r, s) = P_2(r, s)$$

This is the only requirement for the applicability of Prescott's test, which can therefore be justified under Gart's model with any distribution of subject effects, provided that the distribution is the same in each group. This latter assumption is justified by the randomization of subjects to groups.

3.4   Modelling binary data from more complex designs

We now consider the construction of appropriate models for more complex designs. We have already met the situation with the 2×2 trial in which there are baselines (Section 2.9) and covariates (Section 2.10). In the next two chapters we will meet higher-order cross-over designs with more than two periods and with more than two treatments. We now describe the construction, in general, of models for binary data from such trials and we give a simple illustration using the complete data from Example 3.1, that is, including the observations from both centres.

3.4.1   A general model for multivariate binary data

The model (3.1) can be generalized for any number of periods using a multivariate form of the same logistic model (Cox, 1972; Bonney,

1987). For p correlated binary random variables $\{Y_1, \ldots, Y_p\}$ this takes the form

$$P(Y_1 = y_1, Y_2 = y_2, \ldots, Y_p = y_p)$$

$$= \exp\left[\beta_0 + \sum_{j=1}^{p} y_j \beta_j + \sum_{j=2}^{p} \sum_{k=1}^{j-1} y_j y_k \beta_{jk} \right] \qquad (3.6)$$

where as in (3.1) we code the responses as 1 and -1. As in the bivariate case β_0 is a normalizing term, the β_j are the 'design' terms and the β_{jk} determine the dependence among the p variables. The interpretation of the parameters is an obvious generalization of the bivariate case. Let $j_1, \ldots, j_p$ be any permutation of $1, \ldots, p$. We have

$$2 \sum_{k=2}^{p} r_k s_k \beta_{j_1 j_k} = \text{logit} \left[P(Y_{j_1} = 1 \,|\, Y_{j_2} = r_2, \ldots, Y_{j_p} = r_p) \right]$$

$$- \text{logit} \left[P(Y_{j_1} = 1 \,|\, Y_{j_2} = s_2, \ldots, Y_{j_p} = s_p) \right] \qquad (3.7)$$

and, for comparisons between groups,

$$\beta_{j_1(1)} - \beta_{j_1(2)} = \text{logit} \left[P(Y_{j_1(1)} = 1 \,|\, Y_{j_2(1)} = r_2, \ldots, Y_{j_p(1)} = r_p) \right]$$

$$- \text{logit} \left[P(Y_{j_1(2)} = 1 \,|\, Y_{j_2(2)} = r_2, \ldots, Y_{j_p(2)} = r_p) \right]$$

$$(3.8)$$

where as in equations (3.2) to (3.4) the subscript (i) indicates the group. Note that the model is defined in terms of the joint outcomes from each group, of which there will be 2^p.

Application to cross-over data

The appropriate parameterization can be obtained through the same three steps used in the bivariate case:

1. Assuming independence, equate the logits of the success probabilities from each combination of group and period to the corresponding linear model for the expectation of continuous data.
2. Still under the assumption of independence, combine the probabilities defined by the logit expressions.
3. Introduce the 'dependence' parameters, the β_{jk}.

As a simple example consider the first group from a three-period three-treatment design with the sequence of treatments ABC (such higher-order designs are the subject of Chapter 5). We have the three steps:

1. Equate the logits to the corresponding linear model:

$$\text{logit}\,[P(Y_{11k} = 1)] = \alpha + \pi_1 + \tau_1$$
$$\text{logit}\,[P(Y_{12k} = 1)] = \alpha + \pi_2 + \tau_2 + \lambda_1$$
$$\text{logit}\,[P(Y_{13k} = 1)] = \alpha + \pi_3 + \tau_3 + \lambda_2$$

where π_j, τ_j and λ_j are the effects associated with period j, direct treatment j and the carry-over from treatment j respectively ($j = 1, 2, 3$).

2. Combining these we get eight probabilities for the eight possible outcomes. For example

$$P(Y_{11k} = 0, Y_{12k} = 0, Y_{13k} = 0) = \exp(\xi_1)$$
$$P(Y_{11k} = 0, Y_{12k} = 1, Y_{13k} = 0) = \exp(\xi_1 + \alpha + \pi_2 + \tau_2 + \lambda_1)$$

and

$$P(Y_{11k} = 1, Y_{12k} = 1, Y_{13k} = 1)$$
$$= \exp(\xi_1 + 3\alpha + \pi_1 + \pi_2 + \pi_3 + \tau_1 + \tau_2 + \tau_3 + \lambda_1 + \lambda_2)$$

where ξ_1 is a normalizing term.

3. Finally the dependence terms are introduced.

$$P(Y_{11k} = 0, Y_{12k} = 0, Y_{13k} = 0)$$
$$= \exp(\mu_1 + \sigma_{12} + \sigma_{13} + \sigma_{23}),$$
$$P(Y_{11k} = 0, Y_{12k} = 1, Y_{13k} = 0)$$
$$= \exp(\mu_1 + \alpha + \pi_2 + \tau_2 + \lambda_1 - \sigma_{12} + \sigma_{13} - \sigma_{23}) \qquad (3.9)$$

and

$$P(Y_{11k} = 1, Y_{12k} = 1, Y_{13k} = 1)$$
$$= \exp(\mu_1 + 3\alpha + \pi_1 + \pi_2 + \pi_3 + \tau_1 + \tau_2 + \tau_3$$
$$+ \lambda_1 + \lambda_2 + \sigma_{12} + \sigma_{13} + \sigma_{23})$$

where μ_1 is the appropriate normalizing term for the eight joint probabilities. Note that there are no group-by-dependence parameters, the generalizations of ϕ in the model for the 2×2 trial. These could be introduced if desired but, given randomization, are unlikely to be necessary and with several groups this can lead to the introduction of many extra parameters.

Categorical covariates

The procedure outlined above can be followed for each group in the trial. Some grouping may be associated with categorical covariates as in Example 3.1 when both centres are considered. If we introduce an effect associated with centre γ_m say, for centre m, then we have from group 1 in centre 1, the generalization of model (3.5):

$$P(Y_{1i1k} = 0, Y_{1i2k} = 0) = \exp(\mu_{11} + \sigma)$$
$$P(Y_{1i1k} = 0, Y_{1i2k} = 1) = \exp(\mu_{11} - \sigma + \alpha + \gamma_1 + \pi_2 + \tau_2$$
$$+ (\gamma, \pi)_{12} + (\gamma, \tau)_{12} + \lambda_1)$$
$$P(Y_{1i1k} = 1, Y_{1i2k} = 0) = \exp(\mu_{11} - \sigma + \alpha + \gamma_1 + \pi_1 + \tau_1$$
$$+ (\gamma, \pi)_{11} + (\gamma, \tau)_{11})$$

and

$$P(Y_{1i1k} = 1, Y_{1i2k} = 1) = \exp(\mu_{11} + \sigma + 2\alpha + \gamma_1 + \pi_1 + \pi_2 + \tau_1 + \tau_2$$
$$+ (\gamma, \pi)_{11} + (\gamma, \pi)_{12} + (\gamma, \tau)_{11} + (\gamma, \tau)_{12} + \lambda_1)$$

where Y_{mijk} is the observation from centre m, group i, period j and subject k and μ_{mi} is the normalizing term for group i in centre m. We have introduced interaction terms for centre-by-period, $(\gamma, \pi)_{mj}$ and for centre-by-direct treatment, $(\gamma, \tau)_{mj}$. Other effects could also be introduced if required, for example centre-by-carry-over, group-by-dependence and group-by-centre-by-dependence. In a similar way, the appropriate expressions can be constructed for the other combinations of sequence group and centre. The analysis using likelihood ratio procedures is then straightforward.

Example 3.1 (cont.)

In the example there is no evidence of an interaction between centre and period, but the likelihood ratio statistic for the centre-by-direct treatment interaction is 3·77 on 1 degree of freedom (P = 0·052). There is therefore some slight evidence of a difference in treatment effect between the two centres. A separate examination of the data from centre 1 shows no evidence of a direct treatment effect, although only eight subjects make a preference and so the treatment test is not particularly sensitive. The observed odds-ratio is, moreover, greater than one, in contrast to centre 2, and this is most likely the source of the non-negligible interaction between treatment and centre.

Continuous covariates

It is also possible to introduce covariates measured on a continuous scale. Suppose for example there is a single continuous covariate in a 2×2 trial, to which we wish to relate the treatment effect. We denote by x_{ik} the value of the covariate for the kth subject in group i. In step 1 of the construction of the model we replace α and τ by

$$\alpha + \alpha_x x_{ik} \quad \text{and} \quad \tau + \tau_x x_{ik}$$

respectively, where α_x and τ_x are the covariate regression coefficients. Note that we also relate the covariate to the constant term α. In omitting to do this we would be assuming that the covariate might be associated with the difference in direct treatment effect but not with the basic odds of a success. This may turn out to be the case but should not be built into the model as an initial assumption. Note that there will now be a different expression for the probabilities in each group for each combination of covariate values. This affects the way in which the data are presented for the analysis; obviously the data can no longer be summarized in a simple contingency table without losing the information on the covariates.

Likelihood procedures can still be based on the assumption that the data consist of independent Poisson observations with expectations defined by the log-linear model, but the subjects are now subdivided within each sequence group into sets with the same combination of covariate values. In the extreme case where each subject has a unique combination of values, each set contains a single subject.

3.4.2 Fixed subject effects

We can also generalize the approach using fixed subject effects described at the end of the last section. Again, each subject has an associated parameter in place of α in step 1 above. The sufficient statistics for these parameters are the subject totals. Conditioning on these we are led to discard the outcomes consisting wholly of zeros or of ones and, in place of the σ_{jk} terms in step 3 (p. 121), we have in each group one parameter for each of the outcomes with the same number of ones. For example, the model for the $(0, 1, 0)$ outcome from the sequence ABC takes the form

$$P(Y_{11k} = 0, Y_{12k} = 1, Y_{13k} = 0) = \exp(\mu_1 + \alpha^* + \pi_2 + \tau_2 + \lambda_1 + \theta_{11})$$

where θ_{iq} is the parameter associated with the outcomes containing q ones in sequence group i (in fact the μ_i are redundant in this model). This expression should be compared with (3.9).

3.5 Modelling categorical data

3.5.1 A log-linear model for multivariate categorical data

We now extend the binary model described in the previous two sections to incorporate general categorical outcomes. The principle behind this extension is a very simple one. Where, for binary data, we have defined effects in terms of log odds-ratios (or logits) of conditional probabilities, we now define effects in terms of ratios of conditional probabilities for different categories. With only two categories this reduces to the logit expressions used earlier. As an example, consider a two-period trial with c outcome categories. The effects will now be defined in terms of ratios of the form

$$\ln\left[\frac{P(Y_{iak} = r \mid Y_{ibk} = t)}{P(Y_{iak} = s \mid Y_{ibk} = t)}\right] \tag{3.10}$$

where r, s and t take values from 1 to c. In terms of the joint probabilities this translates into the categorical generalization of (3.6) (for p periods):

$$P(Y_{i1k} = y_{i1k}, Y_{i2k} = y_{i2k}, \ldots, Y_{ipk} = y_{ipk})$$

$$= \exp\left[\mu_i + \sum_{j=1}^{p} \gamma_{ij(y_{ijk})} + \sum_{j=2}^{p}\sum_{m=1}^{j-1} \sigma_{jm(y_{ijk}, y_{imk})}\right]$$

where the subscript $ij(y_{ijk})$ on the term $\gamma_{ij(y_{ijk})}$ identifies that parameter as being associated with the outcome y_{ijk} in period j of group i and will be determined by the various period and treatment effects. The dependence term $\sigma_{jm(y_{ijk}, y_{imk})}$ is associated with the outcome (y_{ijk}, y_{imk}) in periods j and m. The role of these parameters can be seen through ratios like (3.10); for details see Jones and Kenward (1988). There is also a version of the model which uses fixed subject effects and this uses a direct generalization of the approach described at the end of the last section.

3.5.2 Application to cross-over data

Again the appropriate parameterization of the γ terms can be achieved through the three steps described earlier in Sections 3.3

and 3.4, the only difference now being the need to have separate parameters for the different categories for each of the types of effect (period, direct treatment, etc.). This introduces additional redundancy into the parameterization, but this is no different from the redundancy present in most orthodox factorial models used in the analysis of variance. This redundancy will be accounted for automatically in any well-designed computer package for the analysis of log-linear models. In fact, as we now outline, the factorial structure of the problem can be exploited to simplify analyses based on the model.

We note that $\gamma_{ij(r)}$ is present in the model if response r is observed in the jth period in the ith group, $r = 1, \ldots, c$. That is, γ_{ij} is a factor with c levels. To emphasize the relationship between this factorial view and the approach taken earlier we consider again the 2×2 trial with binary data. The γ parameters for group 1, the AB sequence group, can be expressed as

$$\gamma_{11(0)} = \mu_{(0)} + \pi_{1(0)} + \tau_{1(0)}$$
$$\gamma_{11(1)} = \mu_{(1)} + \pi_{1(1)} + \tau_{1(1)}$$
$$\gamma_{12(0)} = \mu_{(0)} + \pi_{2(0)} + \tau_{2(0)} + \lambda_{1(0)}$$
$$\gamma_{12(1)} = \mu_{(1)} + \pi_{2(1)} + \tau_{2(1)} + \lambda_{1(1)}$$

where to conform with the binary models we have taken $r = 0, 1$ rather than $1, 2$. The corresponding log-linear model can be written, for the four outcomes in group 1:

$$L_{11} = \mu_{(0)} + \pi_{1(0)} + \tau_{1(0)} + \mu_{(0)} + \pi_{2(0)} + \tau_{2(0)} + \lambda_{1(0)}$$
$$L_{12} = \mu_{(0)} + \pi_{1(0)} + \tau_{1(0)} + \mu_{(1)} + \pi_{2(1)} + \tau_{2(1)} + \lambda_{1(1)}$$
$$L_{13} = \mu_{(1)} + \pi_{1(1)} + \tau_{1(1)} + \mu_{(0)} + \pi_{2(0)} + \tau_{2(0)} + \lambda_{1(0)}$$
$$L_{14} = \mu_{(1)} + \pi_{1(1)} + \tau_{1(1)} + \mu_{(1)} + \pi_{2(1)} + \tau_{2(1)} + \lambda_{1(1)}$$

Clearly this new parameterization has considerable redundancy. Removing it with the following constraints:

$$\mu_{(0)} = \pi_{1(0)} = \pi_{2(0)} = \tau_{1(0)} = \tau_{2(0)} = \lambda_{1(0)} = \lambda_{2(0)} = 0$$
$$- \pi_{1(1)} = \pi_{2(1)} = \pi$$
$$- \tau_{1(1)} = \tau_{2(1)} = \tau$$
$$- \lambda_{1(1)} = \lambda_{2(1)} = \lambda$$
$$\sigma_{12(0,0)} = - \sigma_{12(0,1)} = - \sigma_{12(1,0)} = \sigma_{12(1,1)} = \sigma$$

and setting $\mu_{(1)} = \alpha$, we obtain the original model for the binary 2×2

trial given in (3.5) with ϕ omitted. This latter parameter could of course have been included if required. Note that many alternative forms of constraint would lead to identical test statistics to those described in Section 3.3.

Now, the $\mu_{(r)}$, $\pi_{j(r)}$, $\mu_{(s)}$, $\pi_{m(s)}$ and $\sigma_{jm(r,s)}$ parameters determine (in the absence of treatment effects) the chance of an r being observed in period j and an s in period m. That is, we can regard $\pi_{j(r)}$ and $\pi_{m(s)}$ as main effects of what we shall call **outcome** factors, and $\sigma_{jm(r,s)}$ is the corresponding **interaction** effect. This greatly simplifies model fitting because we need only introduce these outcome factors and their interaction to account for all the terms in the model apart from those associated with treatments. Therefore, with appropriate computing facilities, it is unnecessary to construct the entire model from first principles (through the three steps used earlier) and the use of the model is not much more involved than an orthodox multifactorial analysis with continuous data. If there is doubt in proceeding this way, however, it is always possible to return to first principles for the analysis, and this can provide a useful check on the results from the shorter method, particularly when the latter is first tried.

3.5.3 Relationship to models for multiway contingency tables

The relationship between this form of model fitting and conventional log-linear modelling for contingency table analysis can be seen more clearly through the following argument. Suppose that we have s sequence groups, p periods and c categories. We can think of the data as comprising a $s \times c \times c \times \cdots \times c$ contingency table, where there are p classifications with c levels, corresponding to the outcomes in the p periods. Period effects and the dependence among the observations are accounted for by fixing all $c \times c$ sub-tables, that is by fitting the 'outcome' factors and their first-order interactions. The group margin must also be fixed to ensure that estimated frequencies in each group match the observed frequencies: quantities that are fixed by the sampling process. In the absence of any effects associated with treatments (including carry-over differences and so on) there should be no association between groups and the 'outcome' classifications. We could test for this by checking for the presence of any association, that is by testing all interactions between the groups and all combinations of the 'outcome' factors, up to the pth order interaction between the groups factor and all the 'outcome' factors. This would be very inefficient, however, as many of the degrees of freedom for association being tested would not be expected to show association even in the presence of treatment effects.

The procedure described above picks out those degrees of freedom that are relevant for the particular comparisons of interest. For example, a direct treatment effect would be expected to manifest itself in a particular set of cross-ratios in the full table, the particular set being determined by the treatment allocation. This set of cross-ratios is precisely equivalent to the set of ratios of conditional probabilities of the form (3.8) which correspond to the treatment parameters; it can be seen that these ratios are also ratios of unconditional joint probabilities from the full contingency table.

Example 3.2 (cont.)

We illustrate the approach using Example 3.2. Recall that this is a 2×2 trial with three (ordered) categories: the simplest possible example of a cross-over with more than two categories. We introduce into the log-linear model a factor G (with two levels) which distinguishes between the two sequence groups, the two 'outcome' factors for periods 1 and 2, $P1$ and $P2$ respectively, and for treatments A and B the two direct treatment factors TA and TB and the two carry-over factors CA and CB. Each of these factors has three levels corresponding to the three response categories, expect for the carry-over factors which have an extra level to represent the absence of a preceding treatment. The allocation of the levels of these factors to the observations is shown in Table 3.3. It is instructive to relate the parameterization implied by this factorial model to the parameterization obtained from first principles through the three steps used in the previous two sections.

Using standard log-linear model procedures we get the likelihood-ratio statistics given in Table 3.4 for comparing different models against the saturated model. The saturated model is the one which has as many independent parameters as observations. These statistics are sometimes called **deviances**. We also give the residual degrees of freedom associated with each model.

To test the carry-over effect we compared the fit of the last two models. We have the deviance difference of 0.871 on $6 - 4 = 2$ degrees of freedom. Comparing this with the χ_2^2 distribution there is clearly

Table 3.3 *The columns of the design matrix for a 2 × 2 trial with 3-category observations*

Outcome	G	P1	P2	TA	TB	CA	CB
(1, 1)	1	1	1	1	1	1	4
(1, 2)	1	1	2	1	2	2	4
(1, 3)	1	1	3	1	3	3	4
(2, 1)	1	2	1	2	1	1	4
(2, 2)	1	2	2	2	2	2	4
(2, 3)	1	2	3	2	3	3	4
(3, 1)	1	3	1	3	1	1	4
(3, 2)	1	3	2	3	2	2	4
(3, 3)	1	3	3	3	3	3	4
(1, 1)	2	1	1	1	1	4	1
(1, 2)	2	1	2	2	1	4	2
(1, 3)	2	1	3	3	1	4	3
(2, 1)	2	2	1	1	2	4	1
(2, 2)	2	2	2	2	2	4	2
(2, 3)	2	2	3	3	2	4	3
(3, 1)	2	3	1	1	3	4	1
(3, 2)	2	3	2	2	3	4	2
(3, 3)	2	3	3	3	3	4	3

Table 3.4 *Likelihood ratio statistics*

Terms included	Deviance	Residual d.f.
$G, P1, P2, P1 \times P2$	17·585	8
$G, P1, P2, P1 \times P2, TA, TB$	3·265	6
$G, P1, P2, P1 \times P2, TA, TB, CA, CB$	2·394	4

no evidence of a carry-over difference. However, when the deviances associated with the first and second models are compared, we get a test statistic for the direct treatment effect of 14·32 on 2 degrees of freedom. This is clearly highly significant. We have very strong evidence of a treatment effect.

We now need to interpret this result. Although each of the two direct treatment factors has three levels, together they contribute only two degrees of freedom to the model. This is expected (any other result would indicate an error in the model) and is a consequence of the elimination of redundant parameters. How we proceed next depends on the way in which the numerical algorithm employed has eliminated the redundant parameters, or equivalently, how the model has been reparameterized to allow for the redundancy. A common method, used for example by GLIM, is to set the parameter corresponding to first level of each factor to zero and then to set to zero any subsequent parameter that is aliased with previous terms in the model. Clearly the order of inclusion of terms is crucial in such a procedure. We have used this method with the example. All the parameters of the second treatment factor TB are aliased when TA is already in the model and are set to zero. The parameters from TA can therefore be interpreted in terms of the $A-B$ difference. Also the parameter associated with the first level of TA has been set to zero and so the remaining two parameters define respectively the odds comparing the probability of category 2 with category 1 and category 3 with category 1. We denote these effects by $\tau_{AB(21)}$ and $\tau_{AB(31)}$ respectively, and from the example we obtain the corresponding estimates -0.748 (s.e. $= 0.768$) and -2.89 (s.e. $= 1.11$). It would seem that the first of these is negligible in comparison with its standard error and so the main treatment effect is manifested in the second odds-ratio. The estimated odds of observing category 3 as compared to category 1 is about 18 (that is, $\exp(2.89)$) times greater for treatment B than for treatment A. It must be emphasized that these are odds based on conditional probabilities; the comparison can be regarded as being between two subjects on the different treatments in one period who are known to have given the same response in the other period. In a sense we are using a form of matching, and generally we would not expect two subjects chosen completely at random to show the same odds, unless the pairs of observations from a subject were independent. As in the binary case we can use the fitted model to calculate such odds and other quantities to aid the presentation and interpretation of the results.

3.5.4 Ordered categorical data

It was mentioned at the start of this chapter that categorical data from clinical trials are very often ordered, indeed, the data just examined are an example of this. We have not taken this into account in the analysis, however. In the present example, with only three categories, the incorporation of this ordering is unlikely to add much to the analysis, but this may not be true in other examples. By working within an orthodox log-linear framework we can directly apply a standard method for modelling ordered categorical data through the present models. For this, a regression is used on the category scores, and for details we refer to Agresti (1984, Chapter 5) and Everitt (1977, Section 5.8). In the example above the factors TA and TB would be decomposed into linear and quadratic components; the generalization with more categories is obvious. The technique is most likely to prove useful when there are more than a very few categories and when the treatment effect is increasing or decreasing with respect to the categories. This would manifest itself as the odds-ratios of categories j vs $j+1$ being all greater or all less than one for the treatment differences. If this were true, at least approximately, then a test on the single degree of freedom corresponding to the linear effect may be far more powerful than an overall test on $c-1$ degrees of freedom.

There are also other approaches to the modelling of ordinal categorical data, for example using proportional odds models (McCullagh, 1980, for example). To apply these to cross-over data, however, we need tractable multivariate versions of the models which can be used with small samples, and these are not yet available. However, this is an active area of research and the situation may well change in the future.

3.5.5   Model checking and goodness of fit

For the previous three sections we have using models for cross-over data and, as in any statistical analysis, it is important to consider the appropriateness and validity of the models used. In principle, an overall measure of the goodness of fit of one of the models used here is provided by the deviance (defined earlier). This is asymptotically equivalent to the classical Pearson's χ^2 statistic:

$$\sum \frac{(\text{observed} - \text{expected})^2}{\text{expected}}$$

This provides a link between some of the likelihood ratio tests and the χ^2 tests described in Section 3.2. However, the justification for these statistics is asymptotic and it is known that the deviance, in particular, may provide a very poor measure of fit in small samples, when cell frequencies are low. In higher-order cross-over trials there may be many zero cells. The deviance differences used to construct the tests for particular effects have a more reliable small-sample

approximation and so these comments mainly concern the assessment
of fit of the model.

It is particularly important, then, that the fit be examined in other
ways and for log-linear models there exist versions of most of the
orthodox regression diagnostics, for example, using standardized
residuals, measures of influence, and so on. These will be of little use
in the binary 2 × 2 trial for which there will be at most two or three
residual degrees of freedom, but should be considered for those
analyses based on the larger contingency tables. McCullagh and
Nelder (1983, Chapter 11) discuss various aspects of model checking
in generalized linear models, which include as a special case the
log-linear models discussed here.

3.6   Other approaches for the binary 2 × 2 trial

3.6.1   Linear contrasts method

In the previous two sections we have used a model in which
comparisons of interest are defined in terms of odds-ratios, for which
direct treatment differences are expressed in statements like '(conditional) odds in favour of a preference for A is x'. This is a convenient
way of expressing a treatment comparison and it has the advantage
of being well defined whatever the underlying probabilities. There
are of course other ways in which one can measure a direct treatment
effect. The odds-ratio approach corresponds to the definition of
comparisons as linear contrasts among the logarithms of the cell
probabilities; an obvious alternative is to construct the comparisons
from contrasts among the untransformed probabilities. For example,
in the absence of a direct-by-period interaction, we can define the
linear analogue of the Mainland–Gart treatment comparison:

$$\tau_{lin} = \tfrac{1}{4}(\rho_{12} - \rho_{13} - \rho_{22} + \rho_{23})$$

In this way we can define a linear analogue of the model (3.5). The
interpretation of a direct treatment difference on this scale takes the
form 'the probability of a preference for drug A is x greater than for
drug B'. One disadvantage of this scale is that the importance of a
difference of size x depends on the sizes of the probabilities. This is
reflected in the fact that such a difference is meaningless if the smaller
probability is greater than $1 - x$. Nevertheless, it is useful to be able
to examine treatment differences on different scales, if only as a

reminder that there is no 'correct' scale on which to make such comparisons. One would hope that clear-cut treatment differences would show up using any reasonable choice of scale and the decision on which scale to use would then be one of how best to present the results.

On the linear scale, likelihood-based procedures do not take the simple form which we have seen for the log-linear model and a different approach to test construction is used. The general approach is described by Grizzle, Starmer and Koch (1969) (for uncorrelated categorical data), and this has been applied to the binary 2×2 cross-over by Zimmerman and Rahlfs (1978) and Le (1984). Earlier work on similar lines was reported by Bennett (1971) and George and Desu (1973). By using particular transformations of the data, Zimmerman and Rahlfs were able to apply the Grizzle *et al.* procedure even though there are pairs of correlated observations from each subject. This is wholly analogous to the reduction of the eight observations to four binomial proportions described in Section 3.3. The estimators of the three linear analogues of the direct treatment, direct-by-period and group-by-dependence interactions from the full model are

$$\hat{\tau}_{\text{lin}} = \tfrac{1}{4}(\rho_{12} - \rho_{13} - \rho_{22} + \rho_{23})$$

$$\hat{\lambda}^*_{\text{lin}} = \tfrac{1}{4}(\rho_{11} - \rho_{14} - \rho_{21} - \rho_{24})$$

$$\hat{\phi}_{\text{lin}} = \tfrac{1}{8}(\rho_{11} - \rho_{12} - \rho_{13} + \rho_{14} - \rho_{21} + \rho_{22} + \rho_{23} - \rho_{24})$$

The variances and covariances of these estimators are very complicated functions of the model parameters but can be written down simply in terms of the raw probabilities $\{\rho_{ij}\}$ which are estimated by the corresponding sample proportions $\{n_{ij}/n_{i.}\}$. Using these it is possible to construct analogues of all the tests described in Section 3.3. For details we refer to Zimmerman and Rahlfs (1978). Surprisingly these tests are not as different from those described earlier as might be expected. The reason is that in the log-linear models the sufficient statistics are linear contrasts among the counts $\{n_{ij}\}$ and the difference between the tests is largely, but not wholly, due to differences in the estimates of the variances of these contrasts. The relationships are closest for those tests in which a single parameter is tested in the presence of all the others. Interestingly Zimmerman and Rahlfs also suggest, as an additional direct treatment test, the analogue of $[\tau | \alpha, \sigma, \pi, \phi]$.

Le (1984) suggests a test for treatments on two degrees of freedom which can be derived from the same model. However, only the difference of the two contrasts proposed lies in the space of the group-by-outcome interaction (the three degrees of freedom of which correspond to τ_{lin}, λ^*_{lin} and ϕ_{lin}) and this corresponds to the τ_{lin} contrast.

It appears that the transformation employed to allow the use of the Grizzle *et al.* procedure is only applicable for, at most, two sequence cross-over designs, and a more general approach is required for other designs. The main drawback of this type of approach for trials with more than two periods or more than two categories of observation is the general sparseness of the resulting contingency table. The observed proportions will then be very poor estimates indeed of the row multinomial probabilities and the use of these in the variance estimate will most likely be unacceptable.

3.6.2 Modelling the marginal probabilities

Up to now we have only considered models for the joint probabilities of the outcomes from each subject. A fundamentally different approach is to model instead the marginal probabilities. Cox and Plackett (1980) describe one approach to this for the 2 × 2 trial, in which they model the logits of the marginal probabilities. We can write Cox and Plackett's model as follows in a way that parallels the definition of the earlier model (3.5). Although we use the same symbols as before for the various parameters, we add the subscript CP to emphasize that these have a different interpretation: they are defined in terms of marginal, not joint, probabilities. Let δ_{ij} be the probability of a success in period j of group i, for example $\delta_{11} = \rho_{13} + \rho_{14}$, $\delta_{12} = \rho_{12} + \rho_{14}$, etc. We then define simple linear models for the log odds (or logits) of δ_{ij}, i.e.

$$\text{logit}(\delta_{11}) = \alpha_{\text{CP}} - \pi_{\text{CP}} - \tau_{\text{CP}}$$

$$\text{logit}(\delta_{12}) = \alpha_{\text{CP}} + \pi_{\text{CP}} + \tau_{\text{CP}} - \lambda_{\text{CP}}$$

$$\text{logit}(\delta_{21}) = \alpha_{\text{CP}} - \pi_{\text{CP}} + \tau_{\text{CP}}$$

$$\text{logit}(\delta_{22}) = \alpha_{\text{CP}} + \pi_{\text{CP}} - \tau_{\text{CP}} + \lambda_{\text{CP}}$$

Although we have simple expressions for the marginal probabilities in this model we cannot write down simple expressions for the probabilities of the joint outcomes. In particular, there is no simple convenient parametric representation of the within-subject dependence structure. This means that the likelihood is not a simple function of the parameters in the model and likelihood ratio and conditional exact tests are not easy to construct. Cox and Plackett therefore use a similar approach to that used above for the linear contrasts method. To begin with, the four logits above are estimated by the corresponding sample logits. The variances and covariances of these are then estimated using functions of the observed counts $\{n_{ij}\}$ and from these appropriate test statistics can be constructed. Cox and Plackett give details.

Just as the linear alternative to the logit scale was used above for modelling the joint probabilities, so a linear version of Cox and Plackett's model is possible. Fidler (1984) uses a modification of such an approach in which linear contrasts among the marginal probabilities are used but in which the second-order moments are also modelled. This does lead to a rather complicated hierarchical definition of the effects and tests, however. As with the other alternative models described in this section, the likelihood for Fidler's model is intractable and Fidler uses conditional exact tests, some of which coincide with the tests described in Sections 3.2 and 3.3. In fact Fidler's model can be written as a particular parameterization of the general bivariate model (3.1). In an extension of his approach, Fidler (1987) shows how, in theory at least, his model could be applied to higher-order cross-over trials. However, the approach is rather involved from a practical viewpoint and it does not appear to fall into a class of models for which existing computational techniques are applicable.

The general problem of modelling marginal probabilities from sequences of correlated binary (and categorical) observations is an active area of research and it is likely that more developments will appear in the near future. Much existing methodology depends on simple estimates of second-order moments to overcome the problem of complicated parametric expressions (as is done in its simplest form in Zimmerman and Rahlfs' and Cox and Plackett's analyses). Such estimates may well be poor in small samples, and are therefore of limited use in many clinical trials. We would regard small sample size as the main problem in the construction of flexible models in this context.

There is a further approach which in one sense combines both the marginal and conditional approaches. In Sections 3.3 and 3.5 we described models with explicit subject effects. Conditional on these effects, the observations from each subject were mutually independent. In these earlier sections we treated these effects as nuisance parameters and eliminated them by conditioning on their sufficient satistics. An alternative way of dealing with the subject effects, which could be applied quite generally (not just with the logit transformation), is to treat them as random and introduce some distributions for them. This idea of random effects is appealing but the resulting computational problems are typically formidable. Cox and Plackett (1980) produced a manageable analysis for the 2 × 2 trial by assuming linearity after a probit rather than a logit transformation, and a normal distribution for the subject effects. Whitehead and Ezzet (1988) consider random effects models for categorical data in a much wider context in which the subject effects are also normally distributed, and describe a very general algorithm for obtaining maximum likelihood parameter estimates and likelihood ratio statistics. In principle, this could be used to analyse binary and categorical data from 2 × 2 and higher-order cross-over trials once the computational complexities have been satisfactorily resolved for routine application.

Appendix   Calculation of exact conditional probabilities

Introduction

Here we explain how to calculate the significance levels of the exact conditional tests described in Section 3.3. These tests were for the binary 2 × 2 trial and were based on the 2 × 4 contingency table of observed counts. We first explain how the conditional exact distributions are derived and then go on to describe various computer algorithms which can be used to enumerate all the different 2 × 4 tables required for the tests. We end by illustrating the methods using the data from centre 2 in Example 3.1.

Constructing the conditional distributions

It will be recalled that the sufficient statistics for the parameters in our model were denoted by $t_\alpha, t_\sigma, t_\pi$, and so on. Conditional on the observed values of t_α, t_σ and t_π, the distribution of the original data is that of a 2 × 4 contingency table with margins equal to those in the observed 2×4 table. So, for example, to test the null hypothesis that $\lambda = 0$ conditional on $\phi = 0$ and the observed values of the sufficient statistics for α, σ, π and τ, we would proceed as follows:

1. Enumerate all the 2×4 tables which have the same margins as the observed table (i.e. condition on the observed values of t_α, t_σ and t_π).
2. Locate within the set of tables found in 1 those tables which give the same value of t_τ as the observed table.
3. For each of the tables in the subset found in 2, calculate the value of the statistic t_λ and the probability of observing that particular table. This probability is derived in Freeman and Halton (1951), for example.
4. Construct the conditional probability distribution of t_λ using the values of t_λ obtained in 3 and the associated probabilities.

Using the conditional distribution so found we can calculate $P(t_\lambda \geqslant \text{observed value of } t_\lambda)$ or $P(t_\lambda \leqslant \text{observed value of } t_\lambda)$, depending on the observed value of t_λ. This probability is the one-sided probability of rejecting the null hypothesis.

The other tests are constructed in a similar way. So for example, if we wished to test the null hypothesis that $\lambda = 0$ conditional on t_ϕ as well as the observed values of $t_\tau, t_\alpha, t_\sigma$ and t_π, we would first enumerate all the 2×4 tables which have the same margins as the observed table and which give the same values of t_τ and t_ϕ as obtained from the observed data.

The same principles as those given above could equally well be applied to the more general situation of r sequence groups and c outcome categories, where both r and c are greater than 2. In order to apply the principles to the more general case we will need to generate all $r \times c$ tables with fixed margins, and methods of doing this are mentioned below.

Enumerating the tables

In order to calculate the exact significance level for a given observed table a computer program is needed which efficiently constructs all possible tables with the given fixed row and column margins, and accurately calculates the conditional probability associated with each table. To generate all the possible 2×4 tables with the same fixed margins as the observed table we wrote a computer program which contained a Fortran version of one of the Algol programs described by Boulton and Wallace (1973). This Algol program generates all possible $2 \times c$ tables with fixed margins, where $c \geqslant 2$. Boulton and Wallace also described an algorithm for constructing all possible $r \times c$ tables with fixed margins, where $r \geqslant 2$. The Boulton and Wallace program used the recursive facilities of Algol which we reproduced using sets of nested DO loops. The accurate calculation of the probabilities was done using a subroutine written by our colleague Dr T.R. Hopkins.

More recently, a number of algorithms which generate all $r \times c$ tables, with $r \geqslant 2$ and $c \geqslant 2$, have been published. An efficient algorithm has been described by Pagano and Halvorsen (1981). Although this algorithm can be used to obtain a total enumeration of all $r \times c$ tables and their associated conditional probabilities, the methods used do not require the total enumeration of all tables. Balmer (1988) described a program for the enumeration of all $r \times c$ tables with fixed margins and the calculation of the conditional probabilities. This program is written in Pascal and makes use of the recursive features of that language. Saunders (1984) described a Fortran program which enumerates all the $r \times c$ tables and calculates the conditional probabilities. This algorithm takes advantage of any equalities among the row totals and is therefore potentially more efficient than the algorithm described by Pagano and Halvorsen (1981).

The main difficulty in using Fortran to enumerate the tables is the lack of recursive facilities to vary dynamically the depth of a sequence of nested DO loops. It should be noted, however, that nested DO loops can be simulated in Fortran using, for example, the programs described by MacKenzie and O'Flaherty (1982) and Gentleman (1975). It should also be noted that if the total number of different tables that must be enumerated is considered to be too large, then sampling methods such as those described by Patefield (1981) may be used.

Example

We end this appendix by showing in more detail the method of calculating two of the significance levels quoted in Section 3.3. The levels were for the test for λ assuming that $\phi = 0$ and the Prescott test for τ and were obtained using the data from centre 2 in Example 3.1.

For the first test we require the distribution of t_λ conditional on the observed value (-8) of t_τ and the observed margins of the table. The conditional distribution so found is given in Figure 3.1, where the values given are t_λ and the probability of observing that value. The observed value of t_λ is 0 and we can see that, by summing the appropriate probabilities, $P[t_\lambda \leqslant 0] = 0.199$.

```
 t_λ       Probability
-12  0.00000066|
-10  0.00002457|
 -8  0.00037259|
 -6  0.00310080|
 -4  0.01595907|**
 -2  0.05412883|*****
  0  0.12559227|************
  2  0.20384377|*******************
  4  0.23426627|**********************
  6  0.19144180|******************
  8  0.11091886|**********
 10  0.04509027|*****
 12  0.01261238|*
 14  0.00235093|
 16  0.00027730|
 18  0.00001897|
 20  0.00000064|
 22  0.00000001|
```

Figure 3.1 *The distribution of* t_λ *given* $\phi = 0$.

```
 t_τ       Probability
-12  0.00025028|
-10  0.00301818|
 -8  0.01658538|**
 -6  0.05505961|*****
 -4  0.12313474|***********
 -2  0.19554009|******************
  0  0.22612488|*********************
  2  0.19183284|******************
  4  0.11843275|***********
  6  0.05184725|*****
  8  0.01525514|**
 10  0.00270194|
 12  0.00021691|
```

Figure 3.2 *The distribution of* t_τ *given* $\lambda = \phi = 0$.

The two-sided probability of rejecting the null hypothesis that $\lambda = 0$ can be taken as 0.398, giving no evidence to reject the null hypothesis.

Similarly we can test the null hypothesis that $\tau = 0$. The conditional distribution of t_τ is given in Figure 3.2. The observed value of t_τ is -8 and $P[t_\tau \leqslant -8] = 0.0198$, giving a two-sided probability of 0.04.

CHAPTER 4

Higher-order designs for two treatments

4.1 Introduction

In this chapter we consider higher-order designs for two treatments. By 'higher-order' we mean that the design includes either more than two sequence groups or more than two treatment periods or both. In Chapter 5 we will consider higher-order designs for more than two treatments.

The main disadvantages of the standard AB, BA design without baselines are that (a) the test for a carry-over effect or direct-by-period interaction lacks power because it is based on between-subject comparisons, and (b) the carry-over effect, the direct-by-period interaction and the group difference are all completely aliased with one another. If higher-order designs are used, however, we are able to obtain within-subject estimators of the carry-over effects or the direct-by-period interaction, and in some designs these estimators are not aliased with each other.

Another feature of the higher-order designs is that it is not necessary to assume that the subject effects are random variables in order to test for a difference between the carry-over effects. Although in principle we could recover direct treatment information from the between-subject variability, it is very unlikely to prove worth while, due to the large differences between the subjects that are typical in a cross-over trial. Consequently we will make the more convenient assumption that the subject effects are fixed and that the within-subject errors are independent with mean zero and variance σ^2. In fact, as long as we use within-subject contrasts, we get the same estimators of the parameters of interest when we use fixed subject effects and independent within-subject errors as when we use the uniform covariance structure.

An important feature of this chapter and the next is the way we determine which effects can be estimated from the within-subject contrasts. In order to do this we first determine how many degrees of freedom (d.f.) are available within subjects and then determine the contrasts that are associated with these d.f.

If a design has s sequence groups and p periods, then there are sp group-by-period means, $\bar{y}_{ij.}$. There are $(sp - 1)$ d.f. between these sp means which can be partitioned into $(s - 1)$ between groups, $(p - 1)$ between periods and $(s - 1)(p - 1)$ for the group-by-period interaction effects. This last set contains the d.f. associated with the effects of most interest, i.e. the direct treatments, direct-by-period interaction, the carry-over effects, and so on. Although this set of d.f. can be partitioned in a number of ways, we will always attempt a partition into three basic sets: (a) the direct treatment effects, (b) the direct-by-period interaction and carry-over effects, and (c) other effects not of direct interest associated with the group-by-period interaction.

For some designs the effects associated with the d.f. in set (b) will be aliased with other effects, and so there will be a choice of which terms to include in our model. For example, it will not always be possible to obtain unaliased estimates of both the direct-by-period interaction and the carry-over effects. Depending on the design, some, none or all the d.f. in set (b) will have aliases. Occasionally some of these d.f. will be confounded with subjects.

Another important feature of this and the next chapter is the way we define the fixed effects in our linear models. It is proved in the appendix to Chapter 7 that the same OLS estimators of the parameters of interest can be obtained in a number of different ways. The way we will use is to include a parameter for each group rather than a parameter for each subject. In this approach the models are specified in terms of the period means in each group and can therefore be easily written down.

In summary then, our approach will be to identify those d.f. which are associated with effects of interest and then to formulate a model which isolates these d.f. We regard the terms in our model as identifying contrasts of interest between the group-by-period means. Also our approach takes account of any marginality requirements induced by our model. So, for example, we would not include an interaction effect in the absence of the corresponding main effects. Further, we would not attempt to interpret a main effect in the presence of its corresponding interaction effect. In connection with this last point we note that it is not unusual in cross-over designs for the carry-over effects to be aliased with the direct-by-period interaction. If the carry-over effects are included in the model and are significant we must satisfy ourselves that it is unlikely that a direct-by-period interaction could have occurred. Only then would it be sensible to estimate the direct treatment difference in the presence of a carry-over difference.

The problem of deciding which design to use to estimate the direct and carry-over effects has been considered by a number of researchers. The designs they have chosen provide minimum-variance unbiased estimators of the effects of interest. In the following sections we will tabulate these designs and some others and look more closely at their properties.

In this chapter and the next we are also going to illustrate the analysis of data from cross-over trials. It should be noted that in these two chapters we are, in effect, assuming that the repeated measurements on each subject have the uniform covariance structure. This leads to OLS estimation and the usual analysis-of-variance tests. We reconsider the uniform covariance assumption in Chapter 7.

4.2 'Optimal' designs

In order to choose an optimal design we must first define the criterion of optimality. The various criteria used to compare cross-over designs with more than two treatments are briefly described in Chapter 5. For two treatments the criterion usually adopted in the literature is that a cross-over design is optimal if it provides minimum-variance unbiased estimators of τ and λ, where $\tau = -\tau_1 = \tau_2$ and $\lambda = -\lambda_1 = \lambda_2$.

Cheng and Wu (1980), Laska, Meisner and Kushner (1983), Laska and Meisner (1985) and Matthews (1987) have proved that if a uniform covariance structure, or our fixed subject effect structure, is adopted, the designs listed in Table 4.1 are optimal. These authors also considered the consequences of assuming that the within-subject errors are not independent, but are autocorrelated. That is, they assumed that the correlation between two repeated measurements depends on how far apart the measurements are in time. Assuming such an error structure provides useful and interesting insights into the properties of the various designs and we

Table 4.1 *Optimal two-treatment designs*

Design 1

Sequence	Period	
	1	2
1	A	A
2	B	B
3	A	B
4	B	A

Design 2

Sequence	Period		
	1	2	3
1	A	B	B
2	B	A	A

Design 3

Sequence	Period			
	1	2	3	4
1	A	A	B	B
2	B	B	A	A
3	A	B	B	A
4	B	A	A	B

Design 4

Sequence	Period				
	1	2	3	4	5
1	A	B	B	A	A
2	B	A	A	B	B

Design 5

Sequence	Period					
	1	2	3	4	5	6
1	A	B	B	A	A	B
2	B	A	A	B	B	A
3	A	A	B	B	B	A
4	B	B	A	A	A	B

will consider a number of alternative structures in Chapter 7. However, as will be seen there, including these structures in the analysis is difficult.

The properties of a number of different two-treatment designs have also been described by Kershner and Federer (1981).

4.3 Balaam's design for two treatments

Design 1 as given in Table 4.1 is a special case of one given by Balaam (1968) for comparing t treatments using t^2 experimental animals. In our version we use only two treatments and assign more than one subject to each sequence group.

Let us denote the mean response for the subjects in period j in group i by $\bar{y}_{ij.}$. There are two means in each group and so there are 4 d.f. for within-group comparisons. One of these is associated with the period difference and another with the direct effect. How we use the remaining 2 d.f. depends on the other effects that we think are important in the trial. Balaam was concerned with obtaining a within-subject estimator of the direct-by-period interaction and so associated one of the remaining d.f. with this effect. He did not make use of the other d.f. and the contrast associated with this was absorbed into the residual SS. If we include a parameter λ for the carry-over effect, then we can interpret the remaining d.f. in a meaningful way. However, we should not forget that λ is completely aliased with the direct-by-period interaction.

In our new parameterization we define $(\tau\lambda)$ to be the direct-by-carry-over interaction. This interaction would be significant if the carry-over effect of a treatment depended on the treatment applied in the immediately following period. Fleiss (1986b) has drawn attention to this possibility, suggesting that the carry-over of A when followed by B may not be the same as the carry-over when A is followed by A.

As usual, we put the following constraints on our parameters:

$$\tau_1 = -\tau_2 = -\tau$$
$$\pi_1 = -\pi_2 = -\pi$$
$$\lambda_1 = -\lambda_2 = -\lambda$$

Let us define the interaction between direct treatment r and carry-over effect m by $(\tau\lambda)_{rm}$ and let us also apply the constraints that

$$(\tau\lambda)_{11} = (\tau\lambda)_{22} = (\tau\lambda)$$

and

$$(\tau\lambda)_{12} = (\tau\lambda)_{21} = -(\tau\lambda)$$

The expectations of the eight group-by-period means are then as given in Table 4.2, where $\gamma_1, \gamma_2, \gamma_3$ and γ_4 are unconstrained parameters for groups $1, 2, 3$ and 4 respectively.

When considering the properties of this design, and those described in the following sections, we will assume that n subjects have been randomly assigned to each group. The achieved design will usually

Table 4.2 *Expectations of $\bar{y}_{ij\cdot}$ for direct-by-carry-over interaction model*

Group	Period 1	Period 2
1 AA	$\gamma_1 - \pi - \tau$	$\gamma_1 + \pi - \tau - \lambda + (\tau\lambda)$
2 BB	$\gamma_2 - \pi + \tau$	$\gamma_2 + \pi + \tau + \lambda + (\tau\lambda)$
3 AB	$\gamma_3 - \pi - \tau$	$\gamma_3 + \pi + \tau - \lambda - (\tau\lambda)$
4 BA	$\gamma_4 - \pi + \tau$	$\gamma_4 + \pi - \tau + \lambda - (\tau\lambda)$

have unequal group sizes and this will, of course, affect the design's properties. However, assuming equal group sizes will emphasize the good and bad features of the designs and will make comparisons between them much easier.

The OLS estimator of $(\tau\lambda)$ is

$$\widehat{(\tau\lambda)} = \tfrac{1}{4}(-\bar{y}_{11\cdot} + \bar{y}_{12\cdot} - \bar{y}_{21\cdot} + \bar{y}_{22\cdot} + \bar{y}_{31\cdot} - \bar{y}_{32\cdot} + \bar{y}_{41\cdot} - \bar{y}_{42\cdot})$$

and has variance

$$V[\widehat{(\tau\lambda)}] = \frac{\sigma^2}{2n}$$

If the direct-by-carry-over interaction is not significant and is dropped from the model, the estimators of $\lambda|\tau$ and $\tau|\lambda$ are as given below:

$$\hat{\lambda}|\tau = \tfrac{1}{2}(\bar{y}_{11\cdot} - \bar{y}_{12\cdot} - \bar{y}_{21\cdot} + \bar{y}_{22\cdot})$$
$$\hat{\tau}|\lambda = \tfrac{1}{4}(\bar{y}_{11\cdot} - \bar{y}_{12\cdot} - \bar{y}_{21\cdot} + \bar{y}_{22\cdot} - \bar{y}_{31\cdot} + \bar{y}_{32\cdot} + \bar{y}_{41\cdot} - \bar{y}_{42\cdot})$$

The variances of these are

$$V[\hat{\lambda}|\tau] = \frac{\sigma^2}{n} \qquad \text{and} \qquad V[\hat{\tau}|\lambda] = \frac{\sigma^2}{2n}$$

Of course, the above estimator of τ is only sensible if we are certain that there is no direct-by-period interaction and we wish to estimate τ adjusted for λ. This is the advantage that this design has over the 2×2 cross-over: we can obtain a within-subjects estimate of τ in the presence of a carry-over effect. We also note that only groups 1 and 2 are used to estimate $\lambda|\tau$.

If the carry-over effect is not significant and can be dropped from the model then the estimator of τ is

$$\hat{\tau} = \tfrac{1}{4}(-\bar{y}_{31\cdot} + \bar{y}_{32\cdot} + \bar{y}_{41\cdot} - \bar{y}_{42\cdot})$$

and has variance

$$V[\hat{\tau}] = \frac{\sigma^2}{4n}$$

If there is no carry-over effect we note that, as in the AB, BA design, only two groups are used to estimate τ.

We will illustrate the analysis of Balaam's design in the next section.

As the analysis of a cross-over trial will almost certainly be done using a computer, it is not necessary to know the formulae for the OLS estimators for the general case of unequal group sizes. However, should these be required, they can be obtained by using the matrix results given in the appendix to Chapter 7. These results are for any number of treatments and periods and so can be used for any of the designs given in this chapter and the next.

4.4   The analysis for Balaam's design

We will illustrate the analysis for Balaam's design by using some data from a trial described by Hunter *et al.* (1970). This trial and the data taken from Taka and Armitage (1983), are described in Example 4.1. It will be noted that in this trial the groups are not all of equal size.

Example 4.1   Amantadine in Parkinsonism

The aim of this trial was to determine if amantadine hydrochloride produced a beneficial effect on subjects suffering from Parkinsonism. Amantadine (treatment A) was compared with a matching placebo (treatment B) on 17 subjects over a period of nine weeks. Each subject's physical signs were evaluated in week 1, prior to receiving A or B, and then at weekly intervals. There were no wash-out periods. Each treatment was administered, in a double-blind fashion, for a period of four consecutive weeks. Subjects were evaluated by using a scoring system. Each of 11 physical signs (drooling saliva, finger dexterity, walking, rising from chair, balance, speech, rigidity, posture, tremor, sweating and facial masking) were scored on a 0–4 point scale. The total of these 11 scores then gave the final score.

For our analysis we will consider a period to be made up of the four weeks on each treatment and we will use the average score over the four weeks as our response measurement. These data are given

Table 4.3 *Average scores for amantadine trial*

Group	Subject	Baseline	Period 1	Period 2
1 AA	1	14	12·50	14·00
	2	27	24·25	22·50
	3	19	17·25	16·25
	4	30	28·25	29·75
2 BB	1	21	20·00	19·51
	2	11	10·50	10·00
	3	20	19·50	20·75
	4	25	22·50	23·50
3 AB	1	9	8·75	8·75
	2	12	10·50	9·75
	3	17	15·00	18·50
	4	21	21·00	21·50
4 BA	1	23	22·00	18·00
	2	15	15·00	13·00
	3	13	14·00	13·75
	4	24	22·75	21·50
	5	18	17·75	16·75

Reprinted from Taka and Armitage (1983), p. 871, by courtesy of Marcell Dekker, Inc.

in Table 4.3, along with the baseline scores taken in week 1. It should be noted that groups 3 and 4 in Table 4.3 correspond to groups 4 and 3, respectively, as given by Hunter *et al.*

We begin our analysis of these data by looking at the subject profiles given in Figure 4.1. For each subject in each group we have plotted the baseline score, the scores for periods 1 and 2, and joined them up. Apart from noticing that most subjects respond with a lower score in period 1 as compared to their baseline and that there does not appear to be a period effect, there is nothing else striking about these plots.

Further information can be obtained from the baseline and period means in each group. These are given in Table 4.4.

The means are more informative and suggest (a) that within groups 3 and 4, A gives a lower score than B; (b) the difference between A and B is greater when the baseline score is high; and (c) in groups 1 and 2 there is no period effect. We now investigate these suggestions further by fitting the model given in Table 4.2. The analysis of variance is given in Table 4.5, where it will be recalled that each SS

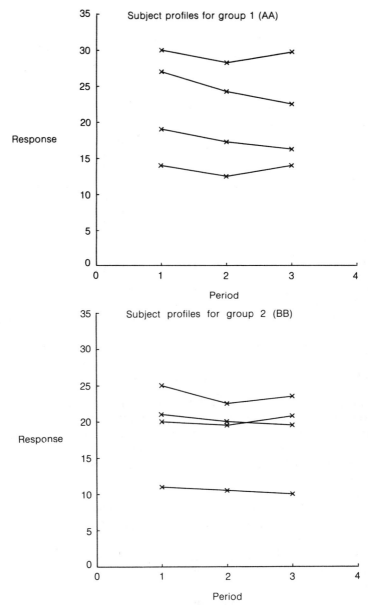

Figure 4.1 *Subject profiles for each group.*

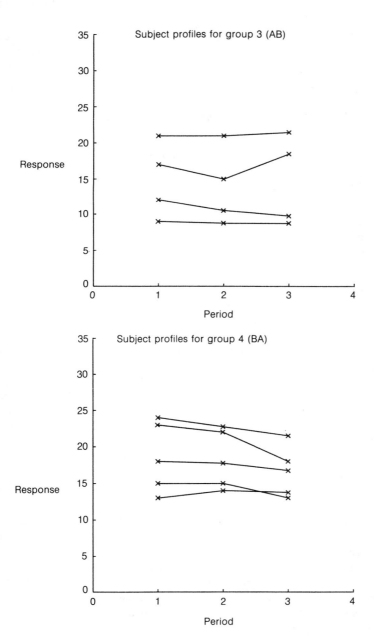

Table 4.4 *The group-by-period means*

Group	Size	Baseline	Period 1	Period 2
1 AA	$n_1 = 4$	22·50	$\bar{y}_{11\cdot} = 20{\cdot}56$	$\bar{y}_{12\cdot} = 20{\cdot}63$
2 BB	$n_2 = 4$	19·25	$\bar{y}_{21\cdot} = 18{\cdot}13$	$\bar{y}_{22\cdot} = 18{\cdot}44$
3 AB	$n_3 = 4$	14·75	$\bar{y}_{31\cdot} = 13{\cdot}81$	$\bar{y}_{32\cdot} = 14{\cdot}63$
4 BA	$n_4 = 5$	18·60	$\bar{y}_{41\cdot} = 18{\cdot}30$	$\bar{y}_{42\cdot} = 16{\cdot}60$

Table 4.5 *The analysis of variance for Hunter et al.'s data*

Source	d.f.	SS	MS	F
Between subjects	16	957·168	59·823	
Within subjects:				
Periods	1	0·411	0·411	
Direct treatments	1	7·434	7·434	6·49
Carry-over	1	0·064	0·064	0·06
Direct × carry-over	1	0·843	0·843	0·74
Residual	13	14·900	1·146	
Total	33	980·820		

in the table is the SS for terms identified in the corresponding Source column adjusted for the effects of all the preceding terms in the table. Therefore, for example, the SS corresponding to Direct × carry-over is the additional SS for $(\tau\lambda)$ given that subjects, periods, direct treatments and carry-overs are already accounted for in the model.

There is insufficient evidence to reject the null hypotheses that $(\tau\lambda) = 0$ and $\lambda = 0$ (P = 0·41 and P = 0·81, respectively), and these parameters can be dropped from the model. (Abeyasekera and Curnow, 1984, argue that carry-over effects should be left in the model even when they are found to be not statistically significant. We, however, will follow common practice and will always remove insignificant effects.) The direct treatment effect, however, is significant at the 5% level (P = 0·02). Using the model without $(\tau\lambda)$ and λ we obtain 1·290 as a point estimate of $\tau_2 - \tau_1$ with a standard error of 0·485 on 15 d.f. A 95% confidence interval is (0·26, 2·32).

As yet we have not made use of the run-in baseline responses that were taken in week 1. We can either (a) include these in our model directly, or (b) use them to provide a covariate adjustment. Let us consider option (a) first.

The model we will use is as defined in Table 4.2 except that: (1) there is a baseline period before period 1 which is modelled as $\gamma_i + \pi_0$, for groups $i = 1, 2, 3$ and 4, where π_0 is the effect of the baseline period; and (2) the three period effects π_0, π_1 and π_2 are such that $\pi_0 + \pi_1 + \pi_2 = 0$.

Using this model the variances of $\widehat{(\tau\lambda)}|\tau, \lambda, \; \hat{\lambda}|\tau, \; \hat{t}|\lambda$ and $\hat{t}$ are, respectively, $3\sigma^2/8n$, $3\sigma^2/7n$, $3\sigma^2/14n$ and $3\sigma^2/16n$. The estimators obtained using baselines have smaller variances and so we have gained in precision. The largest reductions have occurred in the variances of $\lambda|\tau$ and $\tau|\lambda$, which have been reduced by 57%.

When the model including the baselines is fitted to our observed data the conclusions we obtained earlier are not altered. However, our estimate of $\tau_2 - \tau_1$ is now 1·209 with a standard error of 0·406 on 31 d.f. That is, the 95% confidence interval for $\tau_2 - \tau_1$ has been shortened to (0·38, 2·04).

Let us now consider option (b), which uses the scores in week 1 as a covariate. Associated with the scores in each of periods 1 and 2 is the corresponding value of the covariate. The covariate cannot help us obtain improved within-subject estimators of our model parameters, because it will be eliminated in any within-subject contrast. It can be used however, to check for any period-by-covariate, direct-by-covariate or carry-over-by-covariate interaction. The analysis of covariance for our data is given in Table 4.6.

The conclusions that we can draw from Table 4.6 are that there is no evidence to suggest an interaction of the baseline with periods or carry-over, but there is a suggestion ($P = 0.14$) of an interaction

Table 4.6 *The analysis of covariance for Hunter et al.'s data*

Source	d.f.	SS	MS	F
Between subjects	16	957·168	59·823	
Within subjects:				
Periods	1	0·411	0·411	
Direct treatments	1	7·434	7·434	6·62
Carry-over	1	0·064	0·064	0·06
Baseline × period	1	0·168	0·168	0·15
Baseline × direct treatment	1	2·778	2·778	2·47
Baseline × carry-over	1	0·439	0·439	0·39
Residual	11	12·356	1·123	
Total	33	980·819		

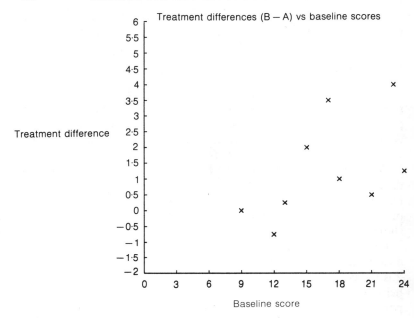

Figure 4.2 *Plot of direct treatment difference (B − A) vs baseline score.*

of direct treatments with baseline. Therefore, although we have no real evidence to suggest an interaction might be present, there is a hint of one which might be worth following up. Had this interaction been significant we would have attempted to discover its cause. This could be done, for example, by plotting for each subject the direct treatment difference against the corresponding value of the covariate and looking for a trend. An increasing trend would indicate that the treatment difference was larger when the response in week 1 was large. A decreasing trend would indicate the reverse.

The plot of the treatment difference (B − A) versus the covariate is given in Figure 4.2. There is certainly the suggestion of an upward trend, suggesting that the direct treatment difference increases as the value of the baseline increases.

4.5   Three-period designs with two sequences

As noted in Section 4.2, the three-period design that is optimal for estimating $\tau|\lambda$ and $\lambda|\tau$ is the one reproduced below, and now labelled as design 3.2.1. We introduce the new labelling to aid the comparison of different designs. We label a design using the code $p.s.i$, where p is the number of periods, s is the number of sequence groups and i is an index number to distinguish different designs with the same p and s.

Design 3.2.1

Sequence	Period		
	1	2	3
1	A	B	B
2	B	A	A

It will be noted that all the optimal designs listed earlier in Section 4.2 are made up of one or more pairs of **dual** sequences. A dual of a sequence is obtained by interchanging the A and B treatment labels. So, for example, the dual of ABB is BAA. From a practical point of view, the only designs worth considering are those which are made up of one or more equally replicated pairs of dual sequences. Designs which have equal replication on each member of a dual pair are called **dual balanced**. Although optimal designs are not necessarily dual balanced, there will always be a dual-balanced optimal design (Matthews, 1988b). Also, as will be seen in Section 4.7, if a design is made up of a dual pair then a simple and robust analysis is possible. This simple analysis can also be extended to designs which contain more than one dual pair, as will be seen in Section 4.9. Therefore, here and in the following, we will only consider designs made up of dual sequences. It will be noted that all the optimal designs listed in Section 4.2 are dual balanced.

The only other three-period designs with two sequences which contain a dual pair are designs 3.2.2 and 3.2.3, which are given below.

Design 3.2.2

Sequence	Period		
	1	2	3
1	A	B	A
2	B	A	B

Design 3.2.3

Sequence	Period		
	1	2	3
1	A	A	B
2	B	B	A

Let us now consider the properties of design 3.2.1 and let $\bar{y}_{ij}$ denote the mean for period j of group i, where $j = 1, 2$ or 3 and $i = 1$ or 2. Within each group there are 2 d.f. associated with the differences between the period means, giving a total of 4 for both groups. Of these, 2 are associated with the period differences, 1 is associated with the direct treatment difference and 1 is associated with direct-by-period interaction. The carry-over effect is aliased with one component of the direct-by-period interaction and so we can, in our model for the within-subject responses, either include a carry-over parameter or an interaction parameter. For convenience, we will include the carry-over parameter.

The expectations of the six group-by-period means are given in Table 4.7, where the period effects are denoted by π_1, π_2 and π_3 and the constraint $\pi_1 + \pi_2 + \pi_3 = 0$ has been applied. The other parameters are as defined previously. For design 3.2.1 the OLS estimators of $\lambda | \tau$ and $\tau | \lambda$ are

$$\hat{\lambda} | \tau = \tfrac{1}{4}[- \bar{y}_{12\cdot} + \bar{y}_{13\cdot} + \bar{y}_{22\cdot} - \bar{y}_{23\cdot}]$$

$$\hat{\tau} | \lambda = \tfrac{1}{8}[- 2\bar{y}_{11\cdot} + \bar{y}_{12\cdot} + \bar{y}_{13\cdot} + 2\bar{y}_{21\cdot} - \bar{y}_{22\cdot} - \bar{y}_{23\cdot}]$$

and

$$\hat{\tau} = \hat{\tau} | \lambda$$

where, as always, we assume that each group contains n subjects. The variances of these estimators are $V[\hat{\lambda} | \tau] = \sigma^2/4n$, $V[\hat{\tau} | \lambda] = V[\hat{\tau}] = 3\sigma^2/16n$ and $Cov[\hat{\tau} | \lambda, \hat{\lambda} | \tau] = 0$.

For the case of unequal group sizes $n_1 \neq n_2$, the estimators of $\hat{\lambda} | \tau$ and $\hat{\tau} | \lambda$ are the same as given above. The formulae for their variances, however, need to be modified in the obvious way. That is,

$$V[\hat{\lambda} | \tau] = \frac{\sigma^2}{8}\left(\frac{1}{n_1} + \frac{1}{n_2}\right) \quad \text{and} \quad V[\hat{\tau} | \lambda] = \frac{3\sigma^2}{32}\left(\frac{1}{n_1} + \frac{1}{n_2}\right)$$

Table 4.7 *The expectations of $\bar{y}_{ij\cdot}$ for design 3.2.1*

Group	Period		
	1	2	3
1 ABB	$\gamma_1 + \pi_1 - \tau$	$\gamma_1 + \pi_2 + \tau - \lambda$	$\gamma_1 - \pi_1 - \pi_2 + \tau + \lambda$
2 BAA	$\gamma_2 + \pi_1 + \tau$	$\gamma_2 + \pi_2 - \tau + \lambda$	$\gamma_2 - \pi_1 - \pi_2 - \tau - \lambda$

Table 4.8 *The variances and covariances for the three-period designs (in multiples of σ^2/n)*

Design	$V[\hat{\lambda}|\tau]$	$V[\hat{t}|\lambda]$	$Cov[\hat{\lambda}|\tau, \hat{t}|\lambda]$
3.2.1	0·2500	0·1875	0·0000
3.2.2	1·0000	0·7500	0·7500
3.2.3	1·0000	0·2500	0·2500

The advantages of using design 3.2.1 can be appreciated if we compare the variances of the estimators obtained from this design with those obtained from designs 3.2.2 and 3.2.3. These variances and covariances are given in Table 4.8, in multiples of σ^2/n. It can be seen that the variances are four times larger in designs 3.2.2 and 3.2.3. Also, the estimators are not uncorrelated in these designs. It should be noted that Matthews (1988b) proved that $Cov[\hat{t}|\lambda, \hat{\lambda}|\tau] = 0$ for any optimal two-treatment design with more than two periods.

In most cross-over trials there will be a run-in baseline measurement on each subject prior to the start of the first treatment period. As with Balaam's design we could either include this baseline in our model as done in Table 4.6 or use it as a covariate. If we include the baseline in our model we find that we get the same estimator of $\lambda|\tau$ but a different estimator of $\tau|\lambda$. Although the new estimator of $\tau|\lambda$ makes use of the baselines, its variance is only slightly reduced: without baselines the variance is $0.1875\sigma^2/n$ as compared to $0.1818\sigma^2/n$ with baselines. In fact, if there had also been a wash-out period between each of the three treatment periods the conclusions would have been the same. The estimator of $\lambda|\tau$ does not change and the variance of $\hat{t}|\lambda$ is only reduced to $0.1765\sigma^2/n$. These variance calculations illustrate a general result proved by Laska, Meisner and Kushner (1983) which states that when three or more periods are used, baselines taken before each period are of little or no use for increasing the precision of the estimators.

The run-in baseline can sometimes be usefully included as a covariate and we will illustrate this in the next section.

Unlike Balaam's design, design 3.2.1 does not provide sufficient d.f. for a direct-by-carry-over interaction to be included in the model. If, however, additional information on the nature of the carry-over effect is available, then our model can be altered to take account of it. For example, if we know that a treatment cannot carry over into

Table 4.9 *Systolic blood pressures from a three-period design with four groups*

Group	Subject	Period			
		Run-in	1	2	3
1 ABB	1	173	159	140	137
	2	168	153	172	155
	3	200	160	156	140
	4	180	160	200	132
	5	190	170	170	160
	6	170	174	132	130
	7	185	175	155	155
	8	180	154	138	150
	9	160	160	170	168
	10	170	160	160	170
	11	165	145	140	140
	12	168	148	154	138
	13	190	170	170	150
	14	160	125	130	130
	15	190	140	112	95
	16	170	125	140	125
	17	170	150	150	145
	18	158	136	130	140
	19	210	150	140	160
	20	175	150	140	150
	21	186	202	181	170
	22	190	190	150	170
2 BAA	1	168	165	154	173
	2	200	160	165	140
	3	130	140	150	180
	4	170	140	125	130
	5	190	158	160	180
	6	180	180	165	160
	7	200	170	160	160
	8	166	140	158	148
	9	188	126	170	200
	10	175	130	125	150
	11	186	144	140	120
	12	160	140	160	140
	13	135	120	145	120
	14	175	145	150	150
	15	150	155	130	140
	16	178	168	168	168
	17	170	150	160	180
	18	160	120	120	140
	19	190	150	150	160
	20	160	150	140	130
	21	200	175	180	160
	22	160	140	170	150
	23	180	150	160	130

(*Continued*)

Table 4.9 (*Continued*)

Group	Subject	Period			
		Run-in	1	2	3
2 BAA	24	170	150	130	125
(*Continued*)	25	165	140	150	160
	26	200	140	140	130
	27	142	126	140	138
3 ABA	1	184	154	145	150
	2	210	160	140	140
	3	250	210	190	190
	4	180	110	112	130
	5	165	130	140	130
	6	210	180	190	160
	7	175	155	120	160
	8	186	170	164	158
	9	178	170	140	180
	10	150	155	130	135
	11	130	115	110	120
	12	155	180	136	150
	13	140	130	120	126
	14	180	135	140	155
	15	162	148	148	162
	16	185	180	180	190
	17	220	190	155	160
	18	170	178	152	174
	19	220	172	178	180
	20	172	164	150	160
	21	200	170	140	140
	22	154	168	176	148
	23	150	130	120	130
4 BAB	1	140	160	145	112
	2	156	156	152	140
	3	215	195	195	180
	4	150	130	126	122
	5	170	130	136	130
	6	170	140	140	150
	7	198	160	160	160
	8	210	140	180	165
	9	170	140	135	125
	10	160	100	129	120
	11	168	148	164	148
	12	200	150	170	134
	13	240	205	240	150
	14	155	140	140	140
	15	180	154	180	156
	16	160	150	130	160
	17	150	140	130	130

itself, and there is no other form of direct-by-period interaction, then our model can be modified so that λ appears only in period 2. The OLS estimators of the parameters are then

$$\hat{\lambda}|\tau = \tfrac{1}{2}[-\bar{y}_{12.} + \bar{y}_{13.} + \bar{y}_{22.} - \bar{y}_{23.}] \quad \text{with } V[\hat{\lambda}|\tau] = \frac{\sigma^2}{n}$$

and

$$\hat{\tau}|\lambda = \tfrac{1}{4}[-\bar{y}_{11.} + \bar{y}_{13.} + \bar{y}_{21.} - \bar{y}_{23.}] \quad \text{with } V[\hat{\tau}|\lambda] = \frac{\sigma^2}{4n}$$

4.6 The analysis for design 3.2.1

In order to illustrate the analysis for design 3.2.1 and another with four sequence groups we will use the data from the trial described in Example 4.2.

Example 4.2   A trial on hypertensive subjects

Ebbutt (1984) described the analysis of design 3.2.1 and another with four sequence groups for the case of equal group sizes. He illustrated his results by using some data from a trial to compare the effects of two treatments on the blood pressure of hypertensive subjects. Subjects were randomly assigned to the four sequence groups ABB, BAA, ABA and BAB. There was a pre-trial run-in period followed by three six-week treatment periods. For ethical reasons there were no wash-out periods. Among other things, the systolic blood pressure of each subject was measured at the end of each period. Ebbutt used the data from only 10 subjects in each group. Table 4.9 gives the systolic blood pressure in each period for all the subjects who completed the trial.

We note that in Table 4.9 groups 1 and 2 make up design 3.2.1 and groups 3 and 4 make up design 3.2.2. Here we will consider the data only from groups 1 and 2 in order to illustrate the analysis of design 3.2.1. The data from all four groups will be considered in Section 4.8.

The period means for groups 1 and 2 are given in Table 4.10. We note that the groups are not of equal size and the period means suggest that blood pressure is lower on treatment B.

Table 4.10 *Period means for each group*

Group	Size	Period		
		1	2	3
1 ABB	$n_1 = 22$	$\bar{y}_{11.} = 157\cdot09$	$\bar{y}_{12.} = 151\cdot36$	$\bar{y}_{13.} = 145\cdot91$
2 BAA	$n_2 = 27$	$\bar{y}_{21.} = 147\cdot11$	$\bar{y}_{22.} = 150\cdot56$	$\bar{y}_{23.} = 150\cdot44$

Table 4.11 *The analysis of variance for groups 1 and 2*

Source	d.f.	SS	MS	F
Between subjects	48	30648·6	638·5	
Within subjects:				
Periods	2	275·9	137·9	
Direct treatments	1	1133·6	1133·6	6·6
Carry-over	1	173·1	173·1	1·0
Residual	94	16192·1	172·3	
Total	146	48423·2		

Ignoring the baseline responses for the moment, the analysis of variance for our two groups is given in Table 4.11. There is no evidence of a carry-over difference but there is strong evidence ($P = 0\cdot01$) of a direct treatment difference and so only τ needs to be retained in the model in addition to the period and group

Table 4.12 *The analysis of covariance for groups 1 and 2*

Source	d.f.	SS	MS	F
Between subjects	48	30 648·6	638·5	
Within subjects:				
Periods	2	275·9	137·9	
Direct treatments	1	1 133·6	1133·6	6·60
Carry-over	1	173·1	173·1	1·01
Baseline × period	2	605·8	302·9	1·76
Baseline × direct treatment	1	80·8	80·8	0·47
Baseline × carry-over	1	21·1	21·1	0·12
Residual	90	15 484·4	172·0	
Total	146	48 423·2		

parameters. A 95% confidence interval for $\tau_1 - \tau_2$ is $5{\cdot}92 \pm 2{\cdot}00 \times 2{\cdot}31 = (1{\cdot}30, 10{\cdot}54)$.

As mentioned in Section 4.4, the baseline responses can be used either (a) formally in the model or (b) as a covariate. We showed in Section 4.5 that formally including the baseline in the model did not result in any significant increase in precision being obtained. Therefore, we do not consider option (a) any further.

If we include the baseline as a covariate, however, then as done for the data given in Example 4.1, we can test for the presence of an interaction with the baseline. The analysis-of-covariance table is given in Table 4.12.

Clearly, there is no evidence in Table 4.12 of any interaction between the periods, direct treatments and carry-over with the baseline. Therefore our previous conclusions are not altered in any way.

4.7   A simple and robust analysis for two-group dual designs

If a design is made up of a pair of dual sequences, as defined in Section 4.5, then a simple and robust analysis is possible. In this analysis we can relax the assumptions made about the covariance structure of the repeated measurements. The analysis uses two-sample t-tests, or, if the data are very non-normal, Wilcoxon rank-sum tests. The analysis is robust in the sense that the only assumptions made are that (a) the responses from different subjects are independent, and (b) the two groups of subjects are a random sample from the same statistical population.

The method of analysis is similar to that described in Section 2.9. That is, we express the estimator of the parameter of interest as a difference between the groups of a particular contrast between the period means. In order to illustrate the method we will use Example 4.2. We first define the contrast for $\lambda|\tau$ and show how a t-test can be constructed, then we do the same for $\tau|\lambda$.

For the kth subject in group 1, $k = 1, 2, \ldots, n_1$, we define $d_{11k} = -y_{12k} + y_{13k}$ and for the kth subject in group 2, $k = 1, 2, \ldots, n_2$, we define $d_{21k} = -y_{22k} + y_{23k}$. We then let $\bar{d}_{11.} = -\bar{y}_{12.} + \bar{y}_{13.}$ and $\bar{d}_{21.} = -\bar{y}_{22.} + \bar{y}_{23.}$. We can then, using the formula for $\hat{\lambda}|\tau$ given in Section 4.5, write

$$\hat{\lambda}|\tau = \tfrac{1}{4}[\bar{d}_{11.} - \bar{d}_{12.}]$$

If $\sigma_1^2 = V[d_{11k}] = V[d_{21k}]$, then

$$V[\hat{\lambda}|\tau] = \frac{\sigma_1^2}{16}\left[\frac{1}{n_1} + \frac{1}{n_2}\right]$$

To estimate σ_1^2 we use the orthodox pooled estimator

$$s_1^2 = \frac{(n_1 - 1)s_{11}^2 + (n_2 - 1)s_{21}^2}{(n_1 + n_2 - 2)}$$

where, s_{11}^2 is the sample variance of d_{11k} and s_{21}^2 is the sample variance of d_{21k}.

To test the null hypothesis that $\lambda = 0$ we calculate

$$t = \frac{\bar{d}_{11\cdot} - \bar{d}_{12\cdot}}{\left[\dfrac{s_1^2}{16}\left(\dfrac{1}{n_1} + \dfrac{1}{n_2}\right)\right]^{1/2}}$$

which on the null hypothesis has the t-distribution with $(n_1 + n_2 - 2)$ d.f.

The d.f. for the above t-statistic are half those for the conventional F-test used in Section 4.6. This loss in d.f. is the price to be paid for making less stringent assumptions. The price, however, as here, is not usually a high one.

To test the null hypothesis that $\tau = 0$ we proceed in exactly the same way, except now the contrasts are $d_{12k} = -2y_{11k} + y_{12k} + y_{13k}$ in group 1 and $d_{22k} = -2y_{21k} + y_{22k} + y_{23k}$ in group 2.

The estimator of $\tau|\lambda$, which equals the estimator of τ in design 3.2.1, can be written as

$$\hat{\tau} = \tfrac{1}{8}[\bar{d}_{12\cdot} - \bar{d}_{22\cdot}]$$

and has variance

$$V[\hat{\tau}] = \frac{\sigma_2^2}{64}\left(\frac{1}{n_1} + \frac{1}{n_2}\right)$$

where σ_2^2 is the variance of the subject contrast for τ.

The values of the two contrasts for each subject are given in Table 4.13, along with the corresponding sample means and variances.

Using the information in Table 4.13 we have that $\hat{\lambda}|\tau = (-5\cdot45 + 0\cdot11)/4 = -1\cdot33$, as before, and that the pooled estimate of σ_1^2 is $332\cdot045$ on 47 d.f. The pooled variance of $\hat{\lambda}|\tau$ is then $1\cdot712$, giving

Table 4.13 *The subject contrasts for* $\lambda|\tau$ *and* τ

Group	Subject	Contrast d_{11k}	Contrast d_{12k}
1 ABB	1	−3	−41
	2	−17	21
	3	−16	−24
	4	−68	12
	5	−10	−10
	6	−2	−86
	7	0	−40
	8	12	−20
	9	−2	18
	10	10	10
	11	0	−10
	12	−16	−4
	13	−20	−20
	14	0	10
	15	−17	−73
	16	−15	15
	17	−5	−5
	18	10	−2
	19	20	0
	20	10	−10
	21	−11	−53
	22	20	−60
	Mean	−5·45	−16·91
	Variance	342·45	913·33

Group	Subject	Contrast d_{21k}	Contrast d_{22k}
2 BAA	1	19	−3
	2	−25	−15
	3	30	50
	4	5	−25
	5	20	24
	6	−5	−35
	7	0	−20
	8	−10	26
	9	30	118
	10	25	15
	11	−20	−28
	12	−20	20
	13	−25	25
	14	0	10
	15	10	−40
	16	0	0
	17	20	40
	18	20	20

(*Continued*)

Table 4.13 (*Continued*)

Group	Subject	Contrast d_{21k}	Contrast d_{22k}
2 BAA	19	10	10
(*Continued*)	20	-10	-30
	21	-20	-10
	22	-20	40
	23	-30	-10
	24	-5	-45
	25	10	30
	26	-10	-10
	27	-2	26
	Mean	$-0\cdot11$	$6\cdot78$
	Variance	323.64	1198·26

a t-statistic of $-1\cdot02$ on 47 d.f. Clearly, there is no evidence ($P = 0\cdot32$) of a difference in carry-over effects.

Repeating the above for τ gives $\hat{\tau} = (-16\cdot91 - 6\cdot78)/8 = -2\cdot96$ and a pooled estimate of σ_2^2 equal to 1070·95. The pooled variance of $\hat{\tau}$ os 1·380, giving a t-statistic for testing $\tau = 0$ of $-2\cdot52$ on 47 d.f. This is significant at the 5% level giving good evidence ($P = 0\cdot016$) to reject the null hypothesis of equal direct effects.

4.8 Three-period designs with four sequences

Although design 3.2.1 is optimal in the sense that it minimizes the variances of the OLS estimators of $\lambda|\tau$ and $\tau|\lambda$, it does have certain disadvantages. For example, the estimators of the carry-over effect and the direct-by-period interaction are aliased with one another, and it is not possible to test for a direct-by-carry-over interaction. The use of additional sequences can overcome these disadvantages and so it is useful to consider the properties of designs with more than two groups.

There are three different four-group designs which can be constructed by using different pairings of the dual designs given in Section 4.5. These new designs are labelled as 3.4.1, 3.4.2 and 3.4.3, and are listed below.

Design 3.4.1

Sequence	Period		
	1	2	3
1	A	B	B
2	B	A	A
3	A	B	A
4	B	A	B

Design 3.4.2

Sequence	Period		
	1	2	3
1	A	B	B
2	B	A	A
3	A	A	B
4	B	B	A

Design 3.4.3

Sequence	Period		
	1	2	3
1	A	B	A
2	B	A	B
3	A	A	B
4	B	B	A

There are 11 d.f. between the 12 group-by-period means and following our usual practice we associate 3 of these with the group effects, 2 with the period effects and 6 with the group-by-period interaction. These last 6 are the ones of most interest to us and we would like to associate them with the direct treatment effects, the direct-by-period interaction and the carry-over effects. However, the 2 d.f. for the direct-by-period interaction are aliased with the d.f. for the first-order carry-over effect and the second-order carry-over effect. The second-order carry-over is the differential treatment effect that lasts for two periods after the treatments are administered. If we choose to include two interaction parameters in our model then there are 3 d.f. left which are associated with uninteresting group-by-period interaction contrasts. If we include parameters for the two different sorts of carry-over effect, however, then we can associate 1 of the remaining 3 d.f. with the interaction between the direct treatments and the first-order carry-over effects. The remaining 2 d.f. are then associated with uninteresting group-by-period interaction contrasts. Whichever parameterization is chosen, the uninteresting d.f. are added to those of the residual SS. Although we choose to include the carry-over parameters, it should be remembered that these parameters are aliased with the direct-by-period interaction parameters and so apparently significant carry-over effects may be caused by the presence of more general interaction effects.

As always we will compare the designs for the special case of $n_1 = n_2 = n_3 = n_4 = n$. The example given in the next section illustrates the analysis for the case of unequal group sizes. General formulae for the case of unequal group sizes can be obtained by referring to the appendix to Chapter 7.

In each of designs 3.4.1, 3.4.2 and 3.4.3 we wish to allocate effects of interest to the 11 d.f. between the group-by-period means. As said earlier, 3 of these are associated with the group effects, 2 are associated with the period effects, 4 are associated with various treatment effects and 2 are associated with the interaction of groups and periods. Let us label the effects associated with these last 6 d.f. as $\tau, \lambda, \theta, (\tau\lambda), (\gamma\pi)_1$ and $(\gamma\pi)_2$, where these refer, respectively, to the direct treatment effect, the first-order carry-over effect, the second-order carry-over effect, the interaction between the direct treatments and the first-order carry-over effects and two particular group-by-period interaction contrasts. These last two contrasts are, of course, not of great interest in themselves and we have included them only in order that the full partition of the 11 d.f. can be seen. It turns out that these two contrasts are orthogonal to each other and to the other effects in the full model.

Let us consider design 3.4.1 in detail. The OLS estimators of $(\gamma\pi)_1$ and $(\gamma\pi)_2$ are

$$(\widehat{\gamma\pi})_1 = \tfrac{1}{4}(-\bar{y}_{11\cdot} + \bar{y}_{12\cdot} + \bar{y}_{31\cdot} - \bar{y}_{32\cdot})$$

and

$$(\widehat{\gamma\pi})_2 = \tfrac{1}{4}(-\bar{y}_{21\cdot} + \bar{y}_{22\cdot} + \bar{y}_{41\cdot} - \bar{y}_{42\cdot})$$

It will be convenient to represent estimators using the notation $\mathbf{c}^T\bar{\mathbf{y}}$ where $\mathbf{c}$ is a vector of contrast coefficients and $\bar{\mathbf{y}} = [\bar{y}_{11\cdot}, \bar{y}_{12\cdot}, \ldots, \bar{y}_{43\cdot}]^T$. So for example,

$$(\widehat{\gamma\pi})_1 = \tfrac{1}{4}[-1, 1, 0, 0, 0, 0, 1, -1, 0, 0, 0, 0]^T\bar{\mathbf{y}}$$

and

$$(\widehat{\gamma\pi})_2 = \tfrac{1}{4}[0, 0, 0, -1, 1, 0, 0, 0, 0, 1, -1, 0]^T\bar{\mathbf{y}}$$

We now consider the remaining effects τ, λ, θ and $(\tau\lambda)$. Whether or not all of these effects need to be included will depend on the particular trial and on the amount of prior knowledge that exists about the nature of the treatment effects. However, for the sake of completeness, we will consider models containing all of the effects τ, λ, θ and $(\tau\lambda)$.

When testing for these effects we begin with $(\tau\lambda)$. If this effect is significant it means that there is evidence of an interaction between the direct treatment and first-order carry-over effects. In the presence of such an interaction it would not be sensible to continue and test for a second-order carry-over effect.

When testing for significant effects we consider them in the order $(\tau\lambda), \theta, \lambda$ and τ. We assume that the model under consideration always contains parameters for the groups and periods.

In the presence of θ, λ and τ the OLS estimator of $(\tau\lambda)$ is

$$\widehat{(\tau\lambda)}|\theta, \lambda, \tau = \tfrac{1}{8}[-1, -1, 2, -1, -1, 2, 1, 1, -2, 1, 1, -2]^{\mathrm{T}}\bar{\mathbf{y}}$$

with

$$V[\widehat{(\tau\lambda)}|\theta, \lambda, \tau] = \frac{3\sigma^2}{8n}$$

If $(\tau\lambda)$ cannot be dropped from the model then we would not test any of the remaining effects. To test τ and λ would break marginality rules and to test θ would not be sensible in the presence of rather unusual first-order carry-over effects.

If $(\tau\lambda)$ can be dropped from the model then

$$\hat{\theta}|\lambda, \tau = \tfrac{1}{8}[1, -5, 4, -1, 5, -4, 7, 1, -8, -7, -1, 8]^{\mathrm{T}}\bar{\mathbf{y}}$$

with

$$V[\hat{\theta}|\lambda, \tau] = \frac{39\sigma^2}{8n}$$

If θ cannot be dropped from the model then we would presumably be interested in estimating $\tau|\theta, \lambda$. The estimator is

$$\hat{\tau}|\theta, \lambda = \tfrac{1}{8}[-1, -1, 2, 1, 1, -2, 1, 1, -2, -1, -1, 2]^{\mathrm{T}}\bar{\mathbf{y}}$$

with

$$V[\hat{\tau}|\theta, \lambda] = \frac{3\sigma^2}{8n}$$

If θ can be dropped from the model then

$$\hat{\lambda}|\tau = \tfrac{1}{26}[-2, -3, 5, 2, 3, -5, -1, -2, 3, 1, 2, -3]^{\mathrm{T}}\bar{\mathbf{y}}$$

with

$$V[\hat{\lambda}|\tau] = \frac{2\sigma^2}{13n}$$

and

$$\hat{t}|\lambda = \tfrac{1}{52}[-8, 1, 7, 8, -1, -7, -4, 5, -1, 4, -5, 1]^{\mathrm{T}}\bar{\mathbf{y}}$$

with

$$V[\hat{t}|\lambda] = \frac{3\sigma^2}{26n}$$

Also

$$Cov[\hat{t}|\lambda, \hat{\lambda}|\tau] = \frac{3\sigma^2}{52n}$$

If λ can be dropped from the model then

$$\hat{t} = \tfrac{1}{16}[-2, 1, 1, 2, -1, -1, -1, 2, -1, 1, -2, 1]^{\mathrm{T}}\bar{\mathbf{y}}$$

with

$$V[\hat{t}] = \frac{3\sigma^2}{32n}$$

A similar derivation can be given for designs 3.4.2 and 3.4.3.

Of most interest to potential users of these three designs is how they differ in terms of the precision with which they estimate the

Table 4.14 *Variances of the estimators (in multiples of σ^2/n)*

Effect	Design 3.4.1	Design 3.4.2	Design 3.4.3
$(\tau\lambda)|\theta, \lambda, \tau$	0·3750	0·1250	0·3750
$\theta|\lambda, \tau$	4·8750	1·9375	1·0000
$\tau|\theta, \lambda$	0·3750	0·4375	0·4375
$\lambda|\tau$	0·1538	0·1935	0·3750
$\tau|\lambda$	0·1154	0·0968	0·1875
τ	0·0938	0·0938	0·0938

various effects. Therefore in Table 4.14 we give the variances of the estimators obtained from each design.

Clearly, no single design is optimal for all effects. As all three designs are equally good at estimating τ in the absence of the other parameters, we might choose to use design 3.4.2 as it has the smallest variance of $\hat{\tau}|\lambda$. However, as design 3.4.1 is better at estimating $\lambda|\tau$ the choice is not clear cut. Our opinion is that in most situations it is not possible from statistical considerations alone to choose the optimal design. Depending on the circumstances, the choice of the design to use will depend on the effects of most interest, the amount of prior knowledge and the practicalities of conducting the trial. We will say more on the choice of an optimal three-period design in Section 4.11.

We conclude this section by analysing the full set of data given in Table 4.9. The analysis of covariance, obtained by including the baseline as a covariate, is given in Table 4.15.

There is some evidence ($P = 0.06$) of an interaction between the direct treatment effect and the baseline response. As this interaction was not evident in groups 1 and 2, we must look to groups 3 and 4 for an explanation. The analysis of covariance for these groups is given in Table 4.16.

The direct treatment-by-baseline interaction is highly significant ($P = 0.02$) in groups 3 and 4, as expected from our earlier remarks. To discover its cause we plot, for each subject, the treatment contrast $d_{32k} = -y_{31k} + 2y_{32k} - y_{33k}$ for group 3, and the treatment contrast

Table 4.15 *The analysis of covariance for all four groups*

Source	d.f.	SS	MS	F
Between subjects	88	82 007·9	931·9	
Within subjects:				
Periods	2	889·9	445·0	
Direct treatments	1	3 491·1	3 491·1	21·35
Carry-over	1	10·4	10·4	0·06
Baseline × period	2	1 264·0	362·0	3·87
Baseline × direct treatment	1	592·2	592·2	3·62
Baseline × carry-over	1	56·1	56·1	0·34
Residual	170	27 796·3	163·5	
Total	266	116 107·9		

Table 4.16 *The analysis of covariance for groups 3 and 4*

Source	d.f.	SS	MS	F
Between subjects	39	51 277·8	1314·8	
Within subjects:				
Periods	2	762·9	381·4	
Direct treatments	1	2 469·2	2469·2	16·17
Carry-over	1	8·8	8·8	0·06
Baseline × period	2	1 174·9	587·4	3·85
Baseline × direct treatment	1	917·1	917·1	6·01
Baseline × carry-over	1	0·7	0·7	0·00
Residual	72	10 991·7	152·7	
Total	119	67 603·2		

$d_{42k} = -y_{41k} + 2y_{42k} - y_{43k}$, for group 4, against the corresponding value of the baseline. These plots are given in Figures 4.3 and 4.4 respectively. It will be noted that $\hat{\tau} = \bar{d}_{32.} - \bar{d}_{42.}$, for these two groups.

Figure 4.3 indicates that there is no relationship between the treatment contrast and the baseline, but in Figure 4.4 we see that the contrast for one subject (subject 13 in group 4) is unusually high, as is that subject's baseline response. If we remove this subject and reanalyse groups 3 and 4, we find that the significant interaction disappears. The analysis of covariance for all four groups, without subject 13 in group 4, is given in Table 4.17. Using the model which

Table 4.17 *The analysis of covariance for groups (without subject 13)*

Source	d.f.	SS	MS	F
Between subjects	87	75 154·1	863·8	
Within subjects:				
Periods	2	696·2	348·1	
Direct treatments	1	2 866·0	2866·0	18·58
Carry-over	1	59·7	59·7	0·39
Baseline × period	2	364·7	182·4	1·18
Baseline × direct treatment	1	91·3	91·3	0·59
Baseline × carry-over	1	2·2	2·2	0·01
Residual	168	25 903·3	154·2	
Total	263	105 137·4		

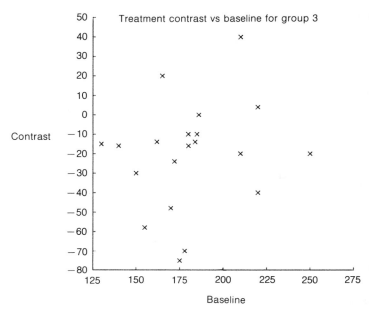

Figure 4.3 *Plot of direct treatment contrast vs baseline for group 3.*

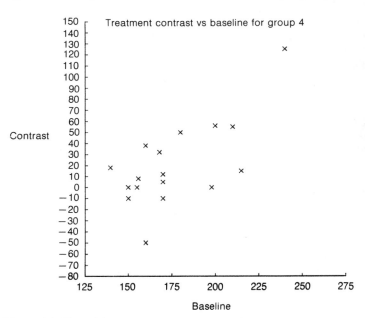

Figure 4.4 *Plot of direct treatment contrast vs baseline for group 4.*

contains terms for the subjects, periods and direct treatments, the estimate of $\tau_1 - \tau_2$ is 7·01 with a standard error of 1·62 on 173 d.f.

4.9 A simple and robust analysis for four-group dual designs

We can extend the simple analysis described in Section 4.7 in an obvious way to more than two groups. To illustrate this extension let us consider again Example 4.2, the full set of data on hypertensives given in Table 4.9. The design for these data is a mixture of designs 3.2.1 and 3.2.2: groups 1 and 2 were on sequences ABB and BAA, respectively, and groups 3 and 4 were on sequences ABA and BAB, respectively. The group sizes are $n_1 = 22, n_2 = 27, n_3 = 23$ and $n_4 = 16$ (with outlier removed).

We first consider the estimation and testing of $\lambda|\tau$. The OLS estimator of $\lambda|\tau$, obtained from design 3.2.1, we label as $[\hat{\lambda}|\tau]_1$, and it is

$$[\hat{\lambda}|\tau]_1 = \tfrac{1}{4}[-\bar{y}_{12.} + \bar{y}_{13.} + \bar{y}_{22.} - \bar{y}_{23.}]$$

The estimator in design 3.2.2, which we label as $[\hat{\lambda}|\tau]_2$, is

$$[\hat{\lambda}|\tau]_2 = \tfrac{1}{2}[-\bar{y}_{31.} + \bar{y}_{33.} + \bar{y}_{41.} - \bar{y}_{43.}]$$

Let

$$d_{11k} = -y_{12k} + y_{13k}$$
$$d_{21k} = -y_{22k} + y_{23k}$$
$$d_{31k} = -y_{31k} + y_{33k}$$
$$d_{41k} = -y_{41k} + y_{43k}$$

be contrasts, respectively, for the kth subject in groups 1, 2, 3 and 4.

The values of contrasts d_{11k} and d_{21k} were given in Table 4.13 and the values of d_{31k} and d_{41k} are given in Table 4.18. Also given in these tables are the contrast means and variances.

We note that

$$[\hat{\lambda}|\tau]_1 = \tfrac{1}{4}[\bar{d}_{11.} - \bar{d}_{21.}]$$

and

$$[\hat{\lambda}|\tau]_2 = \tfrac{1}{2}[\bar{d}_{31.} - \bar{d}_{41.}]$$

The variances of these estimators are

$$V([\hat{\lambda}|\tau]_1) = \frac{\sigma_1^2}{16}\left(\frac{1}{n_1} + \frac{1}{n_2}\right)$$

Table 4.18 *The subject contrasts for groups 3 and 4*

Group	Subject	Contrast d_{31k}	Contrast d_{32k}
3 ABA	1	−4	−14
	2	−20	−20
	3	−20	−20
	4	20	−16
	5	0	20
	6	−20	40
	7	5	−75
	8	−12	0
	9	10	−70
	10	−20	−30
	11	5	−15
	12	−30	−58
	13	−4	−16
	14	20	−10
	15	14	−14
	16	10	−10
	17	−30	−40
	18	−4	−48
	19	8	4
	20	−4	−24
	21	−30	−30
	22	−20	36
	23	0	−20
	Mean	−5.48	−18·70
	Variance	251·26	816·86

Group	Subject	Contrast d_{41k}	Contrast d_{42k}
4 BAB	1	−48	18
	2	−16	8
	3	−15	15
	4	−8	0
	5	0	12
	6	10	−10
	7	0	0
	8	25	55
	9	−15	5
	10	20	38
	11	0	32
	12	−16	56
	14	0	0
	15	2	50
	16	10	−50
	17	−10	−10
	Mean	−3·81	13·69
	Variance	295·10	774·23

and

$$V([\hat{\lambda}|\tau]_2) = \frac{\sigma_2^2}{4}\left(\frac{1}{n_3} + \frac{1}{n_4}\right)$$

where σ_1^2 is the variance of each of the contrasts d_{11k} and d_{21k} and σ_2^2 is the variance of each of the contrasts d_{31k} and d_{41k}.

Using the values given in Tables 4.13 and 4.18 we obtain

$$[\hat{\lambda}|\tau]_1 = -1\cdot336$$

and

$$[\hat{\lambda}|\tau]_2 = -0\cdot833$$

The pooled sample variance of $[\hat{\lambda}|\tau]_1$, obtained using the method explained in Section 4.7, is $1\cdot712$ on 47 d.f. and the pooled sample variance of $[\hat{\lambda}|\tau]_2$ is $7\cdot128$ on 37 d.f. The extra precision obtained by using design 3.2.1 is clearly evident here.

A combined estimator, $[\hat{\lambda}|\tau]_w$, can be obtained by taking a weighted average of our two estimators, where the weights are taken to be inversely proportional to the variances of the estimators. That is, if

$$W_1 = \frac{1}{V([\hat{\lambda}|\tau]_1)}$$

and

$$W_2 = \frac{1}{V([\hat{\lambda}|\tau]_2)}$$

then

$$[\hat{\lambda}|\tau]_w = \frac{W_1[\hat{\lambda}|\tau]_1 + W_2[\hat{\lambda}|\tau]_2}{W_1 + W_2}$$

We do not know W_1 and W_2 and so we replace them with their estimates, $\hat{W}_1 = 1/1\cdot712$ and $\hat{W}_2 = 1/7\cdot128$. This gives

$$[\hat{\lambda}|\tau]_w = 0\cdot81(-1\cdot336) + 0\cdot19(-0\cdot833) = -1\cdot240$$

The estimate of the variance of the combined estimator, again obtained using our estimated weights, is

$$(0\cdot81)^2(1\cdot712) + (0\cdot19)^2(7\cdot128) = 1\cdot381.$$

We should be aware that if the sample sizes are small the weights may be poorly estimated and introduce extra variability into the estimator. This may then make the combined estimator less precise than a simple average.

Just as in Section 2.11, an approximation to the d.f. of the estimated variance of our combined estimator can be obtained using the result given by Satterthwaite (1946). We let

$$a_1 = \frac{W_1}{W_1 + W_2}$$

$$a_2 = \frac{W_2}{W_1 + W_2}$$

$$V_1 = V([\hat{\lambda}|\tau]_1)$$

$$V_2 = V([\hat{\lambda}|\tau]_2)$$

$$V_w = V([\hat{\lambda}|\tau]_w)$$

and let f_1, f_2 and f_w be the d.f. respectively, of $\hat{V}_1, \hat{V}_2$ and $\hat{V}_w$. Then

$$f_w = \frac{(a_1 \hat{V}_1 + a_2 \hat{V}_2)^2}{(a_1 \hat{V}_1)^2/f_1 + (a_2 \hat{V}_2)^2/f_2}$$

Putting our values into this formula gives $f_w = 83 \cdot 03$. Rounding this we have 83 d.f. for $\hat{V}_w$. The t-statistic for testing the null hypothesis that $\lambda = 0$ is then $- 1 \cdot 240/1 \cdot 175 = - 1 \cdot 06$ on 83 d.f. Hence there is insufficient evidence to reject the null hypothesis of equal carry-over effects.

To estimate the treatment effect τ and to test the null hypothesis that $\tau = 0$ (given that $\lambda = 0$) we repeat the steps described above but with the following contrasts:

$$d_{12k} = - 2y_{11k} + y_{12k} + y_{13k}$$

$$d_{22k} = - 2y_{21k} + y_{22k} + y_{23k}$$

$$d_{32k} = - y_{31k} + 2y_{32k} - y_{33k}$$

and

$$d_{42k} = - y_{41k} + 2y_{42k} - y_{43k}$$

Then

$$[\hat{\tau}]_1 = \tfrac{1}{8}[\bar{d}_{12.} - \bar{d}_{22.}]$$

and

$$[\hat{\tau}]_2 = \tfrac{1}{8}[\bar{d}_{32.} - \bar{d}_{42.}]$$

The variances of these estimators are

$$V([\hat{\tau}]_1) = \frac{\sigma_3^2}{64}\left(\frac{1}{n_1} + \frac{1}{n_2}\right)$$

and

$$V([\hat{\tau}]_2) = \frac{\sigma_4^2}{64}\left(\frac{1}{n_3} + \frac{1}{n_4}\right)$$

where σ_3^2 is the variance of each of the contrasts d_{12k} and d_{22k} and σ_4^2 is the variance of each of the contrasts d_{32k} and d_{42k}.

The values of d_{12k} and d_{22k} were given in Table 4.13 and the values of d_{32k} and d_{42k} are given in Table 4.18. Using their means and variances we obtain

$$[\hat{\tau}]_1 = -2\cdot961, \qquad \hat{V}([\hat{\tau}]_1) = 1\cdot380 \text{ on 47 d.f.}$$
$$[\hat{\tau}]_2 = -4\cdot048, \qquad \hat{V}([\hat{\tau}]_2) = 1\cdot324 \text{ on 37 d.f.}$$

Therefore,

$$[\hat{\tau}]_w = 0\cdot49(-2\cdot961) + 0\cdot51(-4\cdot048) = -3\cdot515$$

The estimated variance of $[\hat{\tau}]_w$ is $0\cdot676$ on 83 d.f., where again we have used the approximation to the d.f.

The upper $2\cdot5\%$ point of the t-distribution on 83 d.f. is $2\cdot00$ and our calculated t-statistic is $-3\cdot515/0\cdot822 = -4\cdot276$. There is strong evidence to reject the null hypothesis of equal treatment effects. A 95% confidence interval for $\tau_1 - \tau_2$ is $(3\cdot74, 10\cdot32)$.

4.10   A three-period, six-sequence design

If we join together designs 3.2.1, 3.2.2 and 3.2.3 we obtain the following design, which we label as design 3.6.1.

Design 3.6.1.

Sequence	Period		
	1	2	3
1	A	B	B
2	B	A	A
3	A	B	A
4	B	A	B
5	A	A	B
6	B	B	A

The advantage of this design is that it provides unaliased estimators of the carry-over and the direct-by-period interaction effects. However, the design is less attractive from a practical point of view because it requires the management of six different groups of subjects.

We will not give the details of the contrasts that can be estimated using design 3.6.1; the variances of the effects of interest will be given in the next section.

4.11   Which three-period design to use?

Here we compare the three-period designs described in the previous sections with a view to deciding which one to use. Let us suppose that N subjects are available and that they can be equally divided among two, four or six sequence groups. That is, the size of each group is $N/2$ if one of designs 3.2.1, 3.2.2 or 3.2.3 is used, the size is $N/4$ if one of designs 3.4.1, 3.4.2 or 3.4.3 is used, and the size is $N/6$ if design 3.6.1 is used. The variances of the various effects which can be estimated in each design are given in Table 4.19.

If one is interested in estimating all the effects then clearly design 3.6.1 is the one to choose. If $(\tau\lambda)$ is of particular interest then design 3.4.2 is the one to choose. The best design for estimating θ is 3.4.3. However, in most trials θ and $(\tau\lambda)$ are unlikely to be significantly

Table 4.19 *The variances of the estimators (in multiples of σ^2/N)*

Effect	τ	$\tau\|\lambda$	$\lambda\|\tau$	$(\tau\lambda)\|\tau,\lambda,\theta$
Design 3.2.1	0·375	0·375	0·500	—
Design 3.2.2	0·375	1·500	2·000	—
Design 3.2.3	0·375	0·500	2·000	—
Design 3.4.1	0·375	0·462	0·615	1·500
Design 3.4.2	0·375	0·387	0·774	0·500
Design 3.4.3	0·375	0·750	1·500	1·500
Design 3.6.1	0·375	0·463	0·794	0·675

Effect	$\theta\|\tau,\lambda$	$\tau\|\lambda,\theta$	$(\tau\pi)_1$	$(\tau\pi)_2$
Design 3.2.1	—	—	—	—
Design 3.2.2	—	—	—	—
Design 3.2.3	—	—	—	—
Design 3.4.1	19·500	1·500	—	—
Design 3.4.2	7·750	1·750	—	—
Design 3.4.3	4·000	1·750	—	—
Design 3.6.1	5·017	1·088	1·750	1·813

large and so we would choose our design on its ability to estimate $\lambda|\tau$ and $\tau|\lambda$. The design which estimates these effects most efficiently is design 3.2.1.

However, as Ebbutt (1984) pointed out, design 3.4.1 might be preferred because it is harder for the subject and the clinician to break the randomization code. Subjects in design 3.2.1 always receive the same treatments in the last two periods and this feature might bias the clinician's assessment of the subject's response. Also design 3.4.1 does permit additional effects to be tested should they become of interest when the trial is completed. If the trial has to be stopped at the end of the second period then both designs revert to being the standard 2×2 trial. Finally, a point in favour of design 3.4.2 is that if the trial is stopped after the second period, we are left with Balaam's design which permits a within-subjects estimate of λ to be obtained.

Of course, any remarks we make concerning the choice of design to use must depend on the assumptions we make about the parameters in the model. If we change the assumptions then it is quite likely that the 'optimal' design will change too. Fleiss (1986b), it will be recalled, questioned whether it was sensible to always assume that the carry-over of treatment A into treatment B, for example, is the same as the carry-over of treatment A into itself. As a special case of this consider the model in which we set to zero the carry-over of a treatment into itself. The variance of the estimators of $\hat{\tau}|\lambda$ and $\hat{\lambda}|\tau$ are then as given in Table 4.20. (The full model used

Table 4.20 *The variances of the estimators (in multiples of σ^2/N) assuming that a treatment cannot carry over into itself*

Effect	$\tau|\lambda$	$\lambda|\tau$
Design 3.2.1	0·500	2·000
Design 3.2.2	1·500	2·000
Design 3.2.3	0·375	—
Design 3.4.1	0·750	1·500
Design 3.4.2	0·857	3·428
Design 3.4.3	1·714	3·428
Design 3.6.1	0·938	2·250

contains terms for the subjects, periods, direct treatments and carry-overs.) We see that, although design 3.2.1 is still optimal, the best four-sequence design is now design 3.4.1 as opposed to the earlier choices of design 3.4.2 (for direct effects) and design 3.4.1 (for ˜carry-over effects). Also, in design 3.2.3, $\lambda|\tau$ is no longer estimable.

More generally we note that under the extra assumption the variances of the effects are larger than they were previously (with the exception of design 3.2.2). This would have implications when deciding on the ideal size of the trial.

4.12 Four-period designs with two sequences

Trials which include four treatment periods are, by their very nature, likely to be more expensive to conduct than their two- and three-period alternatives. Also, the longer a trial lasts, the greater will be the chance of subjects dropping out for reasons unconnected with the treatments. Therefore, if a four-period trial is to be used it must offer substantial improvements over trials with fewer periods.

It will be recalled that the main reason for using three periods is to obtain a within-subjects estimator of the carry-over effect, λ. However, in order to obtain an estimator which is not aliased with the direct-by-period interaction, a design with six sequences is needed. If it is thought that the monitoring and organization of six different groups of subjects will be difficult, then a four-period design might be attractive if it uses fewer than six sequences. If, on the other hand, a direct-by-period interaction is thought unlikely to occur then a four-period design will be attractive if it provides estimators of τ and λ (and perhaps $(\tau\lambda)$ and θ) which have substantially smaller variances than could be achieved by using three periods.

As in the previous sections we only consider designs made up of dual sequences. We will consider, in turn, the properties of the designs with two, four and six sequences and then return to consider the remarks made above.

Although the optimal design for estimating $\lambda|\tau$ and $\tau|\lambda$ is the four-group design 3 given in Section 4.2, we first consider the properties of the various two-group dual designs. This is because these designs have the attractive and important property of permitting a simple and robust analysis, as illustrated in Section 4.7 for a three-period design. We will also consider using more than four

Table 4.21 *Four-period, two-sequence designs*

Design 4.2.1

Sequence	Period			
	1	2	3	4
1	A	A	B	B
2	B	B	A	A

Design 4.2.2

Sequence	Period			
	1	2	3	4
1	A	B	A	B
2	B	A	B	A

Design 4.2.3

Sequence	Period			
	1	2	3	4
1	A	B	B	A
2	B	A	A	B

Design 4.2.4

Sequence	Period			
	1	2	3	4
1	A	B	A	A
2	B	A	B	B

Design 4.2.5

Sequence	Period			
	1	2	3	4
1	A	A	B	A
2	B	B	A	B

Design 4.2.6

Sequence	Period			
	1	2	3	4
1	A	B	B	B
2	B	A	A	A

Design 4.2.7

Sequence	Period			
	1	2	3	4
1	A	A	A	B
2	B	B	B	A

groups in order to see what practical advantages this might have over the optimal four-group design.

If we discard the sequences AAAA and BBBB then there are seven different two-sequence designs and they are listed in Table 4.21.

In each of these designs there are 6 d.f. within-subjects and 3 of these are associated with the period effects and 3 are associated with

Table 4.22 *Variances (in multiples of σ^2/n) of effects obtained from designs 4.2.1–4.2.7*

Effect	τ	$\tau\|\lambda$	$\lambda\|\tau$	$\theta\|\tau,\lambda$	$\tau\|\lambda,\theta$
Design 4.2.1	0·1250	0·1375	0·2000	—	0·1375
Design 4.2.2	0·1250	0·6875	1·0000	1·0000	0·7500
Design 4.2.3	0·1250	0·1375	0·2000	0·5556	0·3056
Deisgn 4.2.4	0·1667	0·2292	0·2500	—	0·2292
Design 4.2.5	0·1667	0·2292	0·2500	3·0000	1·2500
Design 4.2.6	0·1667	0·1719	0·1875	0·2500	0·1719
Design 4.2.7	0·1667	0·1875	0·7500	1·0000	0·2500

τ, λ and θ. In designs 4.2.1 and 4.2.4, θ is not estimable and in the remaining designs λ and θ are aliased with the direct-by-period interaction. The variances associated with each of the seven designs are given in Table 4.22, where we assume that there are n subjects in each group. Of these designs the one which provides minimum-variance estimators of τ and $\tau|\lambda$ is design 4.2.3. The design which is best for estimating $\theta|\tau, \lambda$ is 4.2.6.

If for some reason θ was of prime interest design 4.2.6 would be the one to use. It should also be noted that although design 4.2.1 provides estimators of τ and λ which have variances equal to those of design 4.2.3, θ is not estimable in design 4.2.1.

4.13 Four-period designs with four sequences

By taking the seven two-sequence designs in pairs we obtain 21 different four-group designs. Each of these provides 12 d.f. within subjects and we can associate 3 of these with the period effects, 4 with τ, λ, θ and $(\tau\lambda)$, respectively and 3 with the direct-by-period interaction effects, which we label as $(\tau\pi)_1$, $(\tau\pi)_2$ and $(\tau\pi)_3$, respectively. The remaining 2 d.f. are associated with uninteresting group-by-period contrasts.

We label the four-group design obtained by joining together designs 4.2.a and 4.2.b as 4.4.ab. Only 7 of the 21 designs provide unaliased estimators of $\tau, \lambda, \theta, (\tau\lambda), (\tau\pi)_1, (\tau\pi)_2$ and $(\tau\pi)_3$, and these are designs 4.4.14, 4.4.16, 4.4.25, 4.4.27, 4.4.35, 4.4.37 and 4.4.67. Assuming that n subjects are in each group, the design which provides minimum-variance estimators of $\tau, \tau|\lambda$ and $\lambda|\tau$ is design 4.4.13. This design is listed below and is seen to be design 3 as given in Section 4.2.

That is, it is the optimal design for four periods. (Consequently, $\text{Cov}\,[\hat{t}\,|\,\lambda,\hat{\lambda}\,|\,\tau] = 0$.)

Design 4.4.13

Sequence	Period			
	1	2	3	4
1	A	A	B	B
2	B	B	A	A
3	A	B	B	A
4	B	A	A	B

However, as is often the case, if other effects are of prime importance then design 4.4.13 is not necessarily the one to choose. The design which minimizes the sum of the variances of the estimators of $(\tau\pi)_1$, $(\tau\pi)_2$ and $(\tau\pi)_3$ is design 4.4.67. However, if $(\tau\lambda)\,|\,\tau,\lambda,\theta$ is of prime interest then design 4.4.13 is again optimal. If $\theta\,|\,\tau,\lambda$ is of prime interest then we would choose design 4.4.36. The variances of the estimators obtained from design 4.4.13, 4.4.36 and 4.4.67 are given in Table 4.23.

In practice, of course, trials are planned to minimize the chances of treatment carry-over and direct-by-period interaction. Under these conditions design 4.4.13 is clearly the one to use. Not only

Table 4.23 *Variances of the estimators (in multiples of σ^2/n)*

Effect	τ	$\tau\,|\,\lambda$	$\lambda\,|\,\tau$	$\theta\,|\,\tau,\lambda$	$\tau\,|\,\lambda,\theta$
Design 4.4.13	0·0625	0·0625	0·0909	0·5238	0·1935
Design 4.4.36	0·0714	0·0719	0·0915	0·1460	0·0840
Design 4.4.67	0·0833	0·0833	0·1429	0·1810	0·0884

Effect	$(\tau\lambda)\,|\,\tau,\lambda,\theta$	$(\tau\pi)_1$	$(\tau\pi)_2$	$(\tau\pi)_3$
Design 4.4.13	0·0909	0·2500	0·5250	—
Design 4.4.36	0·3333	0·1804	—	—
Design 4.4.67	0·1250	0·4219	0·2969	0·2969

does it provide the most precise estimators of τ and λ but it also provides unaliased estimators of nearly all the other effects. If for some reason the fourth period had to be abandoned then design 4.4.13 reduces to the three-period design 3.4.2, which provides the minimum variance estimator of $\tau|\lambda$. If the third and fourth periods are lost then design 4.4.13 reduces to Balaam's design.

4.14   Four-period designs with six sequences

By choosing all possible triples of the seven two-sequence designs listed in Section 4.1.2, we can obtain 35 different six-group designs. We will not list them all here but will refer to a particular design by using the label 4.6.*a.b.c*, which indicates that the design has been formed by joining together designs 4.2.*a*, 4.2.*b* and 4.2.*c*. As usual we assume that there are n subjects in each group.

If our model includes only terms for the groups, periods, direct treatments and carry-over, then the design which provides the minimum-variance estimator of $\tau|\lambda$ is design 4.6.136. The designs which provide minimum-variance estimators of $\lambda|\tau$ are 4.6.146 and 4.6.156. Designs 4.6.136 and 4.6.146 are listed below.

Design 4.6.136

Sequence	Period			
	1	2	3	4
1	A	A	B	B
2	B	B	A	A
3	A	B	B	A
4	B	A	A	B
5	A	B	B	B
6	B	A	A	A

A number of other designs provide values of $V[\hat{\tau}|\lambda]$ which are not much larger than that of design 4.6.136. The index numbers of these designs are 123, 137, 134, 135, 146 and 156.

The variances of the estimated effects obtained from designs 4.6.136 and 4.6.146 are given in Table 4.24. Overall the two designs are very similar in terms of these variances, with no design having the

Design 4.6.146

Sequence	Period			
	1	2	3	4
1	A	A	B	B
2	B	B	A	A
3	A	B	A	A
4	B	A	B	B
5	A	B	B	B
6	B	A	A	A

Table 4.24 *Variances (in multiples of σ^2/n) of effects obtained from designs 4.6.136 and 4.6.146*

Effect	τ	$\tau\|\lambda$	$\lambda\|\tau$	$\tau\|\lambda,\theta$	$\theta\|\tau,\lambda$
Design 4.6.136	0·0455	0·0456	0·0608	0·0641	0·1415
Design 4.6.146	0·0500	0·0500	0·0606	0·0552	0·1301

Effect	$(\tau\lambda)\|\tau,\lambda,\theta$	$(\tau\pi)_1$	$(\tau\pi)_2$	$(\tau\pi)_3$
Design 4.6.136	0·0682	0·4255	0·2420	0·4368
Design 4.6.146	0·1071	0·2269	0·3237	0·1786

minimum variance for all effects. Overall, design 4.6.136 is the one we recommend, unless the direct-by-period interactions are of prime interest. Design 4.6.146 provides estimators of the interactions which have a smaller total variance, although even in this design the precision of estimation is quite low.

We compare the two-, four- and six-group designs in the next section.

4.15 Which four-period design to use?

Here we compare the four-period designs described in the previous sections with a view to deciding which one to use. As done in Section 4.11, we suppose that N subjects are available and that they

Table 4.25 *The variances of the estimators (in multiples of σ^2/N)*

Effect	τ	$\tau\|\lambda$	$\lambda\|\tau$	$(\tau\lambda)\|\tau,\lambda$	$\tau\|\lambda,\theta$
Design 4.2.3	0·2500	0·2750	0·4000	—	0·6112
Design 4.2.6	0·3334	0·3438	0·3750	—	0·3438
Design 4.4.13	0·2500	0·2500	0·3636	0·3636	0·7740
Design 4.4.36	0·2856	0·2876	0·3660	1·3333	0·3360
Design 4.4.67	0·3332	0·3332	0·5716	0·5000	0·3536
Design 4.6.136	0·2730	0·2736	0·3648	0·4092	0·3846
Design 4.6.146	0·3000	0·3000	0·3636	0·6426	0·3312

Effect	$\theta\|\lambda,\tau$	$(\tau\lambda)\|\tau,\lambda,\theta$	$(\tau\pi)_1$	$(\tau\pi)_2$	$(\tau\pi)_3$
Design 4.2.3	1·1112	—	—	—	—
Design 4.2.6	0·5000	—	—	—	—
Design 4.4.13	2·0952	0·3636	1·0000	2·1000	—
Design 4.4.36	0·5840	1·3333	0·7216	—	—
Design 4.4.67	0·7240	0·5000	1·6876	1·1876	1·1876
Design 4.6.136	0·8490	0·4092	2·5530	1·4520	2·6208
Design 4.6.146	0·7806	0·6426	1·3614	1·9422	1·0716

can be equally divided among two, four or six sequence groups. That is, the size of each group is $N/2$ if one of designs 4.2.3, 4.2.6 is used, the size is $N/4$ if one of designs 4.4.13, 4.4.36 or 4.4.67 is used and the size is $N/6$ if design 4.6.136 or design 4.6.146 is used. The variances of the various effects which can be estimated in each design are given in Table 4.25.

If the only effects of interest are τ and λ, then clearly design 4.4.13 is the one to choose. This design is, of course, optimal in the sense considered in Section 4.2. However, this design is not as good at estimating $(\tau\lambda)$ or θ, for example, as design 4.4.67. If all effects are of interest, including the direct-by-period interactions, then design 4.4.67 is a good overall design to use. Also, it is clear from Table 4.25 that there is no real advantage to be gained from using six sequence groups. If only two groups can be used then design 4.2.3 should be used, unless θ is of particular interest, when design 4.2.6 should be used. Design 4.2.3, it will be noted, provides similar variances to the 'optimal' design 4.4.13. Also, it will be recalled that two-group designs consisting of a dual pair permit a simple and robust analysis. This makes designs 4.2.3 and 4.2.6 quite attractive if we suspect a nonparametric analysis might be needed.

As already noted in Section 4.11, we must not forget that the final choice of design will depend on the assumptions we make about the parameters in the model. So for example, if we only retain terms in the model for subjects, periods, direct and carry-over effects and set to zero the carry-over of a treatment into itself, as done in Section 4.11, we find that:

1. Design 4.4.13 is no longer optimal; design 4.4.16 is now optimal for direct effects and design 4.4.36 is optimal for carry-over effects.
2. Of the two-group designs, designs 4.2.1 and 4.2.6 are optimal for direct effects and design 4.2.3 is optimal for carry-over effects.

4.16   Which two-treatment design to use?

When comparing the designs we will assume that N subjects can be made available for the trial. How large N needs to be will depend on (a) how efficient our chosen design is at estimating the effects of interest, and (b) the anticipated size of the within-subject variance σ^2. One design, D1 say, is more efficient at estimating an effect than another design, D2 say, if the variance of the estimated effect is smaller in design D1. Often a reasonable estimate of σ^2 can be made by using results from earlier trials on the treatments or from trials involving similar treatments.

The choice between the designs described in this chapter is complicated slightly because we are comparing designs of different sizes: Balaam's design requires $2N$ measurements to be taken (two for each subject), whereas the designs which use three or four periods require $3N$ and $4N$ measurements, respectively. Therefore, in practice we need to weigh the possible increase in precision obtained from using an extra period against the expense of taking additional measurements on each subject.

Let us assume that the maximum value of N has been decided upon from practical considerations. The next things to be decided are the maximum number of periods and sequences that can be used. The maximum number of periods will depend on the nature of the trial. If the treatments to be compared require a long time before their effect can assessed then the total time for the trial may be too long if more than two or three periods are used. In other trials the treatment effects can be assessed quite quickly and so there is more freedom to use up to four periods. Generally, we can increase the precision with which we estimate the direct treatment and carry-over effects by using more periods. However, this 'replication in time' may not be as cost-effective as using additional subjects. The choice, if we have any, between using more periods or subjects, will depend, among other things, on the relative costs of recruiting subjects and the costs of taking repeated measurements on the subjects. If repeat measurements are costly then we would be inclined to use more subjects and fewer periods. However, if the major cost is one of recruitment, then we would want to keep each subject for as many periods as is practical and ethical. However, we should always bear in mind that the longer a trial lasts, the greater the chance that subjects will drop out. We have not mentioned wash-out periods as they do not help increase the precision of estimation when three or more periods are used. If they are thought to be necessary, to reduce carry-over effects for example, then this needs to be taken into account when calculating the total time of the trial.

The choice of the number of sequences will depend on the effects we wish to estimate or test for. If we are sure that there is no possibility of direct-by-period interactions or second-order carry-over, then fewer sequences will be needed than would otherwise be the case. More sequences may also be thought desirable as a means of disguising as much as possible the randomization code used to allocate subjects to sequences.

Clearly, the choice of design involves many different and sometimes conflicting decisions. In the following we will base our comparison of the designs on the precision with which they estimate the effects of interest. Here we will make the more usual assumption that the carry-over effects do not interact with the succeeding direct treatments.

If only two periods can be used then we have no choice but to use Balaam's design as described in Section 4.3. Compared with the designs with three periods, however, the precision of this design is quite low: using an extra period, for example, reduces the variance of $\hat{\lambda}|\tau$ from $4\sigma^2/N$ to $0.5\sigma^2/N$ if design 3.2.1 is used.

Let us now consider the choice between the three- and four-period designs. If we wish to estimate all the effects, including the direct-by-period interactions, then only designs 3.6.1 and 4.4.67 need to be considered. The extra precision obtained by using design 4.4.67 makes it the natural choice if four periods can be used. The increased precision is not great, however, except for θ. If subjects are cheap to recruit it might be better to increase the number of subjects and use design 3.6.1. Of course, comparisons involving the six-sequence designs are rather academic as we would not seriously plan to conduct a cross-over trial if large carry-over or interaction effects were anticipated.

If direct-by-period interactions are not anticipated but we still need to retain a check on θ and $(\tau\lambda)$, then the choice of design is between 3.4.2 and 4.4.67. The logical choice here is design 4.4.67 unless using four periods poses a problem. However, as will be seen below, design 4.4.67 is not a good overall choice.

If τ and λ are the only anticipated effects (as is usually the case) then our choice is between 3.2.1 and 4.4.13. Excluding cost considerations the natural choice here is 4.4.13 as using the extra period produces a large increase in precision and permits additional effects to be estimated.

One other consideration that might be important is the consequences of the trial having to be stopped before all the periods have been completed.

Let us consider the four-period designs. If only the first three periods of design 4.4.67 are used then the third and fourth sequences become AAA and BBB, respectively. As such sequences provide no within-subject comparisons of the treatments we have lost the advantages of using the cross-over principle. If only the first two periods of design 4.4.67 are used then the design becomes Balaam's design.

If design 4.4.13 is used, however, then its first three periods make up design 3.4.2, which provides good estimators of $\tau|\lambda$ and $\lambda|\tau$. The first two periods of design 4.4.13 also make up Balaam's design. Therefore, we would prefer design 4.4.13 over design 4.4.67 if the possibility of the trial ending prematurely was a serious consideration.

Of the three-period designs, design 3.2.1 is the natural choice.

If we had to pick a single design to recommend then we would probably choose design 4.4.13. However, if it was important to use only two groups, in order to use the robust analysis for example, then design 3.2.1 would be a good choice. Its four-period competitor is design 4.2.3 which provides a more precise estimate of $\tau|\lambda$.

However, compared with an increase of 33% in the number of measurements entailed in adding the fourth period, the increase in precision is probably not cost-effective. If design 4.2.3 is used, however, it is worth noting that its first three periods make up design 3.2.1. In other words, if we did change our mind about using four periods then stopping early would not be a problem.

CHAPTER 5

Designs and analyses for three or more treatments

5.1 Introduction

The aims of this chapter are as follows:

1. to review the large number of designs which have been proposed in the literature;
2. to compare them with a view to recommending which ones should be used; and
3. to illustrate how data from such designs might be analysed.

For almost the whole of this chapter it is assumed that the response to be analysed is continuous. The analysis appropriate for binary and categorical responses which was introduced in Chapter 3 is illustrated in Section 5.9 using a three-treatment example.

As most of the literature on three or more treatments assumes that the only treatment effects present are the direct and the first-order carry-over effects, we too will do the same. The t treatments will be labelled as $A, B, C, \ldots$, and the corresponding direct treatment effects will be denoted by $\tau_1, \tau_2, \tau_3, \ldots, \tau_t$. The corresponding carry-over effects will be denoted by $\lambda_1, \lambda_2, \lambda_3, \ldots, \lambda_t$.

The full model we will use in this chapter contains terms for the general mean, the subjects, the periods, the direct treatment effects, and the first-order carry-over effects. To simplify the notation we will now let τ_i denote the direct effect of treatment i in the presence of all the other effects in the full model. In particular, if carry-over effects are in the model, then τ_i will denote the direct effect of treatment i adjusted for the carry-over effects (and all the other effects). Similarly, λ_i denotes the carry-over effect of treatment i adjusted for the treatments (and all the other effects.)

Compared with trials for two treatments, the most fundamental difference that arises when trials for three or more treatments are planned is that we must decide which contrasts are to be estimated with the highest precision.

Quite often we will want to plan the trial so that all pairwise differences between the treatments are estimated with the same precision, that is $V[\hat{\tau}_i - \hat{\tau}_j] = v\sigma^2$, where v is constant for all $i \neq j$. A design which possesses this property is referred to as **variance balanced**. It should be noted that we have been careful in the choice of this term. When used without qualification, the term 'balance' has been a source of confusion in the past, as Preece (1982) has pointed out. In the following the terms 'balance' and 'complete balance' will be used to describe cross-over designs which satisfy certain combinatorial (as opposed to statistical) conditions. See Preece (1982, Section 17) for a useful review of the various definitions of balance that have been used in connection with cross-over designs.

As we shall see, variance-balanced designs cannot be constructed for all values of n and p, where n is the number of subjects and p is the number of periods. As a compromise we may consider using a design which has **partial balance**. In a partially balanced design the value of $V[\hat{\tau}_i - \hat{\tau}_j]$ depends on which treatments i and j are being compared. If the design has two associate classes then there are only two different variances depending on the choice of i and j. If the two variances are not much different then the design has similar properties to one which is variance balanced.

A further possibility when no variance balanced design exists is to use a **cyclic** design. Although these designs can have up to $[t/2]$ different contrast variances, where $[t/2]$ is the greatest integer less than or equal to $t/2$, some have the attractive property that these variances are not very different.

If one of the treatments, A say, is a control or standard treatment, the aim of the trial might be to compare each of B, C, D, etc., with A; the comparisons between B, C, D, etc., being of less interest. In this situation we would want to ensure that the contrasts which involve A are estimated with the highest achievable precision, possibly at the expense of estimating the other contrasts with low precision.

If the treatments are increasing doses of the same drug and we wish to discover the dose which gives the highest response, then we would want to estimate the linear, quadratic, cubic, etc., components of the response function. These components can be expressed as contrasts and we would want the components of most interest to be estimated most precisely. For example, the linear and quadratic components would be of most interest if we were estimating the maximum response, with the higher-order components being of interest only to check on the adequacy of the fitted model.

In another situation we might have four treatments, for example, made up of the four combinations of two different drugs, each present at a low and a high level. The four treatments would then be more appropriately labelled as AB_{11}, AB_{12}, AB_{21} and AB_{22}, where AB_{11} indicates that the treatment is made up of the low level of A and the low level of B, and AB_{21} indicates that the treatment is made up of the high level of A and the low level of B, etc. In this 2×2 factorial structure the contrasts of interest are the interaction and main effects. That is, we would want to discover if the effects of changing A (or B) from its low to its high level depends on the level of B (or A). If it does not then we would want to estimate the average effect of changing A (or B). If the effects of the two drugs are well known when used separately, then the purpose of the trial might be to obtain a precise estimate of the interaction, the main effects being of little interest. Cyclic designs, among others, can also be useful for this situation.

The points made above, concerning the choice of contrasts, should have made it clear that we cannot choose between the large number of available designs until the objectives of the trial have been carefully resolved. In order to choose the most appropriate design we need to know the following details:

1. the contrasts of interest and their relative importance;
2. the maximum number of periods that can be used;
3. the maximum number of subjects that could be made available for the trial.

Having found a design which meets these requirements we can then check that, based on a prior estimate of the within-subject variance, the design is likely to be large enough to detect differences between the treatments of the size we think are important.

The chapter is organized as follows. In Section 5.2 we consider designs which are variance balanced and in Section 5.3 we review some recent work on the optimality of cross-over designs for three or more treatments. In Section 5.4 we compare the different balanced designs for $t \leqslant 9$ and in Sections 5.5 and 5.6 we consider partial balance. In Section 5.7 we consider the case where one treatment is a control to be compared with all the others and in Section 5.8 we consider designs for factorial sets of treatments. In Section 5.9 we give two examples to illustrate the analysis of designs with three or more treatments and in Section 5.10 we briefly describe a Bayesian analysis. The chapter ends with Section 5.11, in which we briefly explain how the methods described in Chapter 3, for binary and categorical data, can be used when there are three or more treatments.

The recommended ways of randomizing the subjects to the treatment sequences are described in Section 5.2.2.

5.2 Variance-balanced designs

5.2.1 Introduction

Variance balance, it will be recalled, means that $V[\hat{\tau}_i - \hat{\tau}_j]$ is the same for all $i \neq j$. Such a design is appropriate when we wish to compare each treatment equally precisely with every other treatment.

Deciding if a cross-over design is variance balanced without calculating all the variances of the pairwise differences between the treatments is not, in general, straightforward. Patterson and Lucas (1962) gave a list of conditions that a variance-balanced design must possess but these referred to designs in which no subject was allowed to receive the same treatment more than once. General conditions can be given, however, in terms of the properties possessed by certain incidence matrices constructed from the design. The direct-by-period incidence matrix, for example, is a $(t \times p)$ matrix $\mathbf{L}$ whose (i,j)th entry is the number of times treatment i occurs with period j. The other incidence matrices that we need are (in the notation of Pigeon and Raghavarao, 1987): (a) the $(t \times n)$ direct-by-subject matrix $\mathbf{M}$, (b) the $(t \times p)$ carry-over-by-period matrix $\mathbf{L}^*$, (c) the $(t \times n)$ carry-over-by-subject matrix $\mathbf{M}^*$, and (d) the $(t \times t)$ direct-by-carry-over matrix $\mathbf{S}$. We also need to define the $(t \times 1)$ vectors $\mathbf{r} = \mathbf{L}\mathbf{1}$ and $\mathbf{s} = \mathbf{L}^*\mathbf{1}$, where $\mathbf{1}$ is a $(p \times 1)$ vector of ones. Then we have (Pigeon, 1984) that a cross-over design is variance balanced if each of the following matrices is completely symmetric: $\mathbf{L}\mathbf{L}^T$, $\mathbf{M}\mathbf{M}^T$, $\mathbf{r}\mathbf{r}^T$, $\mathbf{L}^*\mathbf{L}^{*T}$, $\mathbf{M}^*\mathbf{M}^{*T}$, $\mathbf{s}\mathbf{s}^T$, $\mathbf{L}\mathbf{L}^{*T}$, $\mathbf{M}\mathbf{M}^{*T}$, $\mathbf{r}\mathbf{s}^T$ and $\mathbf{S}$. If each treatment occurs an equal number of times in each period then $\mathbf{L}\mathbf{L}^T$, $\mathbf{r}\mathbf{r}^T$, $\mathbf{L}^*\mathbf{L}^{*T}$, $\mathbf{s}\mathbf{s}^T$, $\mathbf{L}\mathbf{L}^{*T}$ and $\mathbf{r}\mathbf{s}^T$ are completely symmetric.

In order to simplify our description of the different types of variance-balanced designs that have been suggested in the literature, we have divided the designs into groups according to whether $p = t$, $p < t$ or $p > t$.

Plans of all the most useful cross-over designs known up to 1962 were given by Patterson and Lucas (1962).

When we give the plan of a design we will give it in its most convenient form. The design given in the plan must be randomized (see Section 5.2.2) before being used. The efficiencies of a design, which we will define shortly, will be given in the title of the table containing the design.

5.2.2 Designs with $p = t$

Orthogonal Latin squares

If carry-over effects are not present, then variance balance can easily be achieved by using t subjects in an arbitrarily chosen Latin square design. An example of such a design for four treatments is given in Table 5.1. A Latin square is a $t \times t$ arrangement of t letters such that each letter occurs once in each row and once in each column. In our context this means that each subject should receive each treatment and that over the whole design each treatment should occur once in each period. As this design provides only $(t - 1)(t - 2)$ d.f. for the residual SS, a number of randomly chosen Latin squares are needed if t is small. To obtain 10 d.f. for the residual SS for $t = 3$, for example, we would need 15 subjects arranged in 5 randomly chosen squares. Further information on the construction, enumeration, randomization and other properties of Latin squares are given in Kempthorne (1983) and Federer (1955), for example.

Table 5.1 *Latin square design for four treatments (18·18, 12·50)*

Subject	Period			
	1	2	3	4
1	A	B	C	D
2	B	C	D	A
3	C	D	A	B
4	D	A	B	C

In the absence of carry-over effects the Latin square design is optimal in the sense that it not only accounts for the effects of subjects and periods, but it also provides the minimum value of $V[\hat{\tau}_i - \hat{\tau}_j]$, for all $i \neq j$. This minimum value is $2\sigma^2/r$, where r is the replication of each treatment. This minimum value can be used as a yardstick by which other designs can be compared. The **efficiency** (expressed as a percentage) with which a design estimates the contrast $\tau_i - \tau_j$ is defined to be

$$E_t = \frac{2\sigma^2/r}{V[\hat{\tau}_i - \hat{\tau}_j]} \times 100$$

The subscript t is used to indicate that the treatments have not been adjusted for carry-over effects. By definition $E_t = 100$ for the Latin square design. If all pairwise contrasts $\tau_i - \tau_j$ have the same efficiency then E_t defines the efficiency of the design. Designs of the same or of different size can be compared in terms of their efficiencies. Naturally, we should use the most efficient design if at all possible, as this makes the best use of the available subjects.

In the presence of carry-over effects we define efficiency exactly as above but with $V[\hat{\tau}_i - \hat{\tau}_j]$ now denoting the difference between two direct treatments adjusted for carry-over effects. We label this efficiency as E_d to distinguish it from E_t which is calculated using the unadjusted effects.

Similarly, we define

$$E_c = \frac{2\sigma^2/r}{V[\hat{\lambda}_i - \hat{\lambda}_j]} \times 100$$

as the efficiency of $V[\hat{\lambda}_i - \hat{\lambda}_j]$. It should be noted that in this definition r is the direct treatment replication. As the carry-over effects appear only in the last $p-1$ periods they have a smaller replication than r. We will keep to the above definition, however, to maintain consistency with Patterson and Lucas (1962).

For information we will always include the values of the efficiencies of a design, in the order E_d, E_c, in the title of the table giving the plan of the design. So, for example, we can see from Table 5.1 that the efficiencies of the design given there are $E_d = 18 \cdot 18$ and $E_c = 12 \cdot 50$.

Let us now return to the design given in Table 5.1. Although this design has maximum efficiency in the absence of carry-over effects, it is not as efficient at estimating the direct treatment effects as it could be. To achieve the highest possible efficiency the design must be **balanced**. Here the term 'balance' refers to the combinatorial properties possessed by the design. In a balanced design, not only does each treatment occur once with each subject, but, over the whole design each treatment occurs the same number of times in each period and the number of subjects who receive treatment i in some period followed by treatment j in the next period is the same for all $i \neq j$. The design in Table 5.1 is not balanced because treatment A is followed three times by treatment B but treatment B is never followed by treatment A.

For the remainder of this section it can be taken (with some exceptions which we will point out) that when we refer to a design as balanced it is also variance balanced.

Balance can be achieved by using a complete set of **orthogonal** Latin squares. Orthogonal Latin squares are defined in John (1971, Chapter 6), for example. This use of orthogonal squares was first pointed out by Cochran, Autrey and Cannon (1941), and the designs given by them for three and four treatments are reproduced in Table 5.2 and 5.3, respectively. Here, and in the following, different squares are separated in the tables by lines. In Table 5.2, for example, we can see that each treatment follows every other treatment twice. A complete set of $t \times t$ orthogonal Latin squares contains $t - 1$ squares and complete sets exist for values of t that are prime or are powers of a prime. A notable exception is $t = 6$. To use a complete set at least $t(t - 1)$ subjects are needed for the trial, and this can be a disadvantage for large t if subjects are difficult or expensive to recruit.

Table 5.2 *Orthogonal Latin square design for three treatments (80·00, 44·44)*

Subject	Period		
	1	2	3
1	A	B	C
2	B	C	A
3	C	A	B
4	A	C	B
5	B	A	C
6	C	B	A

Table 5.3 *Orthogonal Latin square design for four treatments (90·91, 62·50)*

Subject	Period			
	1	2	3	4
1	A	B	C	D
2	B	A	D	C
3	C	D	A	B
4	D	C	B	A
5	A	D	B	C
6	B	C	A	D
7	C	B	D	A
8	D	A	C	B
9	A	C	D	B
10	B	D	C	A
11	C	A	B	D
12	D	B	A	C

Randomization

As with all the designs in this book, we must, having chosen the treatment sequences, randomly assign them to the subjects. The simplest way to randomize a cross-over trial is to

1. randomly assign the treatment names to the letters A, B, C, ..., etc.; and
2. randomly assign the treatment sequences to the subjects.

If the trial is a large one it may include subjects from a number of different treatment centres. If this is the case then after step 1 above, step 2 would be undertaken for each centre separately.

Sometimes only a single replicate of the design is used, but it is made up of a number of smaller, self-contained, sub-designs, e.g. the orthogonal squares design is made up of $t - 1$ Latin squares. If the single replicate is to be assigned to subjects from different centres then after step 1 above each sub-design (or sets of sub-designs, if there are more sub-designs than centres) should be randomly assigned to a different centre and then step 2 undertaken at each centre.

In some circumstances a single replicate will be used at a single centre but the subjects within the centre can be subdivided into groups that correspond to another source of systematic variability, e.g. the subjects may be recruited sequentially in batches. If the single replicate is made up of sub-designs then each sub-design could be randomly assigned to a different batch.

Obviously, the precise form the randomization will take will depend on the design and the circumstances in which it is to be used. The basic rule is that, if at all possible, we randomly allocate the subjects to sequences in a way which will take account of any other known sources of systematic variation. Doing this can lead to an increase in precision obtained at the analysis stage. For example, if an orthogonal squares design is used and the individual Latin squares are associated with a systematic source of variability then a component of the residual SS due to the period-by-square interaction can be isolated and removed, leaving a more representative residual SS. In addition, and perhaps of more importance in clinical trials, is that we can test for a treatment-by-square interaction. If this interaction is not negligible we would need to estimate the treatment effects using each square separately.

Williams designs

Although using orthogonal Latin squares has additional advantages, as we will note below, they require more subjects than is necessary to achieve balance. Williams (1949) showed that balance could be achieved by using only one particular Latin square if t is even and by using only two particular squares if t is odd. For more than three treatments, therefore, the designs suggested by Williams require fewer subjects than those based on complete sets of orthogonal squares. Although Williams (1949) described the steps needed to construct one of his designs, a more easily remembered algorithm was given by Sheehe and Bross (1961). Bradley (1958) also gave a simple algorithm, but only for even values of t, and Hedayat and Afsarinejad (1978) gave a formula for deciding on $d(i, j)$ where $d(i, j)$ is the treatment to be applied in period i on subject j.

The steps in Sheehe and Bross's algorithm are as follows:

1. Number the treatments from 1 to t.
2. Start with a cyclic $t \times t$ Latin square. In this square the treatments in the ith row are $i, i + 1, \ldots, t, 1, 2, \ldots, i - 1$.
3. Interlace each row of the cyclic Latin square with its own mirror image (i.e. its reverse order). For example, if $t = 4$, the first row

Table 5.4 *Balanced Latin square design for four treatments (90·91, 62·50)*

Subject	Period			
	1	2	3	4
1	A	D	B	C
2	B	A	C	D
3	C	B	D	A
4	D	C	A	B

of the cyclic square is 1, 2, 3, 4. Its mirror image is 4, 3, 2, 1. When the two sequences are interlaced we get 1, 4, 2, 3, 3, 2, 4, 1.

4. Slice the resulting $t \times 2t$ arrangement down the middle, to yield two $t \times t$ arrangements. The columns of each $t \times t$ arrangement correspond to the periods, the rows are the treatment sequences, and the numbers within the square are the treatments.

5. If t is even we choose any one of the two $t \times t$ arrangements. If t is odd we use both arrangements.

The design for $t = 4$ obtained by using this algorithm and choosing the left-hand square is given in Table 5.4. The efficiencies of this design are, of course, the same as those given for the orthogonal squares design given in Table 5.3. However, the Williams design requires fewer subjects, and this may be an advantage in certain circumstances. For example, if sufficient power can be obtained using only 16 subjects then the Williams design, replicated four times, could be used: designs based solely on complete sets of orthogonal squares, however, require multiples of 12 subjects.

To see the gain in efficiency obtained by using a Williams design, rather than an arbitrarily chosen Latin square, compare the efficiencies of the designs given in Tables 5.1 and 5.4.

Although a design with nine periods will not usually be contemplated in a clinical trial, it is of interest to note that for $t = 9$, a balanced design which uses only nine subjects has been reported by Hedayat and Afsarinejad (1978), who attribute it to K.B. Mertz. The efficiencies of this design are $E_d = 98·59$ and $E_c = 86·42$. To achieve the same efficiencies the corresponding Williams design would require 18 subjects.

Sometimes, we may need to decide between using a number of

replicates of a Williams design and using a complete set of orthogonal squares. One advantage of using the complete set is that, as Williams (1950) proved, they are balanced for all preceding treatments. That is, they are balanced for first-, second-,..., $(p-1)$th-order carry-over effects. Using the complete set therefore enables other effects to be conveniently tested should they be of interest. The disadvantage of using a complete set is that it consists of $t(t-1)$ different sequences and so the chance of a sequence being incorrectly administered through mishap is increased. Also the loss of subjects from the complete set is likely to be more damaging as its combinatorial structure is more complex.

Minimal designs

Hedayat and Afsarinejad (1975) considered the construction of **minimal balanced** (MB) designs. These are balanced designs which use the minimum possible number of subjects. They referred to a cross-over design for t treatments, n subjects and p periods as an $RM(t, n, p)$ design. They noted that for even values of t, MB $RM(t, t, t)$ designs exist and can be constructed using the method of Sheehe and Bross (1961), for example. For odd values of t, they noted that no MB $RM(t, t, t)$ is possible for $t = 3, 5$ and 7 but such a design does exist for $t = 21$. Hedayat and Afsarinejad (1978) later added that MB $RM(t, t, t)$ designs for $t = 9$, 15 and 27 had been found and gave the plans of them.

For all odd values of t and $n = 2t$, MB $RM(t, 2t, t)$ designs exist and are the Williams designs, which again can be easily constructed using the Sheehe and Bross algorithm. In addition, Hedayat and Afsarinejad (1975) showed how to construct MB $RM(t, 2t, p)$ when t is a prime power. Methods of constructing MB designs for $p < t$ were described by Afsarinejad (1983). However, these designs are not varianced balanced except in a few special cases.

5.2.3   Designs with $p < t$

Designs obtained from orthogonal squares

All the designs described in the previous section are such that each subject receives every treatment. In practice this may not be possible for ethical or practical reasons. Even if all treatments could be administered, it is sometimes desirable to use a smaller number to decrease the chances of subjects dropping out of the trial. A number of balanced designs for $p < t$ have been suggested in the literature and we will describe and compare them in the following subsections. As in the previous section we will include the efficiencies of the design in the title of the table containing the design.

The simplest method of obtaining a balanced design with $p < t$ is to delete one or more periods from the full design obtained from a complete set of orthogonal Latin squares. This method was first suggested by Patterson (1950) and described in more detail by Patterson (1951, 1952). If we remove the last period from the design given in Table 5.2, for example, we will get a design for three periods with efficiencies $E_d = 71 \cdot 96$ and $E_c = 41 \cdot 98$

Although more than one period can be removed we should always ensure that the design we use has at least three periods. This is because designs with two periods have low efficiencies and should be avoided if possible. Two-period designs can, however, form a useful basic design to which extra periods are added. Extra-period designs are described below. Designs obtained from complete sets of orthogonal squares are also balanced for second-order carry-over effects and this property is retained when periods are removed.

Table 5.5 *One of Patterson's incomplete designs for seven treatments (79·84, 57·03)*

Subject	Period			
	1	2	3	4
1	A	B	D	G
2	B	C	E	A
3	C	D	F	B
4	D	E	G	C
5	E	F	A	D
6	F	G	B	E
7	G	A	C	F
8	A	G	E	B
9	B	A	F	C
10	C	B	G	D
11	D	C	A	E
12	E	D	B	F
13	F	E	C	G
14	G	F	D	A

Designs obtained from Youden squares and other methods

Patterson (1951) noted that a design which uses $4t$ subjects can always be constructed when a $4 \times t$ Youden square exists. (John, 1971, for example, gives a definition of a Youden square.) Patterson also gave a design for $t = 7$ which uses 14 subjects. This design, which is given in Table 5.5, can be divided into two blocks of seven subjects, as indicated. This design is also of the cyclic type: the sequences for subjects 2 to 7 are obtained by cycling the treatments for subject 1, and the sequence for subjects 9 to 14 are obtained by cycling the treatments for subject 8. In this cycling the treatments are successively changed in the order ABCDEFGA, etc. A number of the incomplete designs given by Patterson and Lucas (1962) for other values of t can be constructed using this cyclic method of construction.

Patterson (1952) extended his earlier results and gave designs which use fewer than $t(t - 1)$ units for the special case of prime $t = 4n + 3$, where n is a positive integer. In addition to the design given here in Table 5.5, he also gave a design for $t = 7$ which uses 21 subjects.

Designs obtained from balanced incomplete block designs

A number of different types of cross-over design can be constructed by starting with a non-cross-over incomplete block design. In this design the experimental units are grouped into b homogeneous blocks of size $p < t$. (We added the qualification 'non-cross-over' to ensure that it is clear that the incomplete block designs we are referring to are the traditional ones which have been used, in agriculture for example, for many years. In these designs each experimental unit in a block receives a single treatment.) Patterson (1952) noted that balanced cross-over designs can be constructed by starting with a **balanced incomplete block design** (BIB design). In a BIB design each treatment is replicated the same number of times and each pair of treatments occur together in the same block α times, where α is a constant integer. An example of a BIB for $t = 4$, $b = 4$ and $p = 3$ is (123), (124), (134) and (234). Each block of the design is enclosed by brackets and it can be seen that each pair of treatments occurs together in two blocks. To build a balanced cross-over design we take each block of the BIB in turn and construct a balanced cross-over design for the p treatments in that block. These blocks are then joined together to give a balanced cross-over design for t

treatments, p periods and bp subjects. If we take the BIB used as our example above then the corresponding balanced cross-over design we need for each block is the one given earlier in Table 5.2. We replace each block of the BIB with this three-treatment design and relabel the treatments where necessary. For example, the treatments in the third block are (134) and so in the balanced cross-over design for three treatments which corresponds to this block, we relabel 1 as A, 2 as C and 3 as D, to get the six sequences to be included in the final cross-over design for four treatments and three periods. The complete design for 24 subjects is given in Table 5.6.

Table 5.6 *Incomplete design for four treatments obtained using a BIB ($71 \cdot 96$, $41 \cdot 98$)*

Subject	Period		
	1	2	3
1	A	B	C
2	B	C	A
3	C	A	B
4	A	C	B
5	B	A	C
6	C	B	A
7	A	B	D
8	B	D	A
9	D	A	B
10	A	D	B
11	B	A	D
12	D	B	A
13	A	C	D
14	C	D	A
15	D	A	C
16	A	D	C
17	C	A	D
18	D	C	A
19	B	C	D
20	C	D	B
21	D	B	C
22	B	D	C
23	C	B	D
24	D	C	B

It should be noted that a design which uses 12 subjects and which has the same efficiencies as the design in Table 5.6 can be obtained by removing the last period from the orthogonal squares design for four treatments.

Other designs with $p < t$

For completeness we mention some other designs that have been suggested in the literature. These designs are generally not as efficient as the ones mentioned previously and so we do not devote much space to them here.

The two-period Balaam design described in Chapter 4 is a special case of the design suggested by Balaam (1968) for two or more treatments. The sequences in this more general design consist of all possible pairings of one treatment with another, including the pairing of a treatment with itself. These designs consist, as Balaam pointed out, of the first two periods of the designs suggested by Berenblut (1964). Balaam introduced his designs for use in animal experiments where a wash-out period is used to eliminate any carry-over effects. The designs are such that they permit a within-subject test of the direct-by-period interaction. In our situation where carry-over effects are included in the model, the Balaam designs, like all designs which use only two periods, do not have high efficiencies. We have included them partly for completeness and partly to draw attention to them again in the following section where $p > t$.

A different type of design, known as the switch-back, was introduced by Lucas (1957) for use in cattle feeding trials. He assumed that there were no carry-over effects or direct-by-period interaction. These designs are an extension of those described by Brandt (1938) for two treatments. These earlier designs used the two different sequences ABAB... and BABA.... That is, in the third period the animal switches back to the treatment it received in the first period, then switches back to the treatment it received in the second period, and so on. In Lucas's extension the design lasts for three periods and the treatment applied in the third period is the same as the treatment applied in the first period. In general, these designs consist of all possible $t(t-1)$ pairings of the treatments, which make up the sequences in the first two periods. Lucas also gave, for odd t, designs which use only $t(t-1)/2$ animals. However, these are not balanced for the adjusted treatment effects in our model. A feature of the Lucas designs is that they can be divided into blocks of t subjects.

More recently, Oman and Seiden (1988) gave a method of construction and the analysis of variance for switch-back designs as used in the context of cow lactation experiments.

Extra-period designs with $p < t$
Extra-period designs are obtained by adding an additional period to an existing cross-over design. In this extra period each subject receives the treatment he or she received in the last period of the original design. Adding the extra period has the effect of increasing the efficiency of estimation of $\lambda_i - \lambda_j$ and of causing the carry-over effects to become orthogonal to both subjects and direct effects. The origins of the idea of adding extra periods are described in the next section, when extra-period designs for $p > t$ are considered. If $p < t - 1$ then adding an extra period still gives a design with $p < t$.

If we add an extra period to one of Balaam's two-period designs we find that $E_d = E_c$. This feature has not, to our knowledge, been noted before. If it were not for their low efficiencies the extra-period Balaam designs would therefore be ideal for the situation where exactly the same precision is required for both carry-over and direct effects. Also the orthogonality of the carry-over and direct effects makes the design quite easy to analyse. These extra-period designs are therefore a possible alternative to the tied-double-change-over designs to be described below.

5.2.4 Designs with $p > t$

Extra-period designs
In general the balanced designs described in the previous sections are such that the efficiency E_c of the carry-over effects is much lower than the efficiency E_d of the direct effects. This, as Lucas (1957) pointed out, is mainly the result of the carry-over effects being non-orthogonal to the direct effects and subjects. This non-orthogonality can be removed, and the efficiency of the carry-over effects increased, if we use a design in which each carry-over effect occurs the same number of times with each subject and the same number of times with each direct effect. The simplest way to achieve this is to (a) take a balanced design for p periods, and (b) repeat in period $p + 1$ the treatment a subject received in period p. The advantages of adding an extra period were first noted by F. Yates in a seminar

Table 5.7 *Balanced extra-period design for three treatments (93·75, 75·00)*

Subject	Period			
	1	2	3	4
1	A	B	C	C
2	B	C	A	A
3	C	A	B	B
4	A	C	B	B
5	B	A	C	C
6	C	B	A	A

in 1947 and by Patterson (1951) at the end of a paper concerned mainly with the analysis and design of trials with $p < t$. Lucas (1957), however, gave the first formal description of adding an extra period.

Extra-period designs for $t = 3$ and 4 are given in Tables 5.7 and 5.8. The design for $t = 3$ is obtained by adding an extra period to the complete set of orthogonal squares and the design for $t = 4$ is obtained by adding an extra period to the Williams square, where now the square is written in standard order (i.e. the first row and column are in alphabetical order).

The change in the relative sizes of E_d and E_c which results from adding the extra period can be illustrated by comparing the efficiencies of the extra-period designs in Tables 5.7 and 5.8 with the efficiencies of their parent designs in Tables 5.2 and 5.4, respectively. The increase in efficiency arises because the extra-period designs are **completely balanced**, i.e. each treatment follows every other treatment, including itself, the same number of times. Therefore, each

Table 5.8 *Balanced extra-period design for four treatments (96·00, 80·00)*

Subject	Period				
	1	2	3	4	5
1	A	B	C	D	D
2	B	D	A	C	C
3	C	A	D	B	B
4	D	C	B	A	A

carry-over effect occurs the same number of times with each direct effect. As with the term 'balance' we will take it as understood that complete balance implies variance balance.

Apart from increasing efficiency, extra-period designs also have the advantage of permitting a more convenient analysis because the direct effects are orthogonal to the carry-over effects. In other words, the estimates of the direct effects are the same whether or not the carry-over effects are present in the fitted model.

Trials which use extra-period designs are, however, by their very nature, going to take longer to complete than trials which use the minimum number of periods. They are also likely to be more expensive and as a consequence may prove useful only when carry-over effects are strongly suspected and need to be estimated with relatively high efficiency. If carry-over effects are not present then the extra-period designs are not as efficient at estimating the direct effects as their parent designs. This is because the direct effects are not orthogonal to subjects in the extra-period designs. Also, some bias may creep into the process of measuring the response if those undertaking the measuring realize that the last two treatments administered to each subject are the same.

As we noted earlier, balanced designs for $p < t$ can also be constructed by adding an extra period. Also, repeating twice the treatment used in the last period of a balanced design will increase the efficiency with which the second-order effects are estimated. This has been noted by Linnerud, Gates and Donker (1962), for example.

Quenouille, Berenblut and Patterson designs
If we are prepared to use considerably more than $t + 1$ periods then completely balanced designs can also be constructed using a method proposed by Quenouille (1953). An example of one of Quenouille's designs for $t = 3$ is given in Table 5.9. It can be seen that the sequences for subjects 2 to 6 are obtained by cyclically shifting the sequence for subject 1. The sequences for subjects 8 to 12 are similarly obtained from sequence 7 and the sequences for subjects 14 to 18 are similarly obtained from the sequence for subject 13. The design is therefore completely and concisely defined by the three sequences (AABBCC), (AACCBB) and (ABCBAC). Quenouille also gave an alternative set of three sequences for $t = 3$ and three alternative pairs of sequences for $t = 4$. One pair of sequences for $t = 4$, for example, is (AABBCCDD) and (ACBADBDC). By cyclically shifting each of

Table 5.9 *Quenouille design for* $t = 3$ *(100·00, 80·56)*

Subject	Period					
	1	2	3	4	5	6
1	A	A	B	B	C	C
2	C	A	A	B	B	C
3	C	C	A	A	B	B
4	B	C	C	A	A	B
5	B	B	C	C	A	A
6	A	B	B	C	C	A
7	A	A	C	C	B	B
8	B	A	A	C	C	B
9	B	B	A	A	C	C
10	C	B	B	A	A	C
11	C	C	B	B	A	A
12	A	C	C	B	B	A
13	A	B	C	B	A	C
14	C	A	B	C	B	A
15	A	C	A	B	C	B
16	B	A	C	A	B	C
17	C	B	A	C	A	B
18	B	C	B	A	C	A

these sequences in turn, a design for four treatments using sixteen subjects and eight periods is obtained.

Berenblut (1964) showed that designs like those of Quenouille, which have direct effects orthogonal to carry-over effects and subjects, can be obtained by using t treatments, $2t$ periods and t^2 different sequences. Therefore, for $t = 4$ for example, they require fewer subjects than the designs suggested by Quenouille. A set of instructions for constructing a Berenblut design was given by Namboodiri (1972), and are somewhat easier to understand than the original set of instructions given by Berenblut (1964). The design for $t = 4$ obtained using these instructions is given in Table 5.10.

Berenblut (1967a) described how to analyse his designs and Berenblut (1967b) described a design appropriate for comparing equally spaced doses of the same drug which uses only eight subjects and four periods. This design is not balanced but does have the property that the linear, quadratic and cubic contrasts of the direct effects are orthogonal to the linear and cubic contrasts of the

Table 5.10 *Berenblut's design for t = 4 (100·00, 85·94)*

Subject	Period							
	1	2	3	4	5	6	7	8
1	A	D	C	B	B	C	D	A
2	B	A	D	C	C	D	A	B
3	C	B	A	D	D	A	B	C
4	D	C	B	A	A	B	C	D
5	D	D	B	B	A	C	C	A
6	A	A	C	C	B	D	D	B
7	B	B	D	D	C	A	A	C
8	C	C	A	A	D	B	B	D
9	C	D	A	B	D	C	B	A
10	D	A	B	C	A	D	C	B
11	A	B	C	D	B	A	D	C
12	B	C	D	A	C	B	A	D
13	B	D	D	B	C	C	A	A
14	C	A	A	C	D	D	B	B
15	D	B	B	D	A	A	C	C
16	A	C	C	A	B	B	D	D

carry-over effects. This design would be useful for comparing equally spaced doses of the same drug when carry-over effects are thought most unlikely; but if present they can be detected by a comparison of the low and high dose levels.

Berenblut (1968) noted that his (1964) designs are such that in addition to the properties already described, the direct-by-carry-over interaction is orthogonal to the direct and carry-over effects. He then described a method of constructing designs for $t = 4$ and 5 which have the same properties as his (1964) designs but require only $2t$ subjects. Each of these designs is constructed by combining two suitably chosen Latin squares. These designs are appropriate when the treatments correspond to equally spaced doses, the direct effects have a predominantly linear component, and the carry-over effects are small in comparison to the direct effects and proportional to them. The designs are such that (a) the linear component of the carry-over effect is orthogonal to the linear, quadratic, etc., components of the direct effect, and (b) the linear direct-by-linear carry-over interaction is orthogonal to each component of the direct effect.

Patterson (1970) pointed out that although Berenblut's (1964) design, when used for four equally spaced treatments, is suitable for the estimation of the direct and carry-over effects, other designs may be preferred for the estimation of the linear direct-by-linear carry-over interaction. He gave a method of constructing a family of designs which contained within it the designs of Berenblut (1964), and also showed how the subjects in his designs could be divided into blocks of eight or four, with a minimum loss of information due to confounding. He also noted that Berenblut's (1967b) design which uses eight subjects has low efficiency for estimating the linear-by-linear interaction and suggested that if economy of subjects and periods is important then it is better to reduce the number of treatment levels to three and to use one of his or Berenblut's designs for three treatments. Patterson (1973) described a way of extending Quenouille's (1953) method so that a larger collection of designs can be obtained.

Federer and Atkinson's designs
Federer and Atkinson (1964) described a series of designs for r periods and c subjects, where $r = tq + 1$, $c = ts$, $sq = k(t - 1)$ and q, s and k are positive integers. These designs, which they called tied-double-change-over designs, are such that the variances of the direct and carry-over effects approach equality as the number of periods increases. If the number of periods is kept to a minimum then these designs require $t(t - 1)$ subjects and $(t + 1)$ periods.

Atkinson (1966) proposed a series of designs for the situation where the effect of consecutive applications of a treatment is the quantity of interest. The designs are obtained by taking a Williams design and repeating each column (i.e. period) k times, where $k \geqslant 2$. The effect of repeating periods is to increase the efficiency of estimation of the carry-over effects at the expense of the direct effects. It should be noted that, unlike Atkinson, we are assuming that the design consists of all $2t$ periods. The analysis given by Atkinson assumed that the data from the first $k - 1$ periods would not be used.

5.3 Optimality results for cross-over designs

Here we briefly review some recent results concerning the optimality of cross-over designs with three or more treatments. In the general (i.e. not necessarily cross-over) design case, optimality criteria are usually defined in terms of functions of the information matrix of the design or the variance–covariance matrix V of $(t-1)$ orthogonal and normalized contrasts between the t treatments. A good design is one which makes V 'small' in some sense. Different ways of defining 'small' have led to different optimality criteria:

1. the D-optimal design minimizes the determinant of V;
2. the A-optimal design minimizes the average variance of the $(t-1)$ orthonormal contrasts; and
3. the E-optimal design minimizes the maximum variance of the $(t-1)$ orthonormal contrasts.

Kiefer (1975) subsumed these criteria and others into his criterion of **universal** optimality: the universal (U)-optimal design is also D-, A- and E-optimal. Later, Hedayat and Afsarinejad (1978) considered the optimality of **uniform** cross-over designs. In a uniform design each treatment occurs equally often in each period and for each subject, each treatment appears in the same number of periods. They proved that uniform balanced designs are U-optimal for the estimation of the direct effects and for the first-order carry-over effects. (These designs, it will be realized, are the ones we described earlier in the section on minimal balanced designs.) Consequently, the Williams designs, and the MB $RM(t,t,t)$ designs which exist, are U-optimal. The rest of this short review is based mainly on Matthews (1988a, Section 3.2).

Cheng and Wu (1980) extended Hedayat and Afsarinejad's results and in particular were able to prove, for i a positive integer, that (a) balanced uniform designs are U-optimal for the estimation of first-order carry-over effects over all $RM(t,it,t)$ designs where no treatment precedes itself, and (b) if a design is obtained from a balanced uniform design by repeating the last period, then it is U-optimal for the estimation of direct and carry-over effects over all $RM(t,it,t+1)$ designs.

Result (b) of Cheng and Wu is particularly useful because it provides a more rigorous justification for the extra-period designs suggested by Lucas (1957). Kunert (1984) proved that if a balanced uniform $RM(t,t,t)$ design exists then it is U-optimal for the estimation of the direct treatment effects.

Cheng and Wu were also able to prove that a strongly balanced uniform $RM(t,n,p)$ design is U-optimal for the estimation of direct and carry-over effects. Their 'strongly balanced' corresponds to our earlier definition of 'completely balanced'.

Finally, we note that Sen and Mukerjee (1987) extended some of the results of Cheng and Wu to the case where the direct-by-carry-over interaction parameters are also included in the model. They proved that completely balanced uniform designs were also U-optimal for the estimation of the direct effects in the presence of these interaction parameters. This follows from the orthogonality of the direct effects, the carry-over effects and the interaction parameters.

Before we leave this section we should emphasize that when planning a trial there will be a number of different criteria that we will want the design to satisfy. Optimal design theory concentrates our attention on a particular aspect of the design, e.g. average variance, and ignores the rest. Therefore the investigator who is planning the trial should try to achieve what we term **practical optimality**. This requires taking into account such things as

1. the likelihood of drop-outs if the number of periods is large;
2. whether or not the staff who will run the trial will be able to successfully administer the treatments correctly if the design plan is at all complicated;
3. whether the clinicians involved in the trial will find it difficult to interpret the results from a rather complicated design.

Although this list could be extended, it is long enough to make the point that in the planning of a trial every aspect must be carefully considered and the various, often conflicting, objectives reconciled. Also, as noted in Chapter 4, if we change the assumptions made by our model we should not be surprised if the optimal design changes too.

5.4 Which variance-balanced design to use?

It should be clear from Section 5.2 that there are a great many balanced designs to choose from. In Table 5.11 we give the efficiencies of a selection of designs for $t \leqslant 9$. The purpose of Table 5.11 is to illustrate the features of the designs which were noted in Section 5.2 and to provide information that can be used to choose a design for particular values of t, p and n. Obviously, by taking m copies of a particular design we get a design with the same efficiencies as the original design but for mn subjects. In Table 5.11 the designs have been identified using the following abbreviations: PLNN – design

Table 5.11 A selection of balanced designs

		3 treatments		
Design	p	n	E_d	E_c
PL1	2	6	18·75	6·25
BAL	2	9	25·00	12·50
WD	3	6	80·00	44·44
LSB	3	6	21·67	18·06
PL30(EP)	3	6	66·67	55·56
BAL(EP)	3	9	44·44	44·44
WD(EP)	4	6	93·75	75·00
FA(1, 2)	4	6	75·00	60·00
ATK	6	6	86·21	69·44
BER	6	9	100·00	80·55
QUE	6	18	100·00	80·55
FA(2, 1)	7	3	76·53	66·96
ATK	7	6	92·60	81·03

		4 treatments		
Design	p	n	E_d	E_c
PL3	2	12	22·22	8·33
BAL	2	16	25·00	12·50
PL4	3	12	71·96	41·98
PL32(EP)	3	12	59·26	51·85
LSB	3	12	21·16	18·52
BAL(EP)	3	16	44·44	44·44
BIB	3	24	71·96	41·98
WD	4	4	90·91	62·50
PL33(EP)	4	12	83·33	68·75
OLS	4	12	90·91	62·50
WD(EP)	5	4	96·00	80·00
OLS(EP)	5	12	96·00	80·00
FA(1, 3)	5	12	87·11	72·59
ATK	8	4	83·64	71·88
BER	8	16	100·00	85·94
FA(2, 3)	9	12	88·89	80·00

(*Continued*)

Table 5.11 (Continued)

5 treatments				
Design	p	n	E_d	E_c
PL7	2	20	23·44	9·38
BAL	2	25	25·00	12·50
PL36(EP)	3	20	55·66	50·00
PL8	3	20	67·90	40·74
LSB	3	20	20·83	18·75
BAL(EP)	3	25	44·44	44·44
PL9	4	20	85·38	59·76
PL37(EP)	4	20	78·13	65·63
WD	5	10	94·74	72·00
PL38(EP)	5	20	90·00	76·00
OLS	5	20	94·74	72·00
FA(1, 1)	6	5	13·89	11·90
WD(EP)	6	10	97·22	83·33
OLS(EP)	6	20	97·22	83·33
FA(1, 4)	6	20	97·06	76·27

6 treatments				
Design	p	n	E_d	E_c
PL12	2	30	24·00	10·00
BAL	2	36	25·00	12·50
PL41(EP)	3	30	53·33	48·89
LSB	3	30	20·61	18·89
BAL(EP)	3	36	44·44	44·44
PL13	5	30	91·00	69·76
WD	6	6	96·55	77·78
PL42(EP)	6	30	93·33	80·56
WD(EP)	7	6	97·96	85·71

(Continued)

Table 5.11 (*Continued*)

Design	p	n	E_d	E_c
			7 *treatments*	
PL16	2	42	24·30	10·42
BAL	2	49	25·00	12·50
PL17	3	21	63·82	39·51
LSB	3	42	20·44	18·98
PL43(EP)	3	42	51·85	48·15
BAL(EP)	3	49	44·44	44·44
PL19	4	14	79·84	57·03
PL44(EP)	4	21	72·92	62·50
PL46(EP)	5	14	84·00	72·00
PL21	5	21	88·49	68·27
PL48(EP)	6	21	90·74	78·70
PL23	6	42	93·89	76·00
WD	7	14	97·56	81·63
PL23(EP)	7	42	95·24	83·67
OLS	7	42	97·56	81·63
WD(EP)	8	14	98·44	87·50

Design	p	n	E_d	E_c
			8 *treatments*	
WD	8	8	98·18	84·38
WD(EP)	9	8	98·76	88·89

Design	p	n	E_d	E_c
			9 *treatments*	
M	9	9	98·59	86·42
M(EP)	10	9	99·00	90·00

NN from Patterson and Lucas (1962); BAL – Balaam (1968); WD – Williams (1949); OLS – Orthogonal Latin squares; FA(q, s) – Federer and Atkinson (1964) with parameters q and s; LSB – Lucas (1957); ATK – Atkinson (1966); BER – Berenblut (1964); QUE – Quenouille (1953); BIB – constructed using a balanced incomplete block design; M – Mertz's design as quoted by Hedayat and Asfarinejad (1978); (EP) – design is of the extra-period type.

Table 5.11 illustrates quite clearly some of the points already made in Sections 5.2 and 5.3:

1. The two-period designs, the switch-back designs and Balaam's designs have low efficiencies and should be avoided if at all possible.
2. For $p = t$, the minimal balanced designs are optimal and for $p = t + 1$, the corresponding extra-period designs are optimal. (This, of course, illustrates the optimality results of Cheng and Wu, 1980.)
3. For $p \neq t$ or $p \neq t + 1$, the choice of design depends on p and n. So, for example, if $3 \leqslant p < t \leqslant 7$ and we ignore any restrictions on n, good choices of design, in the notation (t, p, n, design), are: $(4, 3, 12, \text{PL4})$; $(5, 4, 20, \text{PL9})$; $(5, 3, 20, \text{PL8})$; $(6, 5, 30, \text{PL13})$; $(6, 3, 30, \text{PL41 (EP)})$; $(7, 6, 42, \text{PL23})$; $(7, 5, 21, \text{PL21})$; $(7, 4, 14, \text{PL19})$; $(7, 3, 21, \text{PL17})$.

If no balanced design can be chosen to fit in with our particular choice of t, p and n, and there is no possibility of changing this choice, then the partially balanced designs which we describe in the next section may provide useful alternatives.

5.5 Partially balanced designs

It sometimes happens that, although a balanced design is required, it is not possible to construct one for the available number of subjects and the chosen values of t and p. In these circumstances a useful compromise is to use a partially balanced (PB) design. Even if a balanced design can be constructed, PB designs may be preferred as they are such that $p < t$ and they usually require far fewer subjects. The characteristic feature of a PB design is that $V[\hat{t}_i - \hat{t}_j]$ (and $V[\hat{\lambda}_i - \hat{\lambda}_j]$) depends on the pair of treatments, i and j, being compared. In balanced designs these variances are constant.

Before we can sensibly explain how to construct PB cross-over designs, we must first define what is meant by a **PB incomplete block design** (PBIB, for short) as used in non-cross-over experiments. Incomplete block designs, it will be recalled, were defined in Section 5.2 when BIB designs were described, and are such that the experimental units are grouped into b homogeneous blocks of size p, where $p < t$. One way of characterizing a PBIB is in terms of how many associate classes it has. If a PBIB has m associate classes then there will be m different values for $V[\hat{t}_i - \hat{t}_j]$ (where $\hat{t}_i$ and $\hat{t}_j$ here refer to treatment estimators in the non-cross-over design). For convenience we will refer to these designs as PBIB(m) designs. The simplest and potentially most useful designs are the PBIB(2) designs and these have been extensively catalogued by Clatworthy (1973). In these designs the treatments are assigned to the blocks in such a way that each treatment occurs 0 or 1 times in each block, and each pair of treatments occurs together in the same block either α_1 times or α_2 times where $\alpha_1 \neq \alpha_2$. If we assume that $\alpha_1 > \alpha_2$, then the pairs of treatments that occur together in α_1 blocks are first associates and the other pairs are second associates. The efficiency of comparisons between first associates is higher than that of comparisons between second associates. Clatworthy's catalogue not only gives the plans of a great many PBIB(2) designs but also the corresponding efficiencies, E_1 and E_2, of treatment differences between first and second associates, respectively, and $\bar{E}$ the **average efficiency** of the design. The average efficiency is defined as

$$\bar{E} = \sum_{i=1}^{t-1} \sum_{j=i+1}^{t} \frac{2E_{ij}}{t(t-1)}$$

where E_{ij} is the efficiency of the estimated difference between treatments i and j.

The average efficiency is a useful measure for comparing designs which have two or more associate classes. Unless a design with a particular pattern of pairwise efficiencies is required, the design of choice will be the one with the highest average efficiency.

Also given by Clatworthy is the association scheme of each design, which specifies which pairs of treatments are first associates and which pairs are second associates.

To illustrate the above points let us look at the design labelled as S1 in Clatworthy's catalogue. This design is for $t = 6$, $b = 3$ and $p = 4$ and is of the group-divisible type. The blocks of the design are (ADBE), (BECF) and (CFAD) and its association scheme can be written as

$$
\begin{array}{cc}
A & D \\
B & E \\
C & F
\end{array}
$$

The treatments in the same row of this scheme are first associates and those in the same column are second associates.

The above definition of a PBIB(2) is extended in an obvious way to PBIB(m) designs. A more formal definition of a PBIB(m) and numerous related references can be found in Raghavarao (1971, Chapter 8).

In the following we describe PB cross-over designs which have been suggested by three different pairs of authors. In Section 5.6 we give some advice on which PB design to use.

The PB designs of Patterson and Lucas

In this method, which was first described by Patterson and Lucas (1962), we take a PBIB(2) from Clatworthy's catalogue and replace each block of the design by a balanced cross-over design for p

Table 5.12 *PB design constructed from PBIB(2) design S1*

Subject	Period			
	1	2	3	4
1	A	D	B	E
2	D	E	A	B
3	B	A	E	D
4	E	B	D	A
5	B	E	C	F
6	E	F	B	C
7	C	B	F	E
8	F	C	E	B
9	C	F	A	D
10	F	D	C	A
11	A	C	D	F
12	D	A	F	C

treatments. This is the same method that was used in Section 5.2 to construct balanced cross-over designs using BIBs.

To illustrate the method let us take the PBIB(2) design S1 which was described in the previous subsection. Each block of this design contains four treatments and so we need to find a balanced cross-over design for four treatments. Such a design was given earlier in Table 5.4 (now written in standard order). We replace each block of the PBIB(2) design with the design given in Table 5.4, and relabel the treatments so that they correspond to those in the block under consideration. The complete cross-over design is then as given in Table 5.12. If we always use a Williams design as our balanced design then the final cross-over design for p periods will require bp subjects if p is even, and $2bp$ subjects if p is odd. The efficiencies of the design in Table 5.12 are $E_{d1} = 90 \cdot 91$, $E_{d2} = 78 \cdot 29$, $E_{c1} = 62 \cdot 50$ and $E_{c2} = 56 \cdot 51$, where E_{d1} (E_{c1}) is the efficiency of the estimated difference between two first-associate direct (carry-over) effects and E_{d2} (E_{c2}) is the efficiency of the estimated difference between second-associate direct (carry-over) effects. Naturally, the association scheme of the parent PBIB(2) design will also apply to the cross-over design constructed from it and the efficiencies of the final design will reflect those of the parent design used to construct it.

In a similarly way to that done in the previous subsection we define $\bar{E}_d$ as the average efficiency of the direct treatment comparisons and $\bar{E}_c$ as the average efficiency of the carry-over comparisons.

In the left-hand part of Table 5.13 we give the efficiencies of some PB cross-over designs, which can be obtained by using Clatworthy's catalogue, and which have $t \leqslant 9$ and $n \leqslant 60$. As with the balanced designs, if necessary, the treatments in the last period can be repeated in an extra period to increase the relative efficiency of the estimated carry-over effects.

It will be recalled that if periods are removed from a balanced design which is made up of a complete set of orthogonal Latin squares, the depleted design is still balanced. We can therefore repeat the above construction procedure using a depleted design obtained from a complete set of Latin squares. Unfortunately, as the complete set of squares for p periods requires $p(p-1)$ subjects, the final cross-over design will be very large if p is bigger than 3 or 4. When $p = 3$ in the original set of squares, however, we can apply the procedure, as done by Patterson and Lucas, to construct a number

Table 5.13 *Some PB cross-over designs for $t \leqslant 9$*

t	p	n	PBIB(2)	$\bar{E}_\mathrm{d}$	$\bar{E}_\mathrm{c}$	t	p	n	Generating sequence	$\bar{E}_\mathrm{d}$	$\bar{E}_\mathrm{c}$
5	3	30	C12	66·85	40·59						
6	3	24	SR18	63·57	39·73	6	3	12	(034)(051)	58·42	34·22
6	3	36	R42	64·55	39·88	6	4	12	(0132)(0314)	81·32	57·44
6	4	12	S1	80·82	57·71	6	5	6	(01325)	85·86	65·64
6	4	24	R94	81·56	57·96						
6	4	36	SR35	81·87	58·06						
6	4	48	R96	81·98	58·10						
						7	3	14	(031)(045)	62·42	35·57
						7	4	14	(0136)(0641)*	79·84	57·03
						7	5	7	(02315)	80·29	61·11
8	3	48	R54	61·68	39·02	8	3	16	(041)(065)	54·59	31·99
8	4	24	S6	75·77	55·42	8	4	16	(0214)(0153)	77·28	54·87
8	4	32	SR36	76·93	55·80	8	5	8	(01325)	78·67	59·06
8	4	40	R97	78·04	56·18						
8	4	48	SR38	77·99	56·16						
8	6	24	S18	91·71	74·59						
9	3	36	LS7	56·39	38·18	9	3	18	(038)(067)	54·74	31·18
9	3	54	SR23	60·28	38·67	9	4	18	(0142)(0526)	74·36	53·61
9	4	36	LS26	76·27	55·40	9	5	9	(01325)	76·36	56·83
9	6	18	S21	89·36	73·15						
9	6	36	LS72	90·20	73·59						
9	6	54	SR65	90·44	73·72						

*This design is actually variance balanced and is included only for completeness.

of PB cross-over design which require only two periods. Of course, as already noted in Section 5.2, two-period designs have low efficiencies and should, if possible, be avoided. However, these two-period designs provide yet another set of designs to which an extra period can be added.

The cyclic PB designs of Davis and Hall

Davis and Hall (1969) proposed a series of PB cross-over designs which were obtained from cyclic incomplete block designs (CIBDs). A CIBD is constructed by cyclically developing one or more generating sequences of treatments. For example if for $t = 6$ a generating sequence is (0132), where 0 represents treatment A, 1 represents treatment B, and so on, then the blocks generated are (0132), (1243), (2354), (3405), (4510) and (5021). We see in this example that the entries in a block are obtained by adding 1 to the entries of the previous block, subject to the restriction that numbers above 5 are reduced modulo 5. In our notation the blocks of the design are then (ABDC), (BCED), (CDFE), (DEAF), (EFBA) and (FACB). Davis and Hall's method is to consider the blocks of the CIBD as the treatment sequences to be applied to the subjects. From the large number of CIBDs available in the literature they selected those which required fewer units than the PB designs of Patterson and Lucas and which had comparable efficiencies. A feature of the selected designs is that, although there may be up to $[t/2]$ associate classes, the efficiencies of the estimated differences between pairs of treatments do not differ very much from each other.

As an example, we give in Table 5.14 the design obtained when the generating sequences are (0132) and (0314). The first sequence which was used as our illustration in the previous paragraph does not generate a useful cross-over design when used alone: when used in conjunction with the second sequence, however, a useful design results. This design has three associate classes.

In the right-hand part of Table 5.13 are given the generating sequences and average efficiencies for the designs given by Davis and Hall for $t \leqslant 9$. We can see that the cyclic designs generally require fewer subjects to achieve comparable efficiencies. Davis and Hall also note that cyclic designs can be analysed after any number

Table 5.14 *PB cyclic design generated by (0132) and (0314)*

Subject	Period			
	1	2	3	4
1	A	B	D	C
2	B	C	E	D
3	C	D	F	E
4	D	E	A	F
5	E	F	B	A
6	F	A	C	B
7	A	D	B	E
8	B	E	C	F
9	C	F	D	A
10	D	A	E	B
11	E	B	F	C
12	F	C	A	D

of

Table 5.15 *Numbers of treatments, periods and subjects*

Series	No. of treatments	No. of periods	No. of subjects
R1	$t = 2q$ ($q \geqslant 4$ and even)	$q + 1$	$2q$
R2	$t = 3q$ ($q \geqslant 3$ and odd)	$q + 1$	$6q$
T1	$t = q(q-1)/2$ ($q \geqslant 5$ and odd)	$q - 1$	$q(q-1)$
T2	$t = q(q-1)/2$ ($q \geqslant 4$ and even)	$q - 1$	$2q(q-1)$

of periods and that further periods may be added if required. These extra periods, they suggest, should be chosen to maximize $\bar{E}_d$ or $\bar{E}_c$. Alternatively, of course, a single extra period can be added by the usual method of repeating the treatment in the last period.

The partially balanced designs of Blaisdell and Raghavarao
Blaisdell (1978) and Blaisdell and Raghavarao (1980) described the construction of four different series of PB cross-over design. Two of the series, which they labelled as R1 and R2, have three associate classes and the other two, which they labelled as T1 and T2, have two associate classes. The association scheme of the R1 and R2 designs is the rectangular scheme defined by Vartak (1955) and the association scheme of the T1 and T2 designs is the triangular scheme defined by Bose and Shimamoto (1952). The number of treatments, periods and subjects required by each of the four series are given in Table 5.15.

It can be seen that the R1 designs are for $8, 12, 16, \ldots$ treatments, the R2 designs are for $9, 15, 21, \ldots$ treatments, the T1 designs are for $10, 21, 36, \ldots$ treatments and the T2 designs are for $6, 15, 28, \ldots$ treatments. As it is unusual for clinical trials to compare large numbers of treatments, it is clear that the four series of designs are of limited usefulness in the clinical trials context. The average efficiencies $(\bar{E}_d, \bar{E}_c)$ of the designs for $t = 6, 8$ and 9 are, respectively, $(63 \cdot 57, 39 \cdot 73)$, $(80 \cdot 38, 51 \cdot 26)$ and $(70 \cdot 94, 41 \cdot 28)$.

5.6 Which partially balanced design to use?

The main reasons for considering PB designs are

1. to fill in some of the gaps where no balanced design exists for given values of t, p and n; and
2. to provide reasonable alternatives when a balanced design for particular values of t and p requires too many subjects.

With regard to 1 we can see that there are PB designs for $t = 8$ and 9 which do not require 8 or 9 periods. (Of course we can always get balanced designs for $t = 8$ or 9 which require fewer than 8 or 9 periods by deleting periods from a complete set of orthogonal Latin squares, but this would require a large ($t(t-1)$) number of subjects.)

Table 5.16 *A selection of PB designs*

t	p	n	Design
5	3	30	PL
6	3	12	DH
6	3	24	PL
6	4	12	DH
6	4	24	PL
6	4	36	PL
6	4	48	PL
7	3	14	DH
7	5	7	DH
8	3	16	DH
8	3	48	PL
8	4	16	DH
8	4	24	PL
8	4	40	PL
8	4	48	PL
8	5	8	BR
8	6	24	PL
9	3	18	DH
9	3	36	PL
9	3	54	PL
9	4	18	DH
9	4	36	PL
9	5	9	DH
9	6	18	PL
9	6	36	PL
9	6	54	PL

With regard to 2 we can see that for $t = 7$, for example, the PB designs require fewer subjects than their balanced counterparts.

In Table 5.16 we have listed our recommendations for which type of PB design to use. The chosen design has the highest value of $\bar{E}_d$ for the given values of t and p. The abbreviations in the table refer to the authors who suggested the designs (PL = Patterson and Lucas, DH = Davis and Hall, BR = Blaisdale and Raghavarao). By looking back to Table 5.13 details of the PL and DH designs can be obtained. As with the balanced designs, m copies of a design can be taken to obtain a design for mn subjects, unless a more efficient design for mn subjects is already given in Table 5.16. So, for example, the PL design for $t = 6$, $p = 3$ and $n = 24$ is more efficient than taking two copies of the DH design for the same values of t and p.

Of course, as always when deciding on the design to use we must take other things into account as well as the efficiency of the designs. The DH designs, it will be recalled, can be analysed easily after any number of periods. On the other hand, the PL designs have only two associate classes and therefore permit a simpler pairwise comparison of the treatment effects to be made.

5.7 Comparing test treatments with a control

Pigeon (1984) and Pigeon and Raghavarao (1987) proposed some designs for the situation where one treatment is a **control** or standard and is to be compared with t test treatments (i.e. there are $t + 1$ treatments in the trial). The characteristic feature of these **control**

Table 5.17 *A control balanced design for*
$t = 3$

Subject	Period		
	1	2	3
1	X	A	B
2	X	B	C
3	X	C	A
4	A	X	C
5	B	X	A
6	C	X	B
7	A	C	X
8	B	A	X
9	C	B	X

balanced designs is that pairwise comparisons between the control and the test treatments are made more precisely than pairwise comparisons between the test treatments. The precision of comparisons between the test treatments has been sacrificed in order to achieve high precision on comparisons with the control.

An example of a control balanced design for $t = 3$ is given in Table 5.17 where X denotes the control treatment and A, B and C denote the test treatments. If τ_x is the direct effect of the control treatment and λ_x is the corresponding carry-over effect, then the variance properties of the control balanced designs are (for $i \neq j \neq x$):

$$V[\hat{\tau}_x - \hat{\tau}_i] = c_1\sigma^2, \qquad V[\hat{\tau}_i - \hat{\tau}_j] = c_2\sigma^2,$$
$$V[\hat{\lambda}_x - \hat{\lambda}_i] = c_3\sigma^2, \qquad V[\hat{\lambda}_i - \hat{\lambda}_j] = c_4\sigma^2$$

where c_1, c_2, c_3 and c_4 are such that $c_1 < c_2 < c_3 < c_4$. The values of c_1, c_2, c_3 and c_4 for the design in Table 5.17 are 0·372, 0·491, 0·648 and 0·818, respectively.

A number of methods of constructing control balanced designs were described by Pigeon and Raghavarao, and their paper should be consulted for details.

We can change each of the control balanced designs into an extra-period design with similar variance properties by repeating the treatment given in the last period. This has the effect of making the direct and carry-over effects orthogonal and reducing the variances of the carry-over effects.

Table 5.18 *Variances of contrasts in Pigeon's designs*

t	p	n	c_1	c_2	c_3	c_4
3	3	9	0·3720	0·4909	0·6477	0·8182
3	3	21	0·1666	0·1896	0·2882	0·3214
3	3	30	0·1147	0·1367	0·1989	0·2308
4	3	28	0·1540	0·2037	0·2608	0·3333
4	3	38	0·1159	0·1440	0·1957	0·2368
4	3	36	0·1174	0·1741	0·1992	0·2812
4	4	16	0·1665	0·1995	0·2395	0·2832
4	4	36	0·0775	0·0844	0·1110	0·1203
5	3	20	0·2628	0·3482	0·4368	0·5625
5	3	30	0·1704	0·2698	0·2839	0·4286
5	4	40	0·0784	0·1044	0·1118	0·1461
5	5	25	0·0972	0·1110	0·1272	0·1445

The values of c_i, $i = 1, 2, 3$ and 4, for some of the control balanced designs for up to five test treatments are given in Table 5.18.

5.8 Factorial treatment combinations

It is not unusual in drug-trial work to administer treatments that are made up of combinations of more than one drug. Among the reasons for doing this are: to determine if a combination of drugs is more efficacious than using a single drug; to investigate the joint actions of drugs that are usually prescribed for different conditions; and that one drug is being used to combat an unpleasant side-effect of another. In this section we will consider treatments that are made up of all possible combinations of the chosen drug dose levels. In the terminology of factorial experiments, each drug is a **factor** and can be administered at a number of different **levels**. A treatment made up by combining one dose level from each of the drugs is called a **factorial treatment combination.**

To take our brief introduction to factorial experiments a little further, consider, as an example, a trial in which the four treatments are: (1) no treatment, (2) drug A at a fixed dose, (3) drug B at a fixed dose, and (4) drugs A and B together at the same fixed doses as in treatments (2) and (3). Here the two factors are the drugs A and B and each factor takes the levels: no dose or the fixed dose for that drug. A standard way of labelling the treatment combinations is to use 0 to indicate that the factor (i.e. drug) is being used at its lower level (i.e. no dose in our example) and to use a 1 to indicate that the factor is being used at its higher level (i.e. at the fixed dose level). The four treatments, in the order listed above, can then be denoted by 00, 10, 01 and 11, respectively. In a different trial, the labels 0 and 1 might represent low dose and high dose rather than absence and presence.

Clearly this system of labelling can be extended to more than two factors and/or to more than two levels. For example, if there are three drugs, the first of which can be administered at three equally spaced doses (no dose, low dose, high dose) and the second and third can be administered at two doses (no dose, fixed dose), then the first factor has three levels and the other two factors have two levels. If we label the levels of the first drug as 0, 1 and 2, and label the levels of the other two drugs as 0 and 1, then the 12 factorial treatment combinations are 000, 001, 010, 011, 100, 101, 110, 111, 200,

201, 210 and 211. By convention we would call this trial a $3 \times 2 \times 2$ factorial. The trial used as our example at the beginning of this section is a 2×2 factorial.

In a factorial experiment the contrasts between the treatments that are of most interest are the main effects and interactions of the factors. In order to explain these terms a little more fully let us again refer to our 2×2 example. It will be recalled that the four treatment combinations are 00, 10, 01 and 11. Let us denote the corresponding direct effects of these combinations as τ_1, τ_2, τ_3 and τ_4, respectively. The three direct contrasts of interest are then as follows:

1. the main effect of drug A $= \frac{1}{2}(-\tau_1 + \tau_2 - \tau_3 + \tau_4)$;
2. the main effect of drug B $= \frac{1}{2}(-\tau_1 - \tau_2 + \tau_3 + \tau_4)$;
3. the interaction of drugs A and B $= \frac{1}{2}(\tau_1 - \tau_2 - \tau_3 + \tau_4)$.

By convention we label these contrasts as A_d, B_d and $A_d \times B_d$, respectively, where the 'd' indicates that we are taking contrasts of the direct effects.

We can see that the main effect A_d is a measure of the change brought about by changing the levels of drug A, averaged over the levels of drug B, i.e. $A_d = \frac{1}{2}[(\tau_2 - \tau_1) + (\tau_4 - \tau_3)]$. Similarly, B_d is a measure of the change brought about by changing the levels of drug B averaged over the levels of drug A. The interaction $A_d \times B_d$ is a measure of how changing the levels of A depends on the level chosen for B, i.e. $\frac{1}{2}(\tau_4 - \tau_3) - \frac{1}{2}(\tau_2 - \tau_1)$. (Of course, $A_d \times B_d$ is also a measure of how changing the levels of B depends on A.)

The attraction of the factorial experiment is that it allows us the possibility of detecting interactions, and in the absence of interactions, to obtain information on the separate effects of each drug (i.e. the main effects) using a single trial.

Let us now consider the carry-over effects. In our 2×2 example there are four treatments and we would, as usual, include the carry-over effects $\lambda_1, \lambda_2, \lambda_3$ and λ_4 in our fitted model. If there is evidence of carry-over differences then we can obtain a better understanding of these by looking at the carry-over main effects and interactions. These contrasts, which are labelled using the subscript c, are as follows:

4. $A_c = \frac{1}{2}(-\lambda_1 + \lambda_2 - \lambda_3 + \lambda_4)$;
5. $B_c = \frac{1}{2}(-\lambda_1 - \lambda_2 + \lambda_3 + \lambda_4)$;
6. $A_c \times B_c = \frac{1}{2}(\lambda_1 - \lambda_2 - \lambda_3 + \lambda_4)$.

That is, they correspond exactly to the contrasts used for the direct effects.

A crucially important feature of the factorial experiment is that there is a well-defined structure among the treatment combinations. For example, the treatments can be subdivided into sets which have the same level of a particular factor, e.g. $(00, 01)$ and $(10, 11)$ in our 2×2 example. When there is structure we are usually no longer interested in all pairwise differences between the treatments but in particular differences or particular contrasts. Naturally we will want a design which estimates the contrasts of interest with as high an efficiency as possible. For example, if the separate effects of the two drugs in our 2×2 experiment are well known and it is their joint effect that is of interest, then the main effects are of much less interest than the interaction. A design which estimates the interaction with as high an efficiency as possible would then be the design of choice. In order to achieve high efficiency of estimation of the contrasts of interest we will usually be happy to accept a low efficiency on the contrasts of little or no interest. If this is the case then the balanced and completely balanced designs will not be the most suitable designs. In these designs the main effects and interactions are estimated with equal efficiency.

The type of design we seek for factorial experiments must take account of the structure of the treatments, the need to estimate effects with different efficiencies, and the need to retain a sufficient degree of balance to keep the data analysis relatively simple. The designs which come closest to satisfying these requirements are the ones which possess **factorial structure**. A design is said to possess factorial structure if and only if

1. estimates of the direct treatment contrasts belonging to different factorial effects are orthogonal;
2. estimates of the carry-over contrasts belonging to different factorial effects are orthogonal;
3. estimates of direct treatment contrasts and estimates of carry-over contrasts belonging to different factorial effects are orthogonal.

This definition is taken from Fletcher and John (1985) and is a generalization of one given by Cotter, John and Smith (1973) for non-cross-over designs.

The attractiveness of factorial structure is enhanced by the availability of a large number of cross-over designs that possess this

Table 5.19 *Generalized cyclic design for the 2 × 2 factorial*

Subject	Period		
	1	2	3
1	00	01	11
2	01	00	10
3	10	11	01
4	11	10	00

structure. Fletcher and John (1985) showed that the generalized cyclic designs (GC/n designs, for short) of John (1973) provide a flexible class of cross-over designs that possess factorial structure.

Fletcher (1987) considered the construction of cross-over designs using GC/n designs and gave a list of suitable designs for up to six periods for the 2 × 2, 2 × 3, 2 × 4, 3 × 3, 4 × 4, 2 × 2 × 2 and 3 × 3 × 3 factorial experiments. Fletcher's designs are such that the main effects are estimated with a higher efficiency than the interactions. An example of one of Fletcher's (1987) designs for the 2 × 2 factorial is given in Table 5.19.

Lewis, Fletcher and Matthews (1988) constructed cross-over designs for factorial experiments by joining together one or more **bricks**. A brick is made up of one or more GC/n cross-over designs. By combining different bricks, designs that have different patterns of efficiencies can be obtained. Jones (1985) used a similar technique to construct block designs for non-cross-over experiments. Lewis *et al.* gave a selection of designs for the 2 × 2, 2 × 3, 2 × 4, and 3 × 3 factorials that used three or four periods. In some of these designs the interactions are estimated with higher efficiencies than the main effects.

From a historical point of view we should note that Seath (1944) described a three-period 2 × 2 factorial for comparing two different diets for dairy cows. Also, Patterson (1952) showed that designs for 2 × 2 and 2 × 2 × 2 experiments could be obtained by using some or all of the subjects from a balanced design constructed from a set of mutually orthogonal Latin squares. Patterson also showed how confounding can be introduced into the design by arranging the subjects into blocks which correspond to the Latin squares or rectangles.

5.9 Examples of data analysis

In this section we illustrate the analysis of data from cross-over trials with three or more treatments. The assumptions we make about the covariance structure of the data are the orthodox ones used in Chapter 4, that is, fixed subject effects and independent within-subject errors. The designs in the two examples we use were both planned to be variance balanced. However, as often happens in real trials, unforeseen difficulties in recruitment, for example, meant that the achieved designs were not quite balanced.

Example 5.1

The aim of this trial was to compare drug A alone, drug B alone and drugs A and B in combination in terms of how well they control mild to moderately severe hypertension. We will refer to the combination as drug C.

After a run-in period of two weeks, during which the subjects were given placebo tablets, the subjects were randomly allocated to one of the six possible treatment sequences: ABC, ACB, BAC, BCA, CAB and CBA. Each treatment period lasted four weeks and there were no wash-out periods. A total of 23 subjects completed the trial. One of the responses measured on each subject at the end of each period was systolic blood pressure (mm Hg). The subjects were recruited from four different centres and prior to the first treatment period a run-in baseline measurement was taken on each subject. The values recorded in the trial are given in Table 5.20.

Let us for the moment ignore the information on the centres and baselines. The model fitted to the data includes parameters for the subjects, periods, direct treatments and the first-order carry-overs. The resulting analysis of variance is given in Table 5.21. It will be recalled that as in Chapter 4 the SS for each set of parameters (subjects, periods, etc.) corresponds to the SS for that set after all the preceding sets of parameters in the table have been included in the model.

There is no evidence ($P = 0.84$) of a difference between the carry-over effects but there is very strong evidence of a difference between the direct effects. The estimated differences (after dropping carry-over effects) between the direct effects are $\hat{\tau}_1 - \hat{\tau}_2 = 26.35$, $\hat{\tau}_1 - \hat{\tau}_3 = 12.22$ and $\hat{\tau}_3 - \hat{\tau}_2 = 14.13$, each with a standard error of

Table 5.20 *Data for Example 5.1 – Systolic blood pressures*

Centre	Subject	Sequence	Run-in	1	2	3
				Period		
1	1	CAB	250	206	220	210
	2	ABC	192	174	146	164
	3	ACB	194	192	150	160
	4	BAC	224	184	192	176
	5	BCA	148	136	132	138
2	1	ABC	170	145	125	130
	2	CAB	185	160	180	145
	3	BCA	165	145	154	166
3	1	ABC	210	230	174	200
	2	BCA	210	194	210	190
	3	CBA	205	180	180	208
	4	BAC	190	140	150	150
	5	ACB	255	194	208	160
	6	CAB	200	188	200	190
	7	ABC	210	240	130	195
	8	BCA	194	180	180	190
	9	CBA	260	210	160	226
	10	ACB	170	175	152	175
	11	BAC	200	155	230	226
	12	ACB	204	202	160	180
	13	BAC	235	180	185	190
	14	CBA	200	185	180	200
4	1	CBA	175	190	145	160

Table 5.21 *Analysis of variance for Example 5.1 (ignoring centres and baselines)*

Source	d.f.	SS	MS	F
Between subjects	22	30 646	1393	
Within subjects:				
Period	2	1 395	698	
Direct treatments	2	7 984	3992	13·83
Carry-over	2	98	49	0·17
Residual	40	11 546	289	
Total	68	51 670		

Table 5.22 *Analysis of variance for Example 5.1 (including centres and baselines)*

Source	d.f.	SS	MS	F
Between subjects:				
Baselines	1	17 334	17 334	33·79
Centres	3	2 788	929	1·81
Centre × Baseline	2	2 323	1 162	2·26
Residual	16	8 202	513	
Within subjects:				
Periods	2	1 396	698	
Centre × Period	6	1 384	231	
Baseline × Period	2	187	93	
Centre × Baseline × Period	4	962	240	
Direct treatments	2	7 282	3 641	7·71
Centre × Direct	4	479	120	0·25
Baseline × Direct	2	669	334	0·71
Centre × Baseline × Direct	2	631	315	0·67
Carry-over	2	193	97	0·20
Centre × Carry-over	2	84	42	0·09
Baseline × Carry-over	2	204	102	0·22
Residual	16	7 555	472	
Total	68	51 670		

4·91 on 42 d.f. All three differences are significantly different at the 5% level (at least), indicating that drug B produces a lower blood pressure than A or C. Drug A produces the highest blood pressure and the combination drug C is intermediate between A and B. A study of the standardized residuals from the full model did not reveal anything untoward.

Let us now consider how the information on centres and baselines can be incorporated into the analysis. This extra information cannot explain any more of the variability between the subjects, but it can be used to partition the between-subjects SS into various components. The extra information is also useful for checking for interactions within subjects between the treatment effects and the centres and baselines. The sort of analysis of variance we can obtain by incorporating centres and baselines into our model is shown in Table 5.22. The terms in the model are fitted sequentially and so choosing to include the terms in a different order will result in different values for the SS. Whether we would, in practice, include so many interaction terms would depend on the particular trial being analysed. We have included those shown in Table 5.22 mainly for illustration. If we first look to the within-subject information we see that none of the interactions between centres, baselines and the other effects are significant. Hence our earlier conclusions are not altered in any way and so we would use the simpler model given earlier to describe our results. If we had discovered an interaction between the treatment effects and centres, for example, then that would require a careful analysis of the data from each centre separately. Similarly, interactions with baselines would require further investigation. In conclusion then, as far as the within-subjects information is concerned, including centres and baselines in the model is useful for checking whether there are any interactions between the treatment effects and centres and baselines.

If we now turn to the between-subject information, we can see that there is no evidence of an interaction between centres and baselines, but there is very strong evidence of a relationship between the observations for the active treatment periods and the baselines. After allowing for this, however, there is no evidence of a difference between the centres.

Example 5.2

The objectives of this trial were to compare the effects of three drugs A, C and D and a placebo drug B on blood flow, cardiac output and an exercise test for claudication, on subjects with intermittent claudication. The trial was a single-centre, double-blind trial in which each treatment period lasted a week and there was a one-week wash-out period between the active periods. There was no run-in period. One of the observations taken at the end of each treatment period was the left ventricular ejection time (LVET) measured in milliseconds (ms). The treatment sequences used in the trial and the LVET values recorded on each subject are given in Table 5.23. It will be noted that no sequence occurs more than once.

From Table 5.24 we can see that there is no evidence ($P = 0.61$) of any differences between the carry-over effects but there is very good evidence ($P = 0.003$) of a difference between the direct effects. We therefore drop the carry-over effects from our model and continue to examine the estimated differences between the direct effects as

Table 5.23 *LVET values (ms) for example 5.2*

Subject	Sequence	Period			
		1	2	3	4
1	BDCA	590	440	500	443
2	ACBD	490	290	250	260
3	CADB	507	385	320	380
4	DBAC	323	300	440	340
5	BADC	250	330	300	290
6	ADCB	400	260	310	380
7	CBAD	460	365	350	300
8	DCBA	317	315	307	370
9	BCDA	430	330	300	370
10	CDAB	410	320	380	290
11	CABD	390	393	280	280
12	ACDB	430	323	375	310
13	BDAC	365	333	340	350
14	ABDC	355	310	295	330

Table 5.24 *Analysis of variance for Example 5.2*

Source	d.f.	SS	MS	F
Between subjects	13	114986	8845	
Within subjects:				
Periods	3	54317	18106	
Direct treatments	3	34327	11442	5·83
Carry-over	3	3661	1220	0·62
Residual	33	64791	1963	
Total	55	272082		

Table 5.25 *Treatment differences for Example 5.2*

Difference	Estimate	s.e.	P
$\tau_1 - \tau_2$	47·3	16·5	0·007
$\tau_3 - \tau_2$	24·5	16·5	0·148
$\tau_4 - \tau_2$	−18·7	16·7	0·270
$\tau_1 - \tau_3$	22·8	16·6	0·179
$\tau_1 - \tau_4$	66·0	16·6	0·000
$\tau_3 - \tau_4$	43·2	16·8	0·014

obtained from this reduced model. In Table 5.25 we list the estimated differences between the direct effects, their associated standard errors (on 36 d.f.) and their significance probabilities P.

The conclusions that we can draw from Table 5.25 are that LVET is greater with A than either B or D; and LVET is greater on C than D.

An examination of the standardized residuals did not reveal anything untowards except perhaps that the variability of the residuals was smaller in period 2 and also smaller on treatment C.

As a general remark we should note that in our use of the standardized residuals we did not take explicit account of the fact that they are correlated. The work of Anscombe and Tukey (1963) and Gentleman and Wilk (1975) indicates that the correlations between the residuals can usually be ignored (at least for graphical procedures). Their work was related to two-way ANOVA models without carry-over effects. Although we have not investigated the statistical behaviour of residuals from models which contain carry-over effects, we assume that the correlations between the residuals can in practice be ignored.

In Chapter 7 we will reanalyse the data from Examples 5.1 and 5.2 under more general assumptions about the covariance structure of the data.

Before we leave the subject of analysis we should perhaps note that apart from a brief mention in the general review by Koch, Amara *et al* (1980), there appears to be hardly any literature on the nonparametric analysis of cross-over designs with three or more treatments. Cornell (1980) suggests that Koch's (1972) analysis can be extended to designs with more than two treatments or periods, but only illustrates the extension for the case of no carry-over effects. Another method, which apparently is used quite a lot in practice, is to replace the observations by their ranks and to proceed as if the ranks were the genuine observations. However, this method, which has its origins in a paper by Conover and Iman (1981), is seriously criticized by Clayton and Hills (1987). In their opinion the use of ranks, which implies using a bounded scale of measurement, is likely to prove inappropriate for linear modelling.

The literature on randomization analyses of cross-over trials is also rather scant. Richards (1980) considered the bias in the randomization analysis of balanced cross-over designs and Shen and Quade (1983) described a randomization test for a three-period, three-treatment cross-over design.

5.10 Bayesian analysis of higher-order cross-over trials

In Chapter 2 we briefly described a Bayesian analysis of the 2×2 cross-over. In this section we briefly describe a Bayesian analysis for trials with more than two treatments. The results reported here are taken from Law (1987), who applied the general results given in Box and Tiao (1973) and Broemeling (1985) to the cross-over model. In the usual linear model notation, let $\mathbf{y}$ denote an $N \times 1$ vector of data, $\boldsymbol{\theta}$ an $m \times 1$ vector of unknown parameters and $\mathbf{X}$ a known matrix such that $E(\mathbf{y}) = \mathbf{X}\boldsymbol{\theta}$. The vector $\boldsymbol{\theta}$ will contain parameters for the subjects, periods, direct treatments and carry-overs. The OLS estimator of $\boldsymbol{\theta}$ is $\hat{\boldsymbol{\theta}} = (\mathbf{X}^\mathrm{T}\mathbf{X})^{-1}\mathbf{X}^\mathrm{T}\mathbf{y}$, where $\mathbf{X}^\mathrm{T}\mathbf{X}$ is of full rank due to constraints placed on the parameters. The elements of $\mathbf{y}$ are normally distributed with variance σ^2.

The marginal posterior and conditional distributions of $\boldsymbol{\theta}$ are now obtained assuming a non-informative prior distribution on the parameters $\boldsymbol{\theta}$ and σ^2, and an informative prior on these parameters.

Non-informative prior

From similar considerations to those given in Chapter 2, we take as our non-informative prior for the parameters $\boldsymbol{\theta}$ and σ^2 one that is proportional to $1/\sigma^2$. The marginal posterior distribution of $\boldsymbol{\theta}$ is then

$$p(\boldsymbol{\theta}|\mathbf{y}) = \frac{\Gamma\left(\dfrac{v+m}{2}\right)|\mathbf{X}^\mathrm{T}\mathbf{X}|^{1/2}}{\Gamma\left(\dfrac{v}{2}\right)[\Gamma(\tfrac{1}{2})]^m(vs^2)^{m/2}}$$
$$\times \left[1 + \frac{(\boldsymbol{\theta} - \hat{\boldsymbol{\theta}})^\mathrm{T}\mathbf{X}^\mathrm{T}\mathbf{X}(\boldsymbol{\theta} - \hat{\boldsymbol{\theta}})}{vs^2} \right]^{-(v+m)/2}$$

which is the multivariate t-distribution discovered independently by Cornish (1954) and Dunnet and Sobel (1954). Following Box and Tiao we denote this by $t_m[\hat{\boldsymbol{\theta}}, s^2(\mathbf{X}^\mathrm{T}\mathbf{X})^{-1}, v]$ where $\hat{\boldsymbol{\theta}}$ is the OLS estimator of $\boldsymbol{\theta}$ and s^2 is the usual unbiased estimator of σ^2 on v degrees of freedom.

As the parameters of interest to us (direct treatments, carry-overs, etc.) form only a subset of the parameters in $\boldsymbol{\theta}$ let us consider the partition $\boldsymbol{\theta}^\mathrm{T} = [\boldsymbol{\theta}_1^\mathrm{T}, \boldsymbol{\theta}_2^\mathrm{T}]$, where $\boldsymbol{\theta}_1$ is of dimension $d \times 1$. We also partition $\mathbf{X}^T\mathbf{X}$ and $(\mathbf{X}^T\mathbf{X})^{-1}$ as

$$\mathbf{X}^T\mathbf{X} = \begin{bmatrix} \mathbf{X}_1^T\mathbf{X}_1 & \mathbf{X}_2^T\mathbf{X}_1 \\ \mathbf{X}_1^T\mathbf{X}_2 & \mathbf{X}_2^T\mathbf{X}_2 \end{bmatrix} \quad \text{and} \quad (\mathbf{X}^T\mathbf{X})^{-1} = \begin{bmatrix} \mathbf{C}_{11} & \mathbf{C}_{12} \\ \mathbf{C}_{21} & \mathbf{C}_{22} \end{bmatrix}$$

where $\mathbf{X}_1^T\mathbf{X}_1$ corresponds to the parameters contained in $\boldsymbol{\theta}_1$, etc. The marginal posterior distribution of $\boldsymbol{\theta}_1$ is then the d-dimensional t-distribution $t_d[\hat{\boldsymbol{\theta}}_1, s^2\mathbf{C}_{11}, v]$.

For a single parameter θ_i of $\boldsymbol{\theta}$, the marginal posterior distribution of $(\theta_i - \hat{\theta}_i)/(s(c_{\theta_i})^{1/2})$ is the Student's t-distribution on v d.f., where c_{θ_i} is the diagonal element of $(\mathbf{X}^T\mathbf{X})^{-1}$ corresponding to θ_i, and $v = N - m$.

Also of interest is the conditional distribution of $\boldsymbol{\theta}_2$ given $\boldsymbol{\theta}_1$ and this is the $(m - d)$-dimensional t-distribution (Box and Tiao, 1973, p. 118) $t_{m-d}[\hat{\boldsymbol{\theta}}_{2\cdot 1}, s_{2\cdot 1}^2(\mathbf{X}_2^T\mathbf{X}_2)^{-1}, v + d]$, where

$$\hat{\boldsymbol{\theta}}_{2\cdot 1} = \hat{\boldsymbol{\theta}}_2 - (\mathbf{X}_2^T\mathbf{X}_2)^{-1}\mathbf{X}_2^T\mathbf{X}_1(\boldsymbol{\theta}_1 - \hat{\boldsymbol{\theta}}_1)$$

and

$$s_{2\cdot 1}^2 = (v + d)^{-1}[vs^2 + (\boldsymbol{\theta}_1 - \hat{\boldsymbol{\theta}}_1)^T(\mathbf{C}_{11})^{-1}(\boldsymbol{\theta}_1 - \hat{\boldsymbol{\theta}}_1)]$$

It will be noted that we will, for example, be interested in the conditional posterior distribution of the subject, period and treatment parameters conditional on setting the carry-over parameters equal to zero. The effect of setting the carry-over parameters to zero can then be assessed by comparing the conditional marginal distribution of a treatment parameter θ_i, say, with its unconditional marginal distribution.

Informative prior
When considering the use of prior information we should be aware that it is unlikely that we will have prior estimates of every element in $\boldsymbol{\theta}$. For instance, it is unreasonable to suppose that any information will be available *a priori* about subject effects. Hence, we seek a method of including prior information on $\boldsymbol{\theta}_r$, an r-dimensional subset of the parameter vector $\boldsymbol{\theta}$.

In order to do this we take the joint prior distribution of $\boldsymbol{\theta}_r$ and σ^2 to be proportional to $p(\boldsymbol{\theta}_r|\sigma^2) \times p(\sigma^2)$, i.e. $p(\boldsymbol{\theta}_r, \sigma^2) \propto p(\boldsymbol{\theta}_r|\sigma^2)p(\sigma^2)$.

If we now take as our priors (Broemeling, 1985, Chapter 1)

$$p(\sigma^2) \propto \left(\frac{1}{\sigma}\right)^{2(\alpha + 1)} \exp\left[-\frac{\beta}{\sigma^2}\right]$$

and

$$p(\boldsymbol{\theta}_r|\sigma^2) \propto \left(\frac{1}{\sigma}\right)^r \exp\left[-\frac{(\boldsymbol{\theta}_r - \tilde{\boldsymbol{\theta}}_r)^{\mathrm{T}}\mathbf{P}_r(\boldsymbol{\theta}_r - \tilde{\boldsymbol{\theta}}_r)}{2\sigma^2}\right]$$

i.e. $\boldsymbol{\theta}_r|\sigma^2$ has mean $\tilde{\boldsymbol{\theta}}_r$ and variance-covariance matrix $\sigma^2\mathbf{P}_r^{-1}$. It can be shown that the marginal prior density of $\boldsymbol{\theta}_r$ is the multivariate t-distribution $t_r[\tilde{\boldsymbol{\theta}}_r, (\beta/\alpha)\mathbf{P}_r^{-1}, 2\alpha]$.

Also if we use the above two priors, it can be shown that

$$E(\sigma^2) = \frac{\beta}{\alpha - 1}$$

$$V(\sigma^2) = \frac{\beta^2}{(\alpha - 1)^2(\alpha - 2)}$$

$$E(\boldsymbol{\theta}_r) = \tilde{\boldsymbol{\theta}}_r$$

and

$$V(\boldsymbol{\theta}_r) = \frac{\beta\mathbf{P}_r^{-1}}{(\alpha - 1)}$$

Prior estimates of the mean and variance of $\boldsymbol{\theta}_r$ and σ^2 can then be inserted into the above expressions in place of the expectations and variances, respectively, to provide values for $\alpha, \beta, \mathbf{P}_r$ and $\tilde{\boldsymbol{\theta}}_r$.

To make use of this prior information we extend $\mathbf{P}_r$ to an $m \times m$ matrix $\mathbf{P}$ by including zeroes in all positions not filled by $\mathbf{P}_r$. Similarly, we extend $\tilde{\boldsymbol{\theta}}_r$ to an m-dimensional vector $\tilde{\boldsymbol{\theta}}$. Law (1987) then shows that the marginal posterior of $\boldsymbol{\theta}$ is the m-dimensional t-distribution $t_m[\boldsymbol{\theta}^*, (\mathbf{D}^*)^{-1}, v + r + 2\alpha]$ where

$$\boldsymbol{\theta}^* = (\mathbf{X}^{\mathrm{T}}\mathbf{X} + \mathbf{P})^{-1}(\mathbf{X}^{\mathrm{T}}\mathbf{X}\hat{\boldsymbol{\theta}} + \mathbf{P}\tilde{\boldsymbol{\theta}})$$

$$\mathbf{D}^* = \frac{(\mathbf{X}^{\mathrm{T}}\mathbf{X} + \mathbf{P})}{(s^*)^2}$$

and

$$(s^*)^2 = \frac{1}{(v + r + 2\alpha)}$$
$$\times [2\beta + \hat{\boldsymbol{\theta}}^{\mathrm{T}}\mathbf{P}\tilde{\boldsymbol{\theta}} + \mathbf{y}'\mathbf{y} - (\mathbf{X}^{\mathrm{T}}\mathbf{X}\hat{\boldsymbol{\theta}} + \mathbf{P}\tilde{\boldsymbol{\theta}})^{\mathrm{T}}(\mathbf{X}^{\mathrm{T}}\mathbf{X} + \mathbf{P})^{-1}(\mathbf{X}^{\mathrm{T}}\mathbf{X}\hat{\boldsymbol{\theta}} + \mathbf{P}\tilde{\boldsymbol{\theta}})]$$

As in the case of the non-informative prior, we will be interested in $\boldsymbol{\theta}_1$, a d-dimensional vector containing d of the parameters contained in $\boldsymbol{\theta}$. Therefore we will wish to use the corresponding d-dimensional marginal t-distribution of the parameters contained in $\boldsymbol{\theta}_1$.

5.11 Categorical data

We end this chapter by briefly illustrating how the methods described in Chapter 3 can be applied to three or more treatments, periods or groups. The data we use for our illustration are given in Table 5.26 and were obtained in a trial to compare a placebo treatment (A), a low-dose analgesic (B) and a high-dose analgesic (C) for the treatment of primary dysmenorrhea. The subjects available for the trial were randomized to receive the three treatments in one of the six possible orders: ABC, ACB, BAC, BCA, CAB and CBA. The number of

Table 5.26 *Example of three-category, three-period data*

Outcome	A B C	A C B	B A C	B C A	C A B	C B A	Total
111		2			3	1	6
112	1			1			2
113	1		1				2
121	2						2
122	3		1				4
123	4	3	1		2		10
131			1	1			2
132		2					2
133	2	4	1			1	8
211		1	1			3	5
212			2		1	1	4
213			1				1
221	1			6	1	1	9
222		2	1				3
223	1						1
231				1		2	3
232							0
233		2			1		3
311				1		2	3
312			2		2	1	5
313			3		4	1	8
321				1			1
322				1			1
323							0
331						1	1
332							0
333							0
Total	15	16	15	12	14	14	86

subjects in each sequence group are given in the final (Total) row of Table 5.26. The entries in the body of Table 5.26 are the numbers of subjects in each group who responded with each of the 27 possible outcome sequences. At the end of each treatment period each subject rated the amount of relief obtained as: none, minimal, moderate, complete. In Table 5.26 we have coded these responses as 1 = none or minimal, 2 = moderate and 3 = complete.

In fact, the data used in our Example 3.2 in Chapter 3 were obtained from this data set, for the purposes of providing a small example, by using only the data from the first two periods of groups 2 and 5. The complete set of data were also analysed by Jones and

Table 5.27 *Factor levels for three-period, three-category data (group 4 = BCA)*

Outcome	G	P1	P2	P3	TA	TB	TC	CA	CB	CC
111	4	1	1	1	1	1	1	4	1	1
112	4	1	1	2	2	1	1	4	1	2
113	4	1	1	3	3	1	1	4	1	3
121	4	1	2	1	1	1	2	4	2	1
122	4	1	2	2	2	1	2	4	2	2
123	4	1	2	3	3	1	2	4	2	3
131	4	1	3	1	1	1	3	4	3	1
132	4	1	3	2	2	1	3	4	3	2
133	4	1	3	3	3	1	3	4	3	3
211	4	2	1	1	1	2	1	4	1	1
212	4	2	1	2	2	2	1	4	1	2
213	4	2	1	3	3	2	1	4	1	3
221	4	2	2	1	1	2	2	4	2	1
222	4	2	2	2	2	2	2	4	2	2
223	4	2	2	3	3	2	2	4	2	3
231	4	2	3	1	1	2	3	4	3	1
232	4	2	3	2	2	2	3	4	3	2
233	4	2	3	3	3	2	3	4	3	3
311	4	3	1	1	1	3	1	4	1	1
312	4	3	1	2	2	3	1	4	1	2
313	4	3	1	3	3	3	1	4	1	3
321	4	3	2	1	1	3	2	4	2	1
322	4	3	2	2	2	3	2	4	2	2
323	4	3	2	3	3	3	2	4	2	3
331	4	3	3	1	1	3	3	4	3	1
332	4	3	3	2	2	3	3	4	3	2
333	4	3	3	3	3	3	3	4	3	3

Kenward (1987), but after recoding the data to provide a binary response.

Following the approach described in Section 3.5 we model these data by setting up a group factor G which has six levels, outcome factors $P1$, $P2$ and $P3$ for the periods, factors TA, TB and TC for the direct treatments and factors CA, CB and CC for the first-order carry-overs. Each of these factors has three levels except the carry-over factors which have four levels. For example, the levels taken by the factors which correspond to the observations in group 4 are given in Table 5.27. The levels corresponding to the observations in each of the other groups can be obtained in a similar way.

The full model we fit to the data will contain the following terms:

$$G + P1 + P2 + P3 + P1 \times P2 + P1 \times P3 + P2 \times P3 + TA + TB$$
$$+ TC + CA + CB + CC$$

It will be noted that the dependencies between the repeated responses on each subject are accounted for by the two-factor interactions $P1 \times P2$, $P1 \times P3$ and $P2 \times P3$. The data we use to fit our model will consist of the 162 zero and nonzero observed counts given in the body of Table 5.26.

When the carry-over parameters are dropped from the model the difference in deviance is 2·95 on 4 d.f., which is not significant at the 5% level. There is no evidence therefore of any difference between the carry-over effects. When the direct treatment parameters are dropped (after dropping the carry-over parameters) the difference in deviance is 64·98 on 4 d.f. There is strong evidence of a difference between the treatments. When the dependency parameters $(P1 \times P2 + P1 \times P3 + P2 \times P3)$ are dropped from the model the difference in deviance is 27.07 on 12 d.f. There is strong evidence of dependence between the repeated responses.

To discover the nature of the differences between the treatments we can define parameters $\tau_{CA(31)}$, $\tau_{CA(21)}$, $\tau_{BA(31)}$ and $\tau_{BA(21)}$ in a similar way to that done in Section 3.5. So for example, $\tau_{CA(31)}$ is a parameter which compares C and A in terms of the conditional odds of observing category 3 rather than category 1. The estimated values of these parameters are, respectively, 3·504, 1·855, 2·767 and 1·371 with asymptotic standard errors 0·679, 0·444, 0·616 and 0·405, respectively. All four parameters are significantly different from zero at the 1% level. In other words, both treatments C and B are much more likely to provide relief than the placebo treatment A. The estimated conditional odds-ratios are $e^{\tau CA(31)} = e^{3.504} = 33.25$, $e^{\tau CA(21)} = e^{1.855} = 6.39$, $e^{\tau BA(31)} = e^{2.76} = 15.91$ and $e^{\tau BA(21)} = e^{1.371} = 3.94$. We see that the estimated odds of observing a 3 rather than a 1 are 33 times higher for treatment C as compared to treatment A. The corresponding odds-ratio for treatments B and A is 15.9. Bearing in mind that treatment C is the same analgesic as treatment B, but given at twice the dose, this result is not too surprising.

The rest of the analysis would now proceed as in Section 3.3. That is, we could predict the probabilities of the joint outcomes and use these to calculate marginal probabilities and other features of interest. (See Jones and Kenward (1988) for further details.)

CHAPTER 6

The analysis of repeated measurements within periods

6.1 Introduction and examples

It is common practice in experiments and trials to collect a sequence of observations from each subject, rather than to measure a single response variable. In one sense the cross-over trial is an example of this in which the sequence consists of observations from successive treatment periods. However, a sequence of observations may also be collected while the subject is under the same experimental treatment and we shall use the term **repeated measurements** to refer to such a sequence. Some typical examples of repeated measurements are as follows:

1. Blood lactate levels measured every two minutes from thumb-prick samples during a bicycle exercise test.
2. Concentration of a test drug in the blood, measured every ten minutes after administration during a bio-availability study.
3. Systolic blood pressure measured 2, 4, 8, 24, 48 hours after treatment with a drug.
4. Daily level of anxiety as recorded on a self-administered questionnaire during a two-month period.
5. Lamb weights taken at eight two-weekly intervals during an experiment on growth rate.

In most trials and studies an attempt is made to ensure that measurements are made at the equivalent times on each subject. If all subjects enter the trial at the same time then measurements would be made at approximately the same absolute time. Otherwise the times would be the same relative to some starting point, for example trial entry, clinic visit or start of treatment. A full analysis is potentially difficult if this is not true and we shall concentrate on the more common situation of equivalent times of measurement.

Repeated measurements can be taken in an experiment in which each subject received only one treatment, or during each period of a cross-over trial. It is with the analysis of the latter that this chapter is concerned. There follows two examples of cross-over trials with repeated measurements.

Example 6.1

This trial was used as an example by Ciminera and Wolfe (1953). Its purpose was to compare the effect on blood sugar level of two insulin mixtures (A and B). The two-sequence design

$$
\begin{array}{cccc}
A & B & A & B \\
B & A & B & A
\end{array}
$$

was used. This is the design labelled (4.2.2) in Chapter 4. Twenty-two female rabbits were divided equally, at random, between the two groups. The insulin mixtures were administered by injection at weekly intervals and, for each rabbit, blood samples were obtained at 0, $1\frac{1}{2}$, 3, $4\frac{1}{2}$ and 6 hours after injection. The full data set is given in Table 6.1 (after Ciminera and Wolfe, 1953, Table II) and the simple treatment means are plotted for each time point in Figure 6.1.

Example 6.2

These data are from a three-treatment three-period cross-over trial involving 12 subjects. The effects of three treatments on blood pressure were to be compared. Treatments A and B consisted of the trial drug at 20 mg and 40 mg doses respectively, while treatment C was a placebo. Two complete replicates of the Williams arrangement were used in which all six possible sequences occur. The measurements are of systolic blood pressure (in mm Hg), measured under each treatment at 10 successive times: 30 and 15 minutes before treatment, and 15, 30, 45, 60, 75, 90, 120 and 240 minutes after treatment. These data are presented in Table 6.2 and the corresponding mean treatment profiles are plotted in Figure 6.2.

There are many reasons for collecting repeated measurements and naturally these will determine in any given situation how we

Table 6.1 *Blood sugar levels (mg %) from Example 6.1*

Group 1

Period (treatment)	Hours after injection	Rabbit										
		1	2	3	4	5	6	7	8	9	10	11
1	0·0	77	77	77	81	90	103	99	90	90	90	85
(A)	1·5	52	56	43	56	73	47	47	35	64	35	68
	3·0	35	43	64	22	52	22	52	22	47	12	56
	4·5	56	56	39	35	60	60	47	26	47	26	68
	6·0	64	64	64	39	64	99	81	22	60	68	73
2	0·0	90	85	90	107	94	90	99	94	81	81	94
(B)	1·5	47	52	30	47	60	47	26	8	39	26	56
	3·0	52	60	30	47	60	30	64	30	47	35	68
	4·5	68	81	47	47	77	43	52	26	77	30	73
	6·0	90	94	60	73	90	68	90	43	94	85	90
3	0·0	85	103	99	77	90	85	90	103	77	81	105
(A)	1·5	52	26	39	26	60	56	43	39	56	56	73
	3·0	35	68	39	56	18	56	18	22	26	60	47
	4·5	39	30	73	64	35	77	30	39	64	81	77
	6·0	60	30	90	64	64	94	39	94	94	103	90
4	0·0	94	107	103	116	94	111	111	90	94	90	97
(B)	1·5	60	60	60	52	56	73	56	18	52	22	73
	3·0	60	68	60	26	47	85	43	26	47	52	52
	4.5	77	90	90	68	81	103	90	18	81	85	81
	6·0	94	94	99	120	99	111	111	22	90	90	94

Group 2

Period (treatment)	Hours after injection	Rabbit										
		12	13	14	15	16	17	18	19	20	21	22
1	0·0	103	85	85	85	85	103	90	81	85	85	94
(B)	1·5	26	68	35	35	35	56	52	22	30	47	39
	3·0	22	56	8	47	39	47	35	12	22	33	35
	4·5	39	64	64	77	85	64	35	22	52	77	52
	6·0	68	81	99	68	77	56	39	77	94	107	85
2	0·0	90	94	90	85	85	103	90	81	90	85	94
(A)	1·5	35	52	35	39	47	35	43	12	30	39	26
	3·0	30	43	30	52	56	39	30	2	26	39	30
	4.5	39	47	43	52	77	68	47	30	52	43	39
	6·0	94	56	99	64	81	99	77	77	90	60	81
3	0·0	103	85	73	90	90	90	77	68	85	85	90
(B)	1·5	26	43	22	12	43	35	56	12	39	35	22
	3·0	26	22	12	43	35	18	64	8	22	26	26
	4.5	56	68	56	85	64	64	81	8	56	43	73
	6·0	103	103	103	99	81	94	99	39	90	73	99
4	0·0	111	111	94	92	85	107	111	85	105	90	103
(A)	1·5	68	52	52	52	52	47	60	26	68	43	47
	3·0	52	99	47	73	52	43	68	12	64	35	35
	4·5	77	103	73	99	77	85	107	18	81	81	64
	6·0	103	120	101	101	99	101	111	39	81	90	94

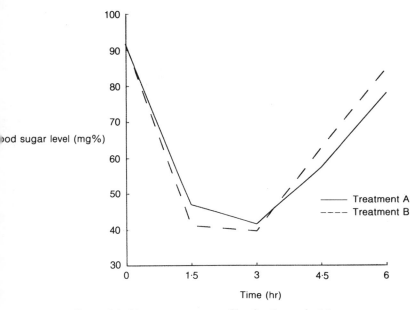

Figure 6.1 *Mean treatment profiles for Example 6.1.*

approach the statistical analysis. Each subject produces a profile of repeated measurements; in a cross-over trial there will be one such profile from each treatment period, and the analysis will usually aim to produce some form of comparison between treatments of the mean profiles.

Repeated measurements can also contain useful information on the form of the carry-over effect, should one exist. It is possible that such an effect may decrease during the treatment period and this might be demonstrated through the analysis of the repeated measurements in the form of a carry-over-by-time interaction. Alternatively, if a carry-over effect in the early part of the treatment period were thought likely, the analysis might be based on the later measurements only.

The difficulty in the analysis of repeated measurements lies in their covariance structure. If we could assume that this was uniform then orthodox methods of analysis (typically ANOVA) could be used. However, we are dealing with a set of short time series and commonly the measurements have a distinctive serial pattern of correlation

Table 6.1 reproduced from Ciminera, J.L. and Wolf, E.K. (1953). An example of the use of extended cross-over designs in the comparison of NPH insulin mixtures. *Biometrics*, **9**, 431–44. With permission from Biometric Society.

Table 6.2 *Systolic blood pressures (mm Hg) from a three-period cross-over trial (Example 6.2)*

Subject	Period	Treatment	Time of measurement (minutes relative to treatment)									
			−30	−15	15	30	45	60	75	90	120	240
1	1	C	112	114	86	86	93	90	106	91	84	102
1	2	B	108	103	100	100	97	103	92	106	106	96
1	3	A	107	108	102	111	100	105	113	109	84	99
2	1	B	101	100	99	81	106	100	100	111	110	96
2	2	A	96	101	101	100	99	101	98	99	102	101
2	3	C	111	99	90	93	81	91	89	95	99	97
3	1	A	105	113	109	104	102	102	111	106	104	101
3	2	C	104	96	84	84	100	91	109	94	108	108
3	3	B	96	92	88	89	91	121	122	135	121	107
4	1	A	112	109	108	92	102	101	101	98	102	106
4	2	B	105	116	105	108	121	103	110	109	113	112
4	3	C	110	112	111	102	99	104	108	102	112	101
5	1	C	96	93	94	96	83	95	88	93	88	93
5	2	A	103	98	97	108	93	101	108	105	104	101
5	3	B	114	97	96	109	102	99	110	105	104	106
6	1	B	115	117	91	102	126	122	128	125	119	117
6	2	C	104	84	88	95	97	115	93	102	90	101
6	3	A	103	97	84	97	92	115	108	114	113	107
7	1	C	82	88	85	87	81	91	87	78	85	81
7	2	B	133	89	93	98	92	94	90	90	94	100
7	3	A	87	83	78	92	80	83	88	88	93	98
8	1	A	124	131	115	119	115	110	108	103	116	109
8	2	C	116	113	109	93	112	89	108	111	107	111
8	3	B	121	120	87	93	94	100	95	100	114	117
9	1	B	118	107	105	111	105	115	137	128	115	114
9	2	A	111	104	112	109	108	114	116	127	117	117
9	3	C	113	107	115	117	105	117	104	110	105	117
10	1	B	111	112	105	111	107	113	105	111	113	101
10	2	C	115	91	111	114	104	105	112	112	102	105
10	3	A	112	110	109	112	110	103	116	106	110	110
11	1	C	120	117	110	110	110	116	115	118	125	125
11	2	A	104	123	119	115	120	120	127	122	125	128
11	3	B	117	113	117	120	125	130	123	128	126	123
12	1	A	134	134	123	118	111	124	125	120	119	115
12	2	B	125	117	129	125	124	126	132	129	125	121
12	3	C	118	110	119	108	105	110	113	117	123	113

which may, in addition, be far from stationary. Such a structure precludes the use of orthodox ANOVA, at least in an unmodified form, and as a consequence a wide variety of techniques have been proposed. Diggle, Donnelly and Kirkby (1985) have produced a bibliography of publications on the subject with about 250 entries.

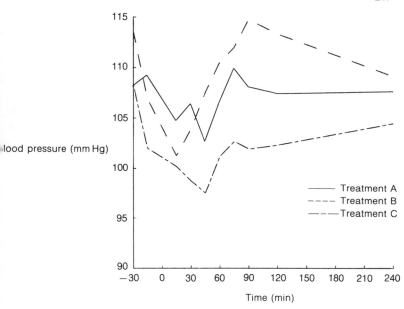

Figure 6.2. *Mean treatment profiles, systolic blood pressure (mm Hg) from Example 6.2.*

Arguably the single most important approach is the one in which the repeated measurements from each individual are reduced to a few summary statistics which can then be analysed separately using standard univariate techniques, like those discussed in previous chapters, or jointly using the multivariate analogues of these techniques. Good discussions of this general approach to the analysis of repeated measurements are given by Rowell and Walters (1976), Salsburg (1981), Yates (1982) and Keen *et al.* (1986). The use of summary statistics has the great advantages of simplicity and robustness and can be understood easily by the statistically less experienced. It is applicable whenever it is possible to summarize the relevant aspects of the profile with a few statistics chosen *a priori*.

There are many forms of summary statistics for repeated measurements. If the profiles are smooth, the overall shape might be summarized by a low-degree polynomial, or if features such as an asymptote are important, a nonlinear function might be more appropriate. The estimated parameters from each subject's fitted curve are the summary statistics. Some other examples of summary statistics that are used are the average over some, or all, of the measurements; area under the profile; maximum or minimum level reached; first time of measurement at which a predefined threshold is passed; level at a given time (or end-point); and change between two particular times. The statistics need not necessarily reflect all the features of the profiles, provided that they contain the information that the experimenter regards as relevant and that they have a meaningful interpretation. It is important to distinguish between features that are chosen beforehand for comparison and those that appear important after examination of the data. The former lead to unequivocal treatment comparisons. The latter may provide important descriptions of profile differences but the statistical significance of such differences may well be less obvious. If only linear contrasts are chosen, some form of multiple comparison procedure may be appropriate, but such analyses belong more properly in the following sections where we discuss techniques that are appropriate when no summary statistics appear appropriate beforehand.

If it is possible to reduce the repeated measurements to a few summary statistics then, for univariate analyses, it is possible to apply all the techniques described in the previous chapters and there is little more to be added here. There is much that can be said about the selection of statistics, in particular about choosing appropriate curves, but this is beyond the scope of the present book. There exist straightforward multivariate versions of the analyses described earlier, typically based on multivariate analysis of variance (MANOVA) and these can be used if joint analyses are required for the summary statistics. For a description of MANOVA see, for example, Morrison (1986, Chapter 5) or Chatfield and Collins (1980, Chapter 8). The main concern now will therefore be with analyses that can be used when no summary statistics are available. The questions that can be answered with confidence by the resulting analyses will necessarily be less specific. To a certain extent description will replace inference.

We shall illustrate the application of two particular methods. The first is the split-plot-in-time ANOVA (Greenhouse and Geisser, 1959; Fleiss, 1986a, Section 8.2) and the second is ante-dependence analysis (Gabriel, 1962; Kenward, 1987), which includes repeated-measurement MANOVA as a special case. For an introduction to these methods and for examples of applications in parallel group trials, the reader should consult the references quoted.

In Section 6.2 we consider how these two approaches can be used with data from two-treatment, two-sequence cross-over designs (including the 2×2 design) and in Section 6.3 these two approaches are applied to other higher-order designs. We cannot of course give a comprehensive coverage of repeated-measurement methodology; this would require at least a book of its own. Our aim is instead to describe in some detail how a couple of techniques are used in the context of cross-over trials, with the intention that this will also point to the way in which other methods can be applied.

6.2 Repeated measurements from two-sequence designs

We have seen several times in earlier chapters how the two-treatment designs form a special class as far as flexibility of analysis is concerned (Sections 2.9, 4.7 and 4.9, for example). We shall see that the same is true now when we come to analyse repeated measurements within the treatment periods. As before, we shall exploit the fact that, for any dual pair of sequences, the same contrast among periods (or sum in one special case) is used in both sequences to estimate an effect. Suppose for the moment that we have only one observation per period, denoted by y_{ijk} for sequence i, subject k and period j. We have seen in Chapter 4 how all estimates of interest can be written in the form

$$\bar{A}_1 \pm \bar{A}_2$$

where $\bar{A}_i$ is a contrast among the period means from sequence i, that is,

$$\bar{A}_i = \sum_{j=1}^{p} a_j \bar{y}_{ij\cdot}, \qquad i = 1, 2, \qquad \text{for } \sum_{j=1}^{p} a_j = 0$$

noting that the coefficients are the same for both sequences. We have met one special case in which the coefficients a_j do not define a contrast, that is for the direct-by-period interaction from the 2×2 design, for which $a_1 = a_2 = \frac{1}{2}$. The procedure described below applies whether a contrast is involved or not, provided that the same coefficients are used in each sequence. For ease of expression, however, we shall continue to refer to contrasts, including tacitly the one exception.

We now introduce repeated measurements in each period. Let y_{ijkm} denote an observation where the additional subscript m, $m = 1, \ldots, q$, identifies the repeated measurements from one period. Also let $\mathbf{y}_m$ denote the set of measurements obtained at the mth time point. The comparisons in which we are interested, for example direct treatment and carry-over, are now comparisons between profiles of repeated measurements. We make these comparisons by reducing, for each effect of interest, the p sequences of q repeated measurements from each subject to a single sequence of q transformed variables. The mth new variable is just the contrast among the p measurements from the mth time defined by the coefficients a_j corresponding to the particular effect. That is, if the effect under examination has associated contrast coefficients $\alpha_1, \ldots, a_p$, we calculate for the (i, k)th subject the new 'repeated measurements'

$$d_{ikm} = \sum_{j=1}^{p} a_j y_{ijkm}, \qquad m = 1, \ldots, q$$

For example, in a 2×2 design, the transformed variable for the direct effect is just $d_{ikm} = \frac{1}{4}(y_{i2km} - y_{i1km})$. Thus, for each effect, each subject provides q derived repeated measurements, and we can apply any of the standard repeated-measurement techniques to these new variables.

The advantage of this procedure is that we need concern ourselves only with the covariance structure of the transformed variables, not with the structure of the original sequence of pq measurements. It is required only that the former structure is the same in both sequences, and we can rely to a certain extent on randomization for this. Several authors have applied this approach to the 2×2 design using different standard methods of repeated measurements analysis: Wallenstein and Fisher (1977; split-plot-in-time ANOVA), Patel and Hearne (1980; repeated-measurement MANOVA), Dunsmore (1981a; split-plot-in-time ANOVA and Bayesian growth-curve analysis).

We now give an illustration using Example 6.1. The appropriate contrast coefficients for this design are, for the direct treatment effect, $\frac{1}{2}(B - A)$, (ignoring carry-over):

$$\tfrac{1}{8}(-1, 1, -1, 1)$$

for the direct treatment effect (adjusted for carry-over):

$$\tfrac{1}{8}(-4, 1, 2, 1)$$

and for the carry-over effect:

$$\tfrac{1}{2}(-1, 0, 1, 0)$$

We could also introduce contrasts for the three degrees of freedom for the direct-by-period interaction, two only of which are estimable within subjects. In this design the carry-over effect is aliased with these two, so we need to make the decision at the beginning whether to examine the interaction, possibly decomposed into the carry-over and remainder, or whether to assume that any interaction, if present, will be due to a carry-over effect and just examine this. Continuing in the same vein as Chapter 4 we shall, in the following, examine only the carry-over effect rather than the full interaction.

Table 6.3 *Carry-over contrasts from Example 6.1*

Rabbit	Group	Hours after injection				
		0·0	1·5	3·0	4·5	6·0
1	1	4·0	0·0	0·0	−8·5	−2·0
2	1	13·0	−15·0	12·5	−13·0	−17·0
3	1	11·0	−2·0	−12·5	17·0	13·0
4	1	−2·0	−15·0	17·0	14·5	12·5
5	1	0·0	−6·5	−17·0	−12·5	0·0
6	1	−9·0	4·5	17·0	8·5	−2·5
7	1	−4·5	−2·0	−17·0	−8·5	−21·0
8	1	6·5	2·0	0·0	6·5	36·0
9	1	−6·5	−4·0	−10·5	8·5	17·0
10	1	−4·5	10·5	24·0	27·5	17·5
11	1	10·0	2·5	−4·5	4·5	8·5
Mean		1·64	−2·27	0·82	4·04	5·64
12	2	0·0	0·0	2·0	8·5	17·5
13	2	0·0	−12·5	−17·0	2·0	11·0
14	2	−6·0	−6·5	2·0	−4·0	2·0
15	2	2·5	−11·5	−2·0	4·0	15·5
16	2	2·5	4·0	−2·0	−10·5	2·0
17	2	−6·5	−10·5	−14·5	0·0	19·0
18	2	−6·5	2·0	14·5	23·0	30·0
19	2	−6·5	−5·0	−2·0	−7·0	−19·0
20	2	0·0	4·5	0·0	2·0	−2·0
21	2	0·0	−6·0	−3·5	−17·0	−17·0
22	2	−2·0	−8·5	−4·5	10·5	7·0
Mean		−2·04	−4·54	−2·45	1·04	6·00

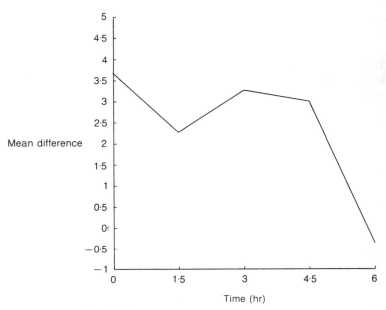

Figure 6.3. *Profile of differences in group means for the carry-over contrasts, Example 6.1.*

The data are transformed as follows:

$$d_{ikm} = \tfrac{1}{2}(-y_{i1km} + y_{i3km})$$

For example, for subject 1, group 1, 0·0 hours, we get

$$d_{111} = \tfrac{1}{2}(-77 + 85) = 4$$

The complete set of transformed data is given in Table 6.3 and the differences between the groups of the means from each time point are plotted in Figure 6.3. There is no clear pattern from this plot that would suggest a carry-over effect, but for a meaningful interpretation we need to consider as well the variability in these mean differences.

The sample variances and correlations of the contrasts are given in Table 6.4. The presence of some small and negative correlations is not surprising given that the data consist of within-subject contrasts, from which overall subject effects have been eliminated. A simple inspection of the variances and correlations suggests that

Table 6.4 *Sample variances (on the diagonal) and correlations (below the diagonal) from the carry-over contrasts for Example 6.1*

Hours					
0·0	36·0				
1·5	−0·16	49·4			
3·0	−0·17	0·27	143·2		
4·5	−0·23	0·31	0·43	147.0	
6·0	−0·00	0·18	0·14	0·72	246·15
Hours	0·0	1·5	3·0	4·5	6·0

the uniform assumption (or full independence) will not hold for these data, however. This is confirmed by a formal goodness-of-fit test (Morrison, 1986, Section 7.3), which gives a value of 42·9 on 13 degrees of freedom. For an approximate χ^2 variable this is clearly significant.

As an illustration we will show both the split-plot and MANOVA/ante-dependence analyses for the carry-over contrasts. In practice of course we would probably be using only one of these techniques, choosing whichever one suited our particular purposes. Remember that now, when we refer to the repeated measurements, we mean the carry-over contrasts calculated from the raw repeated measurements, and so the 'treatment effect' corresponds to a carry-over difference. The first measurement, at 0 hours, was made at the same time as the injection and so cannot contain a treatment effect. Its inclusion among the repeated measurements does not invalidate the results of the analysis, but will dilute to some extent the influence on the test statistic of any real treatment effects which may be present in the remaining measurements. We could either omit the first measurement altogether or use it as a covariate, noting that in the split-plot analysis such a between-subject covariate does not affect the within-subject part of the analysis. The small correlations between the first measurement and its successors suggest that it will make little contribution as a covariate but we shall include it anyway in the split-plot analysis as an illustration.

The split-plot-in-time ANOVA is presented in Table 6.5. Since we are now analysing within-subject contrasts we should not expect there to be a distinct between-subject component in the error variation. Hence the separation of the between-subject stratum in the split-plot

Table 6.5 *Split-plot-in-time ANOVA for the carry-over contrasts from Example 6.1*

Source	d.f.	SS	MS	F
First measurement (covariate)	1	99·508	99·508	0·33
Treatments main effect (Carry-over)	1	176·537	176·537	0·59
Between-subjects residual	19	5 694·739	299·723	
Between-subjects total	21	5 970·784		
Time main effect	3	1 063·437	354·479	3·645
Treatment-by-time-interaction (Carry-over-by-time interaction)	3	45·513	15·171	0·156
Within-subject residual	60	5 835·048	97·251	
Total	87	12 914·782	109·4	

ANOVA does not have its usual motivation. The significance of the separate stratum is now due rather to its validity under a general covariance structure. We know from examining the sample covariance structure of all five repeated measurements that the uniform structure is not appropriate for these data and a similar conclusion is reached if only the structure of the last four measurements is examined. Hence the within-subject analysis is not valid without modification. That is, the within-subject F-ratios must be used with adjusted degrees of freedom. In this example the adjustment can only affect our conclusions about the time main effect, however, because the time-by-treatment F-ratio is equal to 0·16, and modifying the degrees of freedom will only lessen its already negligible statistical significance. The time main effect F-ratio is equal to 3·65. With unmodified degrees of freedom of 3 and 60 this is significant at the 5% level. From the sample dispersion matrix of the last four repeated measurements we estimate ε, the adjustment factor, as 0·70, from which we get the adjusted degrees of freedom of 2·1 and 42. For a definition of ε and its estimate see Greenhouse and Geisser (1959). Note that we can use the original sample dispersion matrix to calculate ε; although the use of the first measurement as a covariate does affect the covariance structure, it leaves ε unchanged. This is obvious when we consider that the introduction of a between-subject covariate does not affect the within-subject sums of squares.

While reducing a little the statistical significance of the observed

Table 6.6 *Analysis of covariance sums of squares for the construction of the goodness-of-fit test statistic for a first-order ante-dependence structure, Example 6.1*

Dependent variate	Covariate	Additional covariates	r_{2m}	e_m	Residual d.f.	b_m
d_3	d_2	d_1	44·88	2614·28	18	0·983
d_4	d_3	d_2, d_1	176·63	2206·21	17	0·926
d_5	d_4	d_3, d_2, d_1	318·27	2011·95	16	0·863

F-ratio, the modification of degrees of freedom does not affect, in this case, the overall conclusion. There is therefore some evidence of an effect associated with time. Since this effect is defined by the sum over groups of the carry-over contrast, this result corresponds to a significant component of the period-by-time interaction, actually the component defined by the period 3 − period 1 difference. The presence of such an effect alone does not of course invalidate the treatment comparison. We can examine the form of the effect through the four between-group means of the carry-over contrasts. These are − 3·41, − 0·82, 2·54 and 5·82 for hours 1·5, 3, 4·5 and 6 respectively. There is a clear positive trend.

We now try ante-dependence analysis with the same data. First we establish the appropriate ante-dependence order. Although the majority of the correlations in Table 6.4 are small, there are enough large values to suggest that the d_{ikm} are not independent. A formal test would confirm this. Hence we check first the fit of the simplest structure that incorporates dependence, the first order. The fact that the first repeated measurement is to be used as a covariate is irrelevant here as it does not enter into the calculations as a dependent variate. The necessary analysis of covariance sums of squares are presented in Table 6.6, where d_m denotes the set of contrasts from the mth

Table 6.7 *Analysis of variance of d_m*

Source	d.f.	SS
Groups	1	g_m
d_{m-1}	1	r_{1m}
$d_{m-2}, \ldots, d_1$	$m-2$	r_{2m}
Residual	$n-m-1$	e_m

time of measurement. The mth row of this table is obtained from the sequential sums of squares in the analysis of variance of d_m (Table 6.7) where n is the total number of subjects. We then have $b_m = e_m/(r_{2m} + e_m)$.

From these we calculate the log likelihood ratio statistic for the goodness of fit of the first-order structure:

$$\Lambda(1,4) = -16 \sum_{m=3}^{5} \ln(b_m) = 3 \cdot 86, \text{ on 6 d.f.}$$

(where $\Lambda(a,b)$ denotes the statistic for the comparison of the ath and bth-order structures). The fit appears to be adequate, so we next compare the profiles under the first-order structure. We take into account the role of the first measurement by omitting the first component, in which it is the dependent variate. The required sums of squares are given in Table 6.8, the mth row of which is obtained from the analysis of variance of $\mathbf{d}_m$ (Table 6.9) and $b'_m = e_m/(h_m + e_m)$.

From these we get the log likelihood ratio statistic for the comparisons of the profiles:

$$\Phi(1) = -19 \sum_{m=2}^{5} \ln(b'_m) = 1 \cdot 58, \text{ 4 on 4 d.f.}$$

This is far from significant and is consistent with the overall

Table 6.8 *Analysis of covariance sums of squares for the construction of the carry-over test statistic under the first-order ante-dependence structure, Example 6.1*

Dependent variate	Covariate	h_m	e_m	Residual d.f.	b'_m
$\mathbf{d}_2$	$\mathbf{d}_1$	44·25	960·91	19	0·956
$\mathbf{d}_3$	$\mathbf{d}_2$	26·87	2659·21	19	0·990
$\mathbf{d}_4$	$\mathbf{d}_3$	13·04	2382·79	19	0·995
$\mathbf{d}_5$	$\mathbf{d}_4$	54·70	2330·24	19	0·997

Table 6.9 *Analysis of variance of* $\mathbf{d}_m$

Source	d.f.	SS
$\mathbf{d}_{m-1}$	1	r_m
Groups	1	h_m
Residual	$n-3$	e_m

conclusions from the carry-over main effect and carry-over-by-time interaction tests in the split-plot analysis. However, note that we learn nothing from this test about the period effect which appeared in the split-plot analysis. In order to examine this effect through ante-dependence analysis, or repeated-measurement MANOVA, we follow the same procedure as before, but test for an overall zero mean at each time point, rather than comparing the group means.

In the absence of a carry-over effect, we apply the same procedures to investigate the direct treatment effect using the contrast coefficients $\frac{1}{8}(-1, 1, -1, 1)$. The corresponding profile of the difference in group means is plotted in Figure 6.4. From this plot we can see a clear positive trend in the group differences among the last four repeated measurements (as expected, the first difference is comparatively close to zero). The initial negative difference at 1·5 hours indicates a greater percentage blood sugar level under A. By the end of the experimental period (6 hours) this difference has reversed and mean level under B is 5·43 mg% higher than under A. Remember that the

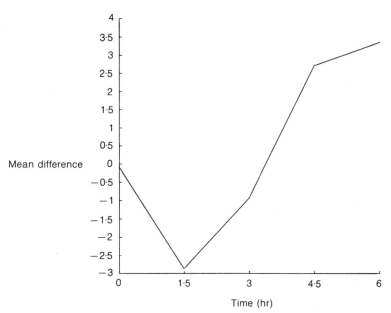

Figure 6.4 *Profile of differences in group means for the direct treatment contrasts, Example 6.1.*

direct contrasts are defined in terms of the B direct effect which is one-half the B − A mean difference. So the heights in Figure 6.4 must be multiplied by two to obtain the corresponding direct differences. It appears from the plot that the main change in direct effect over time occurs between 3 and 4·5 hours, during which period the change is 3·87 mg%. In the other two periods (1·5–3 and 4·5–6 hours) the changes are only 1·71 and 0·59 mg% respectively. It can be noted also that the mean differences are fairly evenly spread about the zero level. This is an example then where we should expect a direct-by-time interaction in the absence of an observed direct main effect. That is, if we used only the mean level over time as a summary statistic, we would miss an important feature of the data. We now see how the formal analyses reflect these impressions from the plot.

The split-plot-in-time ANOVA is presented in Table 6.10 and we estimate the adjustment factor ε as 0·70. Recall that this is the same (to two decimal places) as the value obtained for the carry-over contrasts. If the covariance structure of the repeated measurements were the same within each period, then we would have the same population value of ε, whatever contrast among periods is used. One might expect, at least approximately, such consistency in the covariance structure if the experimental conditions were similar in each period. Hence the similarity of the two estimates of ε is perhaps not unexpected, and is, to a certain degree, encouraging.

As before, the first measurement has been included as a covariate in the split-plot analysis. The direct main effect is quite negligible, whereas the interaction with time has an associated significance

Table 6.10 *Split-plot-in-time ANOVA for the direct treatment contrast from Example 6.1*

Source	d.f.	SS	MS	F
First measurement (covariate)	1	49·621	49·621	2·45
Direct main effect	1	6·076	6·076	0·30
Between-subjects residual	19	384·805	20·253	
Between-subjects total	21	440·502		
Time main effect	3	89·456	29·819	3·55
Direct-by-time interaction	3	147·703	49·234	5·83
Within-subject residual	60	507·137	8·452	
Total	87	1184·798		

probability of 0·006, with modified degrees of freedom of 2·1 and 42·0. This reflects the clear pattern seen in Figure 6.4. If the interaction sum of squares were partitioned into a linear component and a remainder, one would expect most of the variation to lie in the former. However, this really tells us only what we can see from the plot of the profile of group differences.

We note also that there is again some evidence of a time effect, $P = 0·038$. As before, this is a component of the time-by-period interaction. The corresponding means are 0·50, 3·04, 2·69 and 2.68 mg% for hours 1·5, 3, 4·5 and 6 respectively. Unlike the earlier component where a clear trend was apparent over time, we now have a large change between the 1·5 hour measurement and its successors, which themselves differ only little. It is difficult to add more to this simple description of the effect in the absence of further knowledge about the trial.

We now consider the ante-dependence analysis for the same data. We omit the details of the determination of order, which follows the same steps as before, and again leads to the choice of a first-order structure. The analysis of covariance sums of squares for the calculation of the profile statistic are presented in Table 6.11, and as with the carry-over contrasts, the first component, corresponding to the first measurement, has been omitted. Combining the b'_m values we get

$$\Phi(1) = -19 \sum_{m=2}^{5} \ln(b'_m) = 9·05$$

on 4 degrees of freedom. The corresponding probability is 0.059, which is close to statistical significance at 5%. Note, however, that if we had included the first measurement as well, the value of $\Phi(1)$ would

Table 6.11 *Analysis of covariance sums of squares for the construction of the direct treatment test statistic under the first-order ante-dependence structure, Example 6.1*

Dependent variate	Covariate	h_m	e_m	Residual d.f.	b'_m
d_2	d_1	44·604	164·717	19	0·787
d_3	d_2	2·804	116·865	19	0·977
d_4	d_3	47·164	200·621	19	0·810
d_5	d_4	0·710	204·402	19	0·997

have been the same (to two places of decimals) but the degrees of freedom would have increased to 5, with a corresponding significance probability of 0·106. This is an example of the loss of sensitivity that can arise through the inclusion of baseline measurements as dependent variates. The component b'_m values are, after transformation to the corresponding F-statistics.

$$5·15, \quad 0·46, \quad 4·47, \quad 0·07$$

and we see that it is the first and third components that have made the major contribution to the size of the statistic, confirming the impression given from the plot of the profile. When a clear and simple trend dominates the profile difference, however, as in this case, the examination of the individual components is of less value. Arguably the interpretation of the profile difference is then best given in terms of the overall trend.

It may have been noticed that the probability associated with the ante-dependence test is somewhat greater than that of the modified split-plot F-test. However, this does not mean necessarily that the former is the less sensitive in this case. It should be recalled that the ante-dependence test is a simultaneous test of the direct main effect and direct-by-time interaction, and this is reflected in its degrees of freedom, 4 rather than 3. Since, in this example, the main effect is negligible, its inclusion has diluted to some extent the contribution of the interaction effect to the overall statistic. If we calculate the ante-dependence statistic for the interaction alone, that is, using the differences $\mathbf{d}_m - \mathbf{d}_{m-1}$ in place of the original observations, we get $\Phi(1) = 8·69$ on 3 degrees of freedom, with a corresponding probability of 0·033; a value which is much closer to the split-plot result.

6.3 Repeated measurements from higher-order designs

To apply the usual repeated measurements techniques in a straightforward way with data from higher-order designs it is necessary to make a further assumption about the covariance structure. Recall that in the previous section we required only that the dispersion matrix of contrasts among periods was the same in both sequences. We now generalize the requirement made in Chapter 5 for the application of analysis of variance in the situation with a single measurement in each period. There it was assumed that with the inclusion of fixed subject effects the errors were independent with constant variance. We now assume, again with the inclusion of fixed subject effects, that the sequences of repeated measurements from each period are independent and have the same dispersion matrix. This is a multivariate generalization of the uniform covariance structure (at least in its manifestation with fixed subject effects). Arguably this is more likely to hold approximately than the assumption that the sequences of repeated measurements themselves have a uniform covariance structure, an assumption against which there is usually overwhelming empirical evidence.

Typically, but not invariably, the time between periods will be much larger than the time between repeated measurements within a period. The former may be of the order of weeks, or even months, the latter perhaps only minutes or hours. When this is the case, and if the condition being monitored is fairly stable between periods, we might reasonably expect an overall subject effect to be the only cause, or at least the clearly dominant cause, of correlations between periods. The use of baseline measurements within periods as covariates has a similar effect to the use of subject effects in that it should allow for overall subject differences. On the other hand, if the times between periods and between repeated measurements are similar, then we should not expect the assumption to hold between periods if we have doubts about the uniform assumption holding within periods. Taka and Armitage (1983) give an interesting example of a trial in which all measurements were made at one-week intervals regardless of the treatment cross-over, although in this case there did not appear to be evidence of any autocorrelation among the observations. It does not appear to be possible to check the overall assumption in a simple powerful way with small samples. We shall say a little more about this problem in Chapter 7 and we shall see below that in certain circumstances we can have quite strong support for the assumption without formally testing for it.

Once we make the assumption, however, the resulting analysis is simple to perform. We treat each subject/period combination as the unit for analysis and include as design terms subject, period and direct effects and, if desired, direct-by-period interaction and/or carry-over effects. This is the same procedure as used in Chapter 5. The only difference now is that each unit provides a sequence of repeated measurements and we just apply the standard repeated-measurement techniques with the given design terms. We can of course also apply the procedure with the two-sequence designs of the previous section.

We have, in these cases though, the option of the more robust analysis discussed in the previous section.

We now try the method with the second example introduced in Section 6.1, the measurements of systolic blood pressure (Example 6.2), and again we use the split-plot-in-time ANOVA and MANOVA/ante-dependence analyses for illustration. The first two repeated measurements, at -30 and -15 minutes respectively, are taken before the administration of the drugs. We can therefore use either or both of these, or a combination, as covariates. It is not obvious that one choice is better than another, so for simplicity we take the average of the two and use this as a single covariate. It hardly seems worth comparing the various combinations to choose the most effective, a procedure that in this case could be regarded as 'overkill'. This leaves a profile of eight measurements to be compared among the three treatments. Note that all but the last two repeated measurements are made at 15-minute intervals, the final two being preceded by 30- and 120-minute periods respectively.

From the plots of the simple treatment means in Figure 6.2 we can see a rough ordering of the heights of the profiles with treatment C (placebo) the lowest and treatment B (the greater dose of the drug) the highest. The picture is not a simple one, however, and it is not until the measurement at 45 minutes post-dose that this ordering is established. Recall that each subject contributes to each mean profile, so we should not expect large overall subject differences.

We now consider the split-plot-in-time analysis. The full ANOVA table is presented in Table 6.12. Note that the covariate only enters the main-plot analysis. We have also chosen, as in the previous section, to examine the carry-over effect rather than the direct-by-period interaction (the first-order carry-over and the interaction are not aliased in this design so we could if desired have examined both). In the presence of the covariate and carry-over term the effects are not all mutually orthogonal, hence sequential sums of squares have been used. The ordering of fitting corresponds to the ordering of the terms in the table and is a logical one to use. Strictly we should need to change the order if we wished to test for a direct treatment effect in the presence of a carry-over effect. There is a very clear direct main effect, presumably reflecting the ordering apparent in the plots of the mean profiles. Also the interaction F-statistics are all far from statistical significance, especially after adjustment of the degrees of freedom (in this case ε is estimated as 0·66). Hence this analysis provides no

Table 6.12 *Split-plot-in-time ANOVA for Example 6.2. Measurements are of systolic blood pressure (mm Hg)*

Source of variation	d.f.	SS	MS
Pre-dose average (covariate)	1	13 236·29	13 236·29
Subjects	11	10 951·02	995·55
Period main effect	2	373·53	186·76
Direct main effect	2	2 134·54	1 067·27
Carry-over (main effect)	2	264·34	132·17
Subject-by-period residual	17	2 149·15	126·42
Subject-by-period total	35	29 108·87	
Time main effect	7	1 767·66	252·52
Period-by-time interaction	14	38·60	0·81
Direct-by-time interaction	14	880·45	62·89
Carry-over-by-time interaction	14	787·95	56·28
Residual	203	9 720·37	47·88
Total	287	42 805·75	

evidence that the mean profiles are different shapes, implying that the observed differences can be ascribed to random variation. Therefore we summarize the direct treatment differences in terms of the covariate-adjusted means of the eight repeated measurements (not adjusted for carry-over). These are (in mm Hg) as follows:

Treatment	A	B	C
Adjusted mean	106·6	108·6	101·6

The standard error of a difference between two of these is about 1·6 (this differs slightly between pairs because of the covariance adjustment). These means suggest that the main difference among the direct effects is between that of the drug (at either level) and that of the placebo. The use of the drugs is associated with the higher systolic blood pressure.

We turn next to the use of the ante-dependence analysis. As with the split-plot analysis, the underlying linear model can be summarized in the form:

$$\text{SUBJECTS} + \text{PERIODS} + \text{DIRECT TREATMENTS} + \text{CARRY-OVER}$$

First we establish the appropriate ante-dependence order. Omitting the computational details we get the goodness-of-fit-statistics

$\Lambda(1, 8) = 45\cdot36$ and $\Lambda(2, 8) = 26\cdot96$ on 28 and 21 degrees of freedom, respectively. Note that these have been calculated using the refined multiplier described in Kenward (1987). It is clear that the first-order structure is inappropriate whereas the second-order appears to be acceptable.

Under the second-order structure we have ante-dependence statistics for each of the four design terms and, as in the split-plot analysis, these are sequential in definition. The component sums of squares are obtained from analyses of covariance (with sequentially determined sums of squares) of the form given in Table 6.13. This illustration has y_4 as the dependent variate (corresponding to the measurement at $+30$ minutes) and y_3 and $\frac{1}{2}(y_1 + y_2)$ as covariates. Combining the results from the set of analyses of covariance for dependent variates y_3 to y_{10} we obtain the ante-dependence test statistics given in Table 6.14. Only the direct treatment effect is noteworthy, with an associated probability of 0·010.

It is interesting that the subject effect is not large. There is a good reason for this, however. The use of the pre-dose average as baseline

Table 6.13 *Analysis of covariance of* y_4 *with* y_3 *and* $\frac{1}{2}(y_1 + y_2)$ *as covariates (Example 6.2)*

Source	d.f.	s.s
Regression on y_3	1	2809·36
Regression on $\frac{1}{2}(y_1 + y_2)$	1	23·85
Subjects	11	774·13
Periods	2	186·08
Direct treatments	2	17·73
Carry-over	2	102·02
Residual	16	536·96
Total	35	4450·13

Table 6.14 *Ante-dependence* $(\Phi(2))$ *statistics for Example 6.2*

Effect	d.f.	$\Phi(2)$
Subjects	88	111·93
Periods	16	17·62
Direct treatments	16	32·00
Carry-over	16	18·75

can be expected to account for much of the between-subject variation in the analysis of covariance of y_3. The preceding measurements in the remaining analyses of covariance can be expected to have much the same effect. We would in fact have obtained a very similar analysis in the absence of the subject term. This suggests that the assumption made at the beginning of this section concerning the independence between periods of measurements from a subject after allowing for a fixed subject effect may be justified quite strongly (without the need for a subject effect) under an ante-dependence structure when pre-treatment baselines are available. A low-order ante-dependence structure implies independence between a particular repeated measurement and earlier measurements after conditioning on a small number of intervening measurements. Hence, after using the baseline as a covariate, we will get, at worst, mild dependence between the earliest components from one period and the latest from the preceding period (and complete independence under the first-order structure). If the time between periods is much greater than that between repeated measurements it would be surprising if such dependence were anything but negligible. Therefore for this particular situation we can be fairly confident that the required assumption of independence between periods within a subject is a reasonable one.

Finally we look at the components of the direct statistic. We have seen that the split-plot analysis pointed only to a direct main effect. It will be interesting to see how this is reflected in the components. These

Table 6.15 *Components of the direct treatment statistic (Example 6.2)*

Variates	Residual d.f.	F
$y_3 \mid \frac{1}{2}(y_1 + y_2)$	17	1·03
$y_4 \mid y_3, \frac{1}{2}(y_1 + y_2)$	16	1·11
$y_5 \mid y_4, y_3$	16	6·32
$y_6 \mid y_5, y_4$	16	5·96
$y_7 \mid y_6, y_5$	16	0·48
$y_8 \mid y_7, y_6$	16	1·53
$y_9 \mid y_8, y_7$	16	2·38
$y_{10} \mid y_9, y_8$	16	1·04

are presented in Table 6.15, after conversion to the corresponding F-statistics with numerator degrees of freedom equal to 2.

There are two dominant components, associated with y_5 and y_6. The interpretation of these is not wholly straightforward though, and we must be careful not to read too much into them. We can conclude, however, that the first real evidence of a difference is not apparent until 45 minutes post-dose. Recall that this is the time of measurement at which the subsequent strict ordering of the profiles is first established, and it corresponds to a crossing of the profiles for treatments A and B (Figure 6.2). Apart from a drawing together of the profiles for A and C in the latter part of the sequence, there appears from the plots to be little relative change in the relative heights of the profiles after 45 minutes. The overall shape of the profiles may well have been predictable and the observed average changes of limited interest. Clearly it is this later consistent difference in the heights of the profiles which has led to the large direct treatment main effect observed in the split-plot analysis. We cannot infer much from the small ante-dependence components that follow the two large components. These do not necessarily (and in this case probably do not) imply an absence of direct treatment differences at these later times, only that in the presence of the autocorrelations subsequent measurements do not add to the evidence of the established direct treatment effect. We conclude that there is little evidence of differences among the profiles up to 30 minutes post-dose. Thereafter a consistent difference emerges with treatment A (active drug, high dose) corresponding to the highest levels of systolic blood pressure and treatment C, the placebo, the lowest.

CHAPTER 7

Cross-over data as repeated measurements

7.1 Covariance structure

One of the main concerns of the previous chapter was with the covariance structure of a sequence of repeated measurements from a subject. In particular it was seen that statistical analyses that ignore the time ordering of the data, and so make inappropriate assumptions about their covariance structure, are likely to be misleading. Such inappropriate analyses are usually based on ANOVA and make the implicit assumption that the covariance structure is uniform. However, in the earlier chapters of this book, we have tended to ignore the fact that the observations from different periods of a cross-over trial themselves constitute a sequence of repeated measurements. Apart from mentioning some simple robust analyses for data from two-treatment designs, we have used, for continuous data, standard ANOVA-based analyses. If such analyses are commonly invalid for 'ordinary' repeated-measurement data of the type discussed in the previous chapter, are we justified in using them for cross-over data? In this chapter we shall examine this question. It should be noted of course that the problem does not arise with the 2×2 design: a pair of observations does not (in this case) constitute a sequence and the analyses discussed in Chapter 2 require no special assumptions to be made about the covariance structure. With one or two important exceptions the question of covariance structure in cross-over data has only recently received attention and so the contents of this chapter are necessarily more speculative and of less direct practical application (at the moment) than the earlier parts of the book.

It is important at the outset to distinguish those situations in which we need to be concerned about the covariance structure of our data, at least in terms of departures from uniformity. The justification for most standard ANOVA-based analyses can be found in the **randomization** process used in the experimental design. One can think of this as inducing or implying the uniform covariance structure within each error stratum which is used in the analysis. It is known that the 'standard' least squares analysis for Latin squares and their extensions can be justified in this way; see for example, Kempthorne (1983, Section 10.5). Since most higher-order cross-over designs are Latin squares, or close relations, one might infer that this should also provide a justification for analysing cross-over data in the same way. However, the key difference with a cross-over trial is the possibility of carry-over effects and direct-by-period interaction. If constants for carry-over effects or interaction are included then the usual randomization argument cannot be used as a justification for the analysis. Moreover, even if these effects are not included, it may be that the restrictions imposed on the design in terms of balance or orthogonality do not allow sufficient randomization. In general, two of the three factors of a Latin square design need to be randomized to justify the useful analysis and this is not necessarily possible in some of the specialized cross-over designs.

Whatever design is used, and whether or not carry-over effects are to be fitted, the random allocation of subjects to sequences can be used to provide some support from equality of covariance structures between sequences, but not, as we have seen, for properties of the structures within sequences. In conclusion, if we can assume that the possibility of carry-over effects can safely be ignored then we can use an ordinary row-and-column design for a cross-over trial, with full randomization, and, provided that we do not then try to estimate, or allow for, carry-over effects in the analysis, a standard least squares analysis has its usual validity. On the other hand, a strong restriction on randomization in the design or the inclusion of carry-over effects in the analysis mean that we cannot justify a particular within-sequence covariance structure from the design alone. This does not, of course, imply that all least squares analyses of cross-over data in which carry-over effects are estimated are automatically invalid, a notion that seems most unrealistic, only that we need to look elsewhere for the justification for such an analysis.

Tyically a cross-over trial will not have many periods, hence our sequences will be short, commonly three to five observations only. Moreover, such a trial ought to be used only for a relatively stable condition. It is therefore plausible that with well-spaced measurements, the dominant cause of correlations within sequences will often be overall subject effects and that the variability of the response will not change greatly between periods. This would imply an approximately uniform covariance structure. In principle, an attempt could be made to model the structure from the trial data, and test hypotheses about particular forms that it might take. This is almost never done in practice, however, although tests for uniformity are commonplace with repeated-measurement data. As a consequence very little is actually known about the covariance structure of cross-over data. The uniform structure may well be an adequate approximation in many cases, but at the moment it is taken on trust. We shall discuss the estimation of the covariance structure in more detail in Sections 7.4 and 7.6.

One situation in which departures from uniformity are commonplace and well-documented is in dairy research (Hoekstra, 1987; Broster and Broster, 1984). A cross-over trial on milk yield typically covers one period of lactation of a cow, and the lactation curve has a clearly marked rise and fall at the beginning and end, respectively, of this period. Since cows effectively enter the trial at different points on their lactation curves, the components of error associated with these curves (roughly quadratic) show much greater variation than the other components. In other types of cross-over trial such a feature is less likely, unless there is a clear and consistent form of period effect.

Several related questions arise when we consider departures from uniformity of the covariance structure of cross-over data:

1. How misleading will a standard least squares analysis be in the presence of such departures? Is it likely to matter in practice?
2. How should the data be analysed if we wish to allow for possible departures? Are ordinary least squares estimators likely to be very inefficient?
3. How do such departures affect the choice of design? Are the broad conclusions reached earlier from the comparison of designs likely to need much revision?

After introducing notation and some basic formulae in the next section, in Section 7.3 we give a brief discussion of the work that has been produced on design. In the remaining sections we consider the problem of analysis under more general covariance structures. The very general model considered at the end of Section 7.6 is also relevant for some problems tackled in previous chapters, in particular missing values and repeated measurements within treatment periods.

7.2 Notation and basic formulae

We first establish the notation that will apply in the rest of this chapter, and this will be kept, as far as possible, consistent with earlier chapters.

As before we will denote by y_{ijk} the observation in the jth period from the kth subject in the ith sequence group, where $i = 1, \ldots, s$, $k = 1, \ldots, n_i$ and $j = 1, \ldots, p$. We have the linear model for y_{ijk},

$$Y_{ijk} = \mu + \pi_j + \tau_{d[i,j]} + \lambda_{d[i,j-1]} [+ (\pi\tau)_{j,d[i,j]}] + s_{ik} + e_{ijk} \qquad (7.1)$$

where the parameters retain their interpretation from earlier chapters. We have enclosed the interaction term in brackets because it will not feature in most of the discussion in the following sections. This does not mean, however, that it may not be included in any particular analysis as required. The terms s_{ik} are the subject effects and may, depending on the circumstances, be assumed to be either fixed or random. Conventional assumptions for random subject effects are that they should be uncorrelated with constant variance, σ_s^2 say, and independent of the within-subject error terms, the e_{ijk}. Our main departure from earlier chapters lies in the assumptions about the within-subject error terms. For the moment we do not impose any structure on the variances and covariances of the observations from a particular subject and simply denote their $(p \times p)$ dispersion matrix by Δ. We do assume of course that observations from different subjects are independent. In matrix notation we have

$$\mathbf{y}_{(i)k} = (y_{i1k}, \ldots, y_{ipk})^T$$

the vector of observations from the (i, k)th subject, and

$$\mathbf{y}_j = (y_{1j1}, y_{1j2}, \ldots, y_{1jn_1}, y_{2j1}, \ldots, y_{sjn_s})^T$$

the vector of n observations from the jth period $(n = n_1 + \cdots + n_s)$. We denote the dispersion matrix of $\mathbf{y}_{(i)k}$ by Σ. With fixed subject effects, we have $\Sigma = \Delta$ and with random subject effects,

$$\Sigma = \Delta + \sigma_s^2 \mathbf{j}_p \mathbf{j}_p^T \qquad (7.2)$$

where $\mathbf{j}_p$ is a p-dimensional vector of 1's. Setting $\Delta = \sigma_w^2 \mathbf{I}_p$ we get the uniform covariance structure, where $\mathbf{I}_p$ is the $(p \times p)$ identity matrix.

It will be convenient in the following sections to work with the array of means from each combination of sequence and period, where each mean is defined as

$$\bar{y}_{ij} = \frac{1}{n_i} \sum_{k=1}^{n_i} y_{ijk}$$

The ith row of this array, corresponding to the ith sequence, is

$$\bar{\mathbf{y}}_{(i)} = (\bar{y}_{i1}, \ldots, \bar{y}_{ip})^{\mathrm{T}}$$

and the jth column, corresponding to the jth period, is

$$\bar{\mathbf{y}}_j = (\bar{y}_{1j}, \ldots, \bar{y}_{sj})^{\mathrm{T}}$$

with

$$\mathrm{Cov}\,[\bar{\mathbf{y}}_{(i)}\bar{\mathbf{y}}_{(i')}^{\mathrm{T}}] = \begin{cases} n_i^{-1}\mathbf{\Sigma} & i = i' \\ 0 & i \neq i' \end{cases} \quad \text{and} \quad \mathrm{Cov}\,[\bar{\mathbf{y}}_j\bar{\mathbf{y}}_{j'}^{\mathrm{T}}] = \sigma_{jj'}\mathbf{r}^{-\delta}$$

for $\sigma_{jj'}$ the (j,j')th element of $\mathbf{\Sigma}$ and $\mathbf{r}^{-\delta} = \mathrm{diag}\,[n_1^{-1}, \ldots, n_s^{-1}]$. Our direct concern will be with the parameters associated with treatment effects and we therefore separate these from the constant term (μ) and the period effects (π_j), which we shall regard as nuisance parameters. The remaining direct, carry-over and possibly direct-by-period interaction parameters will be associated with the means (or raw observations) through two complementary sets of design matrices. By implication we are working with random subject effects.

The first set, to be denoted $\{\mathbf{A}_{(i)}\}$, $i = 1, \ldots, s$, is defined in terms of the **sequences**. We have

$$E[\bar{\mathbf{y}}_{(i)}] = \boldsymbol{\pi} + \mathbf{A}_{(i)}\boldsymbol{\xi}, \qquad i = 1, \ldots, s, \tag{7.3}$$

where $\boldsymbol{\xi}$, $(g \times 1)$ say, contains the parameters of interest (treatment and so on) and $\boldsymbol{\pi} = (\pi_1^*, \ldots, \pi_p^*)$, for $\pi_j^* = \mu + \pi_j$.

The second set, $\mathbf{A}_j$, $j = 1, \ldots, p$, is defined in terms of **periods**. We have

$$E[\bar{\mathbf{y}}_j] = \pi_j^*\mathbf{j}_s + \mathbf{A}_j\boldsymbol{\xi}, \qquad j = 1, \ldots, p \tag{7.4}$$

The two expressions (7.3) and (7.4) define exactly the same model. We shall find that each has particular notational and computational advantages in different situations.

We now give the expressions for the generalized least squares (GLS) estimator $\hat{\xi}$ of ξ and its dispersion matrix $\mathbf{V}_\xi$. We have two pairs of expressions, obtained through the two representations (7.3) and (7.4). For these we need to define the matrix $\mathbf{H} = \mathbf{r}^\delta - n^{-1}\mathbf{r}\mathbf{r}^{\mathrm{T}}$ where $\mathbf{r} = (n_1, \ldots, n_s)^{\mathrm{T}}$ and $\mathbf{r}^\delta = \mathrm{diag}(n_1, n_2, \ldots, n_s)$. We have

$$\hat{\xi} = \mathbf{V}_\xi \sum_{i=1}^{s} \sum_{i'=1}^{s} h_{ii'} \mathbf{A}_{(i)}^{\mathrm{T}} \mathbf{\Sigma}^{-1} \bar{\mathbf{y}}_{(i')} = \mathbf{V}_\xi \sum_{j=1}^{p} \sum_{j'=1}^{p} \sigma^{jj'} \mathbf{A}_j^{\mathrm{T}} \mathbf{H} \bar{\mathbf{y}}_{j'} \quad (7.5)$$

where $h_{ii'}$ is the (i, i')th element of $\mathbf{H}$ and $\mathbf{V}_\xi$ is the dispersion matrix of $\hat{\xi}$, the inverse of which can be written

$$\mathbf{V}_\zeta^{-1} = \sum_{i=1}^{s} \sum_{i'=1}^{s} h_{ii'} \mathbf{A}_{(i)}^{\mathrm{T}} \mathbf{\Sigma}^{-1} \mathbf{A}_{(i')}$$

$$= \sum_{j=1}^{p} \sum_{j'=1}^{p} \sigma^{jj'} \mathbf{A}_j^{\mathrm{T}} \mathbf{H} \mathbf{A}_{j'} \quad (7.6)$$

for $\sigma^{jj'}$ the (j, j')th element of $\mathbf{\Sigma}^{-1}$.

We can separate the between- and within-subject components of the covariance structure in these expressions by using the equality (7.2). From this, using a standard matrix result, we have

$$\mathbf{\Sigma}^{-1} = \mathbf{\Delta}^{-1} - \frac{1}{\sigma_s^{-2} + \mathbf{j}_p^{\mathrm{T}} \mathbf{\Delta}^{-1} \mathbf{j}_p} \mathbf{\Delta}^{-1} \mathbf{j}_p \mathbf{j}_p^{\mathrm{T}} \mathbf{\Delta}^{-1} \quad (7.7)$$

which can be substituted into (7.5) and (7.6).

We can obtain the corresponding expressions under the assumption of fixed subject effects (or equivalently sequence effects) by taking the limit as σ_s^2 tends to infinity. We have

$$\lim_{\sigma_s^2 \to \infty} \mathbf{\Sigma}^{-1} = \mathbf{\Delta}^{-1} - \frac{1}{\mathbf{j}_p^{\mathrm{T}} \mathbf{\Delta}^{-1} \mathbf{j}_p} \mathbf{\Delta}^{-1} \mathbf{j}_p \mathbf{j}_p^{\mathrm{T}} \mathbf{\Delta}^{-1} \quad (7.8)$$

which again can be substituted into (7.5) and (7.6) to obtain the required expressions.

Finally, the ordinary least squares (within-subject) estimators used in previous chapters can be obtained from these latter by setting $\mathbf{\Delta} = \sigma_w^2 \mathbf{I}_p$, from which we get

$$\lim_{\sigma_s^2 \to \infty} \mathbf{\Sigma}^{-1} = \sigma_w^{-2} [\mathbf{I}_p - p^{-1} \mathbf{j}_p \mathbf{j}_p^{\mathrm{T}}] \quad (7.9)$$

We shall be displaying a number of dispersion matrices in the following sections and in an attempt to make these as informative as possible we shall use a lower-triangular format with **variances** on the diagonal and **correlations** below the diagonal.

7.3 Comparison of designs

When we compared the properties of designs in earlier sections of this book, in particular in Chapters 4 and 5, we were able to report quite extensive and practically useful results. The mathematics on which that work was based is tractable and lends itself to the exploration of different design ideas. The key to this tractability is the assumption of a uniform error structure, or for our purposes, the equivalent assumption of equally variable independent errors with fixed subject effects. This means that when using within-subject information only, as we generally have done, the appropriate methodology falls into the class of ordinary least squares. Hence the expressions for parameter estimators do not involve the unknown dispersion matrix of the observations and the finite-sample dispersion matrices of these estimators are known up to a constant multiplier, the within-sample variance. Provided that we can assume that two competing designs are associated with the same within-subject variance, we can compare their properties without ever knowing the particular value that this variance may take. The measures of comparison need to be calculated once only, and apply in general. When we relax the assumption of a uniform covariance structure this tractability is lost in two ways.

First, there is no longer any obviously 'appropriate' set of estimators. If the dispersion matrix Σ were known then GLS estimators, which are minimum-variance unbiased, would be used. Unfortunately, in practice, Σ rarely is (if ever) known. An alternative would be to estimate Σ from the data and use this in place of the true value. There is no guarantee however that in any particular case such empirical generalized least squares (EGLS) estimators will be more precise than ordinary least squares (OLS) estimators. There are other alternatives, including maximum likelihood (ML) estimators and we shall be looking at these in more detail in later sections of this chapter. Experimental designs are conventionally compared through the dispersion matrices of the associated parameter estimators, so in principle, to compare designs, we should first specify the type of estimator to be used. However, this is probably not too serious a problem in practice. It is plausible that the relative strengths of designs are fairly insensitive to the choice of estimator, at least among the 'better' of the alternatives, and so any convenient form of estimator can be used. Almost invariably GLS estimators are used under the assumption that the dispersion matrix is known.

Second, whichever type of estimators are used, their dispersion matrix will depend on the elements of Σ in a more or less complicated way. Conclusions on the relative merits of designs will have to be conditional on the particular covariance structure and the values of its parameters. Many such structures could be appropriate in different situations. Moreover, it is likely that an analytical expression will exist only for the dispersion matrix of the asymptotic distribution of an estimator. The relevance of these for estimators from small trials requires yet further research, which will probably be obtainable in most cases only through simulation, again making it difficult to draw general conclusions.

It is perhaps not surprising, then, that little work has been done on this problem, and that which has been done has been, with a few important exceptions, of limited practical value. A useful short review is given by Matthews (1988a, Section 4). We shall briefly discuss this work while concentrating on the results which have the most practical relevance.

In order to avoid most of the problems outlined above it has usually been assumed that Σ is known. This allows us to write down directly the GLS estimators and their small-sample dispersion matrix (7.6). This matrix is also the **asymptotic** dispersion matrix of the ML estimators, and of a broad class of EGLS estimators that use a consistent estimator of Σ. Most importantly, it is also necessary to postulate some structure for Δ, and this cannot depend on more than a few parameters if the number of alternative cases is to be kept to a manageable size. Almost without exception it has been assumed that the within-subject errors follow a stationary first-order autoregressive process. That is,

$$e_{ijk} = \begin{cases} f_{i1k} & j = 1 \\ \rho e_{i,j-1,k} + f_{ijk} & j = 2,\ldots,p \end{cases}$$

where the f_{ijk} are uncorrelated with

$$V[f_{ijk}] = \begin{cases} (1-\rho^2)^{-1}\sigma_{\mathrm{w}}^2 & j = 1 \\ \sigma_{\mathrm{w}}^2 & j = 2,\ldots,p \end{cases}$$

This implies that the (j, j')th element of Δ can be written as

$$\delta_{jj'} = \frac{\sigma_w^2}{1 - \rho^2} \rho^{|j - j'|}$$

The variance σ_w^2 enters as a constant multiplier into the elements of Δ and so can remain unspecified for the comparison of designs. Hence, under this structure for Δ, only a single parameter, the autocorrelation ρ, need be introduced as a component of the design comparisons. It is probable that the assumption of a particular structure for Δ has far greater implications for the relative behaviour of the designs than the assumption that the structure is known. The stationary autoregressive structure is a convenient and mathematically tractable way of introducing serial correlation among the within-subject errors, but it must be remembered in the discussion that follows that the results presented apply only under this structure. For the moment we can only conjecture about the wider applicability of these results.

Attempts have been made to extend optimality results to the autoregressive case. Broadly the same classes of designs found to have good properties under the uniform error assumption, and discussed in Chapter 5, are also found to be the better designs, at least with respect to certain specific optimality criteria, under stationary autoregressive errors. One can think of these results as strengthening the case for the use of these designs in practice, rather than providing absolute arguments for their use. The comments made earlier about the limitations of summarizing the qualities of a design with a single measure of 'optimality' apply equally here.

Before reviewing this work we should mention an important related area of research. This is concerned with the optimal design of field experiments under non-uniform patterns of spatial correlation. When only one dimension is considered, the problems have strong similarities to those considered here. The models no longer involve period effects, however, and the experimental layouts fall into the class of block designs. Kiefer and Wynn (1981) review existing work and produce several new results. A more recent reference is Russell and Eccleston (1987). These authors concentrate on so-called 'nearest-neighbour' correlation patterns which reduce in one dimension to the stationary first-order moving-average process. This provides an approximation to the autoregressive process for small ρ. Gill and Shukla (1985), Kunert (1987b) and Azzalini and Giovagnoli (1987) investigate optimality for the same situation under the assumption of autoregressive errors.

Berenblut and Webb (1974) produced some of the first results on optimality among cross-over designs under autoregressive errors. They considered the class of 4×4 Latin squares, without including carry-over effects. Unusually, in defining the autoregressive error structure, they set the variance of f_{i1k} equal to σ_w^2, implying an initially nonstationary process in which the variances of the e_{ijk} increase over time to an asymptote of $\sigma_w^2 (1 - \rho^2)^{-1}$. Arguably, for most situations, this is less realistic than the conventional stationary process. Berenblut and Webb included sequence effects in their model, which leads to the same estimators as would be obtained with fixed subject effects. (This equivalence is demonstrated in the appendix to this chapter.) They show that Williams squares, defined in Subsection 5.2.2, are A-optimal among the class of 4×4 Latin squares, whether period effects are included or not. (See Section 5.3 for the definitions of optimality.)

Kunert (1985) also derived some optimality results in the absence of carry-over effects and with fixed subject effects, but using the conventional stationary covariance structure. By omitting carry-over effects one need not take account of the direction of time, which provides for some mathematical simplification, and as a consequence Kunert was able to restrict attention to two forms of balance. The first is in terms of adjacency, that is, equating the number of times each pair of treatments occupy adjacent periods on the same unit, and the second is in terms of the end-points of the sequences, that is equating the number of times each pair of treatments occupy opposite ends of a subject's sequence. In both types of balance one can ignore the order in which the treatments of a particular pair occur. Kunert showed that for $t > 3$, uniform designs with adjacency balance are E-optimal:

1. among the class of all uniform designs with $p = t$, for ρ in the interval $(-1, 1)$; and
2. among the class of all designs with $t = p = n$, for ρ in the interval $(-(t-1)^{-1}, \frac{1}{2})$, with the upper limit increased to about 0.62 when $t = 4$.

With the additional restriction of balanced end-pairs, Kunert was able to show some universal optimality properties for uniform adjacency balanced designs. Such designs do require rather many units, however.

Bora (1984, 1985) investigated designs with $p < t$ and gave necessary and sufficient conditions for balance under stationary autoregressive errors. He also presented examples of such designs. Bora's models included sequence effects (hence the resulting estimators coincide with those obtained with fixed subject effects) and he considered both the situation with and without carry-over effects (1985 and 1984 respectively). The balanced designs in the former case require pre-trial periods with treatments applied, but no measurements taken, or at least used in the analysis. It is difficult, however, to imagine a situation in which this might be done in practice, although Matthews (1988a) points to their possible value for psychological experimentation in the presence of a learning effect.

The designs discussed so far exclude the important case of two treatments. Laska and Meisner (1985) considered optimal two-treatment designs under both uniform and autoregressive errors. Their results for the uniform-error case were mentioned in Chapter 4. Their use of the autoregressive error structure is not quite straight-forward in that they do not include sequence or subject effects (fixed or random). This implies an equal weighting of between- and within-subject information in the corresponding estimators, which would probably be avoided in practice. Under their model, they demonstrate that if carry-over effects are omitted, then, for all $\rho > 0$ and $p > 2$, the optimal designs have alternating treatments. They used numerical search methods to obtain optimal designs for $p = 3$ and $p = 4$ when carry-over effects are included.

The results of Laska and Meisner were extended by Matthews (1987), who used the stationary autoregressive structure with fixed subject effects. He showed that in the absence of carry-over effects, for $\rho < 0$ the optimal design changes treatment only once and balances as nearly as possible the treatments on each sequence. The latter can be achieved exactly of course with even p, and there will be two possible designs with odd p. The results have a simple practical explanation. Negative values of ρ correspond to higher-frequency oscillations of the within-subject errors, which increase the variances of differences among observations from neighbouring periods. Hence different treatments should be as well spaced as possible. Like-wise, positive values of ρ correspond to low-frequency oscillations, requiring different treatments to be as close as possible. However, the situation changes greatly when carry-over effects are introduced. Matthews was also able to derive analytical solutions for the case with carry-over effects. Interestingly, these results agree with Laska and Meisner's for even p but not for odd p (recall the different assumptions about the subject effects). The optimal designs have different proportions of the available subjects on different dual pairs of sequences, where the actual proportions depend on ρ in a fairly complicated way.

For estimating the direct treatment effect adjusted for carry-over from a three-period design the sequence ABA and its dual make a very small contribution (if any) to the optimal design. For small positive ρ the best design is based almost wholly on ABB and its dual, while for larger positive ρ the sequence AAB and its dual dominate. We know that for uniform errors the optimal design is the single pair based on ABB. It is interesting to note that there is an abrupt change from this pair to that based on AAB (which actually occurs at $\rho = 0.464$). For the estimation of the carry-over effect, still with $p = 3$, the optimal design uses a mixture of pairs from ABA and ABB for negative ρ and solely the ABB pair for $\rho \geqslant 0$. For $p = 4$ the optimal design for the direct treatment effect uses a mixture of the AABB and ABBA pairs, a somewhat greater proportion on the former for negative ρ; equal proportions, as we have already seen in Chapter 4, for zero ρ (that is, under uniform errors); and a rapidly dominating proportion on the latter for increasing positive ρ. Of course, the actual proportions provide only a guide to the choice of design in practice, particularly as ρ will be unknown. It is useful therefore to know how much efficiency is lost through the use of the simpler designs with equally replicated sequences discussed in Chapter 4 for different values of ρ.

We should be quite prepared to use a design which is, in the strict mathematical and rather artificial sense, 'sub-optimal', but which performs well enough under a range of likely covariance assumptions. Tables 7.1 and 7.2, which are reproduced from Matthews (1987, Tables 3a and 3b), contain the relative efficiencies of some of these designs for a range of values of ρ from -0.8 to 0.8. For the three-period case, the single dual pair corresponding to ABB performs reasonably well both for the direct treatment and carry-over effects, provided that ρ is not too large and negative, and this is probably unlikely in practice. The four-sequence design using the dual pairs ABB and AAB is also worth considering as its efficiencies

Table 7.1 *Relative efficiencies of three-period designs, as a percentage of the optimum. Each dual pair is represented by the sequence beginning with A, upper and lower figure for direct treatment and carry-over effects respectively (Reproduced from Matthews, 1987, Table 3a, with permission of the Biometrika Trustees.)*

ρ	AAB	ABA	ABB	ABB ABA	ABB AAB	AAB ABA	ABB ABA AAB
−0·8	19	14	54	56	100	30	72
	14	68	54	93	86	43	89
−0·6	36	20	80	70	99	35	75
	20	50	80	100	77	39	80
−0·4	51	23	93	77	99	40	78
	23	39	73	96	72	36	73
−0·2	64	25	99	80	98	45	80
	25	31	98	89	68	35	68
0·0	75	25	100	81	97	50	81
	25	25	100	81	65	33	63
0·2	85	25	100	82	97	56	83
	25	21	100	74	63	33	60
0·4	95	25	100	82	99	63	87
	25	18	100	69	63	33	58
0·6	100	24	95	80	98	68	87
	25	16	100	64	64	34	57
0·8	99	22	87	74	93	70	85
	25	14	100	61	66	35	57

for the direct treatment effects are not much below (or slightly greater) than those of the ABB design. From the selection of four-period designs included in Table 7.2, the four-sequence design based on AABB and ABBA performs quite well for the full range of ρ for both direct treatment and carry-over effects.

In a modification of the model we have been considering it is possible to use an additional autoregression as a mechanism for introducing carry-over effects. The model (7.1) becomes

$$Y_{ijk} = \rho_2 y_{i, j-1, k} + \pi_j + \tau_{d[i, j]} + s_{ik} + e_{ijk} \qquad (7.10)$$

where we assume as above that the within-subject errors follow a stationary first-order autoregressive process, but now with parameter

Table 7.2 Relative efficiencies of four-period designs, as a percentage of the optimum. Each dual pair is represented by the sequence beginning with A, upper and lower figure for direct treatment and carry-over effects respectively (Reproduced from Matthews, 1987, Table 3b, with permission of the Biometrika Trustees.)

ρ	AABB	ABBA	ABBB	ABAA	ABAB	AABB ABBA	AABB ABAA	ABBA ABBB
−0·8	98 41	50 96	27 53	37 16	7 15	88 75	80 34	49 95
−0·6	98 53	60 94	37 65	41 26	13 16	91 82	81 46	59 97
−0·4	98 66	71 93	50 78	46 40	16 17	95 89	83 62	70 99
−0·2	95 79	81 92	63 89	50 57	18 18	99 95	86 81	80 100
0·0	91 91	91 91	73 97	55 73	18 18	100 100	87 99	87 99
0·2	84 88	97 80	76 89	57 74	18 16	98 91	85 99	89 86
0·4	76 86	100 76	71 83	58 76	16 14	94 86	80 99	87 80
0·6	68 87	100 76	62 79	57 77	15 13	88 85	75 99	81 77
0·8	61 88	100 78	53 75	56 79	14 12	84 85	70 99	77 77

ρ_1 to distinguish it from the coefficient representing the auto-regression on the previous response (ρ_2).

Taka and Armitage (1983) consider this model, in a slightly different, but equivalent, parameterization and without the period effects, for both design and analysis. Following the general form of their experimental data they considered three designs with two treatments and two sequences (dual pairs) and ten periods. The three designs had sequences which changed treatments (1) once in the middle; (2) after approximately every other period; and (3) after every period. Using numerical methods they reached similar conclusions to those of Laska and Meisner (1985) and Matthews (1987) for the case without autoregression on the response and without fixed carry-over effects. Broadly design (1) is to be preferred for negative, and design (3) for positive, autocorrelations. Interestingly the efficiency of design (1) proved to be less sensitive to the value of ρ_1 than to that of ρ_2. As should be expected, the efficiency of design (2), which represents a compromise, is less sensitive to the values of either autocorrelation. Gill and Shukla (1987) also consider the model (7.10), including both period and fixed subject effects. Assuming, as previous authors have done, that the autoregressive parameters (now two) are known, they derive some optimality results. They indicate that among designs which are uniform on periods, with $p = t$, universal optimality requires many subjects, agreeing with Kunert's results under the simple autoregressive structure. They conjecture that among the same class with $n = t$, designs with adjacency balance are universally optimal. Again, the omission of fixed carry-over effects allows the direction of time to be ignored. For p a multiple of t, Gill and Shukla come to similar conclusions to those of Taka and Armitage. That is, with negative ρ_2, treatments should be changed as little as possible, while with positive ρ_2, they should be changed as often as possible.

7.4 Ordinary least squares estimation under a general covariance structure

Even when the uniform errors assumption is relaxed we can still use OLS estimators. They have the advantage of simplicity and remain unbiased under a general covariance structure. They have the disadvantage that they may, although not necessarily, be less efficient than some alternatives. The dispersion matrix of the estimators will of course depend on the unknown covariance structure and so usually this will have to be estimated from the data, and in general the ANOVA methods used in Chapters 4 and 5 will not produce the correct estimates of error, unless the uniform error assumption holds.

Before moving on to consider the problem of appropriate error estimates, it is worth considering whether there are situations for which the ANOVA-based analyses used in Chapters 4 and 5 will be at least approximately valid under non-uniform errors. Matthews (1988c) has looked at this for the case of two-treatment designs (with fixed subject effects), assuming a stationary first-order autoregressive process and a first-order moving-average process. In the latter the elements of Δ are constant on the diagonal, constant on the leading sub-diagonal and zero elsewhere. For moderate positive values of the autocorrelation and moving-average correlation, the least squares analysis is quite acceptable both with respect to efficiency and validity of the error estimate for the three-period designs:

			ABB		ABB
	ABB		BAA		BAA
(i)	BAA	(ii)	AAB	(iii)	ABA
			BBA		BAB

and for the four-period design:

$$\text{ABBA}$$
$$\text{BAAB}$$

This is encouraging, and suggests that the analyses used earlier would not be too misleading for these designs. It must be emphasized, however, that these results are tied to the assumed stationary error structures and cannot be expected to hold in general.

Kunert (1987a) has also considered the validity of the ANOVA analysis, this time under a general covariance structure. His results apply to Williams designs, with a model including fixed subject effects and carry-over effects. He obtains lower bounds on the ratio between the expected value of the estimated variance of the estimators (using the ANOVA analysis) and their true variance, both for direct treatment and carry-over effects. These bounds give a measure of how poorly the estimated variance may approximate the true variance. Interestingly these bounds prove to be fairly moderate in size, indicating that the ANOVA estimates of the variances will not grossly underestimate the true variances. Unfortunately the substitution of the lower bounds as corrections to the ANOVA-based variances produce estimates of error that are too conservative for practical use, and as the true correction is unknown, Kunert's results do not really help in the analysis. For particular designs and certain strict assumptions about the covariance structure this ratio (or correction) can be determined exactly and independently of the covariance parameters, and so be used to correct the OLS variance estimates (Patterson, 1950, 1951, 1971; Lucas 1951) but as Kunert points out, in general one must obtain some estimate of the covariance parameters. This is effectively what we shall do below, although we shall go directly to the variances of the parameter estimates, and not work through the ANOVA-based estimates of these.

Once again the two-treatment designs form a special case. The robust analyses described in Sections 2.9, 4.7 and 4.9 are examples of a general procedure that can be used to provide correct estimates of the variances of OLS estimates under any covariance structure. The general principle should be clear from these examples. Recall that each effect is estimated using a particular contrast among periods. For any covariance structure these contrasts will have the same variance from each subject and it is a trivial matter to calculate this variance from the sample of the subjects' contrasts. The resulting estimated variance is used to obtain the variance of the estimated effect. For details we refer to the previous examples. The procedure can be extended simply in an *ad hoc* way for designs made up of dual pairs of sequences, provided that the effect of interest can be estimated separately from each dual pair. This will usually be possible for the direct treatment effect and first-order carry-over effect, but may well not be true for terms like the direct-by-period interaction and higher-order carry-over effects. When separate estimates do exist, these are obtained from each dual pair, together with their associated estimated variances, and are combined using the inverse variances as weights. It is also necessary to estimate the appropriate degrees of freedom for the estimated variance of the combination. An example of the procedure for a design made up of two dual pairs was given in Section 4.9. When separate estimates are not available the general approaches discussed below will be required.

For higher-order cross-over trials we can of course use the standard ANOVA techniques of Section 5.9 to obtain the OLS estimators of the effects of interest. The new feature which we must consider now is the estimation of the dispersion matrix of these estimators under a general covariance structure, represented by the matrix Σ. We can obtain expressions for the dispersion matrix of the OLS estimators using the results in Section 7.2. First, we have from (7.5) and (7.9) the OLS estimator of ξ:

$$\hat{\xi}_{OLS} = \mathbf{W}^{-1}\left[\sum_{j=1}^{p} \mathbf{A}_j^T \mathbf{H}\bar{\mathbf{y}}_j - p^{-1} \sum_{j=1}^{p} \sum_{j'=1}^{p} \mathbf{A}_j^T \mathbf{H}\bar{\mathbf{y}}_{j'} \right]$$

where

$$\mathbf{W} = \sum_{j=1}^{p} \mathbf{A}_j^T \mathbf{H}\mathbf{A}_j - p^{-1} \sum_{j=1}^{p} \sum_{j'=1}^{p} \mathbf{A}_j^T \mathbf{H}\mathbf{A}_{j'}$$

From this we get the dispersion matrix of $\hat{\xi}_{OLS}$ under a general covariance structure as

$$V[\hat{\xi}_{OLS}] = \mathbf{W}^{-1}\left[\sum_{j=1}^{p} \sum_{j'=1}^{p} \phi_{jj'} \mathbf{A}_j^T \mathbf{H}\mathbf{A}_{j'} \right]\mathbf{W}^{-1} \qquad (7.11)$$

where $\phi_{jj'}$ is the (j, j')th element of

$$\mathbf{\Phi} = [\mathbf{I}_p - p^{-1}\mathbf{j}_p\mathbf{j}_p^T]\mathbf{\Sigma}[\mathbf{I}_p - p^{-1}\mathbf{j}_p\mathbf{j}_p^T]$$

To estimate this we need only an estimate of Σ. We shall consider two ways of obtaining such an estimate. If there is a reasonable amount of replication on each sequence then we can use within-sequence information only. An unbiased estimate of Σ is given by the within-sequence sample dispersion matrix:

$$\mathbf{S} = \frac{1}{n-s} \sum_{i=1}^{s} \sum_{k=1}^{n_i} (\mathbf{y}_{(i)k} - \bar{\mathbf{y}}_{(i)})(\mathbf{y}_{(i)k} - \bar{\mathbf{y}}_{(i)})^T$$

As an illustration we try this for the systolic blood pressure measurements from Example 5.1. This is a three-period three-treatment design in which all six sequences are represented, based at four centres, with 23 subjects altogether. We shall ignore the centres in the following. The presence of such extra between-unit factors does not affect the general principle of the analyses to be described but it can make the dispersion matrix of the estimated effects rather unwieldy and so complicate the presentation. For these data we have the within-sequence sample dispersion matrix:

$$\begin{matrix}
691\cdot91 & & \\
0\cdot46 & 705\cdot60 & \\
0\cdot69 & 0\cdot66 & 756\cdot13
\end{matrix}$$

The differences among the variances and among the correlations are not large, given the moderate degrees of freedom on which they are calculated $(n - s = 17)$, and the uniform covariance assumption should be a reasonable one in this case. One advantage of using this estimate of Σ is that we can test for particular covariance structures using procedures developed for simple sample dispersion matrices. So we can apply, for example, the test for uniformity (Morrison, 1986, Section 7.3). In this case we get a likelihood ratio goodness-of-fit statistic of 4·49 on 4 degrees of freedom. Although this test provides no evidence of departures from uniformity it should be noted that the residual degrees of freedom associated with the dispersion matrix are not large and there are only three repeated measurements. In these circumstances the test is not particularly powerful.

We can substitute this dispersion matrix into (7.11) to obtain an unbiased estimate of the dispersion matrix of the effects of interest. We must of course decide first which effects are to be included in the analysis and how these are to be parameterized. We shall include in ξ the direct treatment and first-order carry-over effects (4 degrees of freedom altogether) and represent these in terms of the $B - A$ and $C - A$ differences. These are the effects that we would obtain from a regression analysis that constrained the first level of each factor to be zero. Other representations could be used if desired, and would suit our present purposes equally well. The OLS estimates of these four effects are:

$\hat{t}_2 - \hat{t}_1$	$\hat{t}_3 - \hat{t}_1$	$\hat{\lambda}_2 - \hat{\lambda}_1$	$\hat{\lambda}_3 - \hat{\lambda}_1$
$-25 \cdot 01$	$-12 \cdot 05$	$3 \cdot 89$	$0 \cdot 35$

Note that these are obtained using within-subject information only, that is with fixed subject or sequence effects in the model. We can now write down the estimated dispersion matrix of these effects, and these are given in Table 7.3(a). The variances within the two pairs of effects (direct treatment and carry-over) are very similar. This reflects the fact that the design is close to balance in the Williams sense; each sequence has replication 4 apart from CAB which has 3. The addition of the extra sequence would produce a Williams design for which all normalized direct treatment contrasts and all normalized carry-over contrasts would have the same variances, irrespective of the covariance structure.

Given the absence of any obvious large departures from uniformity we might expect to get similar estimates of the variances and

Table 7.3 *Estimates of the dispersion matrix of the OLS direct treatment and carry-over effects from Example 5.1.* (1) $\hat{t}_2 - \hat{t}_1$, (2) $\hat{t}_3 - \hat{t}_1$, (3) $\hat{\lambda}_2 - \hat{\lambda}_1$, (4) $\hat{\lambda}_3 - \hat{\lambda}_1$

(a) *Calculated using the within-sequence sample dispersion matrix*

(1)	26·33			
(2)	0·48	26·26		
(3)	0·28	0·17	40·72	
(4)	0·09	0·31	0·51	44·10
	(1)	(2)	(3)	(4)

(b) *Calculated from the standard ANOVA analysis with fixed subject effects*

(1)	31·02			
(2)	0·48	31·39		
(3)	0·42	0·24	54·77	
(4)	0·17	0·44	0·50	58·82
	(1)	(2)	(3)	(4)

(c) *Calculated using both within- and between-sequence information*

(1)	25·96			
(2)	0·48	25·57		
(3)	0·30	0·17	33·97	
(4)	0·09	0·33	0·51	36·98
	(1)	(2)	(3)	(4)

covariances from the OLS analysis. Using the methods of Section 5.9 we obtain the values of these given in Table 7.3(b). The variances from the OLS analysis are somewhat larger than those in Table 7.3(a), but not greatly so. The largest difference is about 30%.

The variances and correlations in Table 7.3(a) are statistically independent of the estimated effects and we can therefore apply asymptotic normal theory directly to produce test statistics and confidence intervals based on these.

Although the method above is convenient to use, it does ignore the information on Σ which is contained in the residuals associated with the sequence-period means. This information becomes increasingly important as the sequence replication decreases and, in the extreme case in which each sequence only occurs once, it is the only information we have about Σ. We can obtain an unbiased estimate of Σ which incorporates this information by equating the sums of squares and cross-products of the residuals with their expectations in terms of the elements of Σ. Patterson (1971) suggested this approach but did not pursue the details for the general case. The vector of residuals from the jth period means is

$$\mathbf{z}_j = \mathbf{r}^{-\delta}\mathbf{H}(\bar{\mathbf{y}}_j - \mathbf{A}_j\hat{\boldsymbol{\xi}})$$

and the sum of cross-products with the residuals from the kth period is

$$R_{jk} = \mathbf{z}_j^{\mathrm{T}}\mathbf{r}^{\delta}\mathbf{z}_k$$
$$= (\bar{\mathbf{y}}_j - \mathbf{A}_j\hat{\boldsymbol{\xi}})^{\mathrm{T}}\mathbf{H}(\bar{\mathbf{y}}_k - \mathbf{A}_k\hat{\boldsymbol{\xi}})$$

Setting $k = j$ gives the expression for the sum of squares $R_{jj} = \mathbf{z}_j^{\mathrm{T}}\mathbf{r}^{\delta}\mathbf{z}_j$. Taking expectations we get

$$E[R_{jk}] = (s-1)\sigma_{jk} - \sum_{u=1}^{p}\sigma_{ju}D_{uk} - \sum_{u=1}^{p}\sigma_{ku}D_{uj} + \sum_{u=1}^{p}\sum_{v=1}^{p}\sigma_{uv}E_{uv,jk}$$

$$(7.12)$$

where

$$D_{ab} = \sum_{u=1}^{p}f_{ua}\operatorname{tr}(\mathbf{V}_{\xi}\mathbf{A}_u^{\mathrm{T}}\mathbf{H}\mathbf{A}_b)$$

and

$$E_{ab,jk} = \sum_{u=1}^{p}\sum_{v=1}^{p}f_{ua}f_{bv}\operatorname{tr}(\mathbf{V}_{\xi}\mathbf{A}_j^{\mathrm{T}}\mathbf{H}\mathbf{A}_k\mathbf{V}_{\xi}\mathbf{A}_v^{\mathrm{T}}\mathbf{H}\mathbf{A}_u)$$

for

$$f_{ab} = \begin{cases} (p-1)p^{-1} & a = b \\ -p^{-1} & a \neq b \end{cases}$$

and $\mathbf{V}_{\xi}$ as defined in (7.6) with $\sigma^{jj'}$ set equal to $f_{jj'}$. We also have the corresponding within-sequence sums of cross-products S_{jk}, the (j,k)th element of $\mathbf{S}$, with expectation $(n-s)\sigma_{jk}$. Adding R_{jk} and S_{jk} and equating the sum with its expectation, we get one of $\frac{1}{2}p(p+1)$

linear equations for the unbiased estimates $\{\tilde{\sigma}_{jk}\}$ of $\{\sigma_{jk}\}$:

$$S_{jk} + R_{jk} = (n-1)\tilde{\sigma}_{jk} - \sum_{u=1}^{p} \tilde{\sigma}_{ju}D_{uk} - \sum_{u=1}^{p} \tilde{\sigma}_{ku}D_{uj} + \sum_{u=1}^{p}\sum_{v=1}^{p} \tilde{\sigma}_{uv}E_{uv,jk}$$

$$j = 1,\ldots,p; \quad k = 1,\ldots,j \quad (7.13)$$

or

$$\mathbf{s}_v + \mathbf{r}_v = \mathbf{Q}\tilde{\sigma}_v$$

where $\mathbf{s}_v, \mathbf{r}_v$ and $\tilde{\sigma}_v$ are vectors of dimension $\frac{1}{2}p(p+1)$ containing the elements S_{jk}, R_{jk} and $\tilde{\sigma}_{jk}$ in a consistent order, and $\mathbf{Q}$ is the $\frac{1}{2}p(p+1) \times \frac{1}{2}p(p+1)$ matrix of coefficients from the equations in (7.13). Assuming that $\mathbf{Q}$ is nonsingular, we have the unbiased estimators of the covariance elements:

$$\tilde{\sigma}_v = \mathbf{Q}^{-1}(\mathbf{s}_v + \mathbf{r}_v)$$

From the elements of $\tilde{\sigma}_v$ we get the unbiased estimator of Σ which we shall label $\tilde{\Sigma}$. Although there is no guarantee in general that $\mathbf{Q}$ will be invertible, this does not appear to be a problem in practice. If there are at least p sequence replicates in a design then the nonsingularity of $\mathbf{S}$ will ensure the existence of a solution, and in our experience solutions also exist for designs with little or no replication of sequences provided that they are of a practically useful size.

Using this method we can get a third estimate of the dispersion matrix for Example 5.1:

560·40		
0·39	649·77	
0·63	0·71	655·70

and substituting this in (7.13) we obtain the dispersion matrix of the estimated effects given in Table 7.3(c). The variances are very similar to those obtained using $\mathbf{S}$. The main difference is in the variances of the carry-over effects which are a little lower using the present method.

The estimates based on $\mathbf{S}$ are adequate in this case and arguably the extra complication of including the between-mean residuals is not justified given the minimal extra information on Σ that they contain. We now consider a second illustration in which the extra effort is necessary. This is provided by Example 5.2, a four-period, four-treatment design with 14 sequences, in which each sequence is replicated once only. Here all the information about Σ is provided by the residuals from the sequence-period means (in this case identical to the residuals from the raw observations). We consider the analysis of one of the measurements from this trial, the left ventricular ejection time. For further details of the trial we refer the reader back to Section 5.9. Using the above method of equating sums of squares and cross-products with their expectations we obtain the following estimate of Σ:

$$
\begin{array}{cccc}
7174{\cdot}2 & & & \\
0{\cdot}67 & 1968{\cdot}3 & & \\
0{\cdot}37 & 0{\cdot}65 & 3781{\cdot}6 & \\
0{\cdot}65 & 0{\cdot}69 & 0{\cdot}47 & 1136{\cdot}3
\end{array}
$$

There are very large changes in variance between the periods, and it is plausible that there is evidence here of a real departure from uniformity. In the light of the small sample size, however, it is difficult to make a firm judgement from a simple inspection and, given the way in which this matrix has been calculated, we cannot apply the test used previously to give a formal check for uniformity. In order to construct such a test we need to use the likelihood methods described in Section 7.6, and we consider there the question of the uniformity of the covariance structure of these data.

As in the previous example we include the direct treatment and carry-over effects in the model for the means and we again parameterize these as differences from the first treatment. The (within-subject) OLS estimates of the six effects are:

$\hat{\tau}_2 - \hat{\tau}_1$	$\hat{\tau}_3 - \hat{\tau}_1$	$\hat{\tau}_4 - \hat{\tau}_1$	$\hat{\lambda}_2 - \hat{\lambda}_1$	$\hat{\lambda}_3 - \hat{\lambda}_1$	$\hat{\lambda}_4 - \hat{\lambda}_1$
$-41{\cdot}79$	$-13{\cdot}19$	$-64{\cdot}79$	$25{\cdot}32$	$22{\cdot}73$	$5{\cdot}39$

From the estimate of Σ we obtain the estimate of the dispersion matrix of these effects given in Table 7.4(a). Again we compare this with the dispersion matrix obtained from the ANOVA analysis of Section 5.9. This is given in Table 7.4(b). The variances of the direct effects are similar, while the ANOVA-based variances of the carry-over effects are about 50% larger than the unbiased estimates. This latter difference is a consequence of the much larger observed variance in the first period. The observations from the first period contribute less to the estimate of the carry-over effects and so this variance should have less influence on the estimates of the variances of these effects. This occurs in the matrix in Table 7.4(a), but not in

Table 7.4 *Estimated dispersion matrix of the direct and carry-over effects from Example 5.2.* (1) $\hat{\tau}_2 - \hat{\tau}_1$, (2) $\hat{\tau}_3 - \hat{\tau}_1$, (3) $\hat{\tau}_4 - \hat{\tau}_1$, (4) $\hat{\lambda}_2 - \hat{\lambda}_1$, (5) $\hat{\lambda}_3 - \hat{\lambda}_1$, (6) $\hat{\lambda}_4 - \hat{\lambda}_1$

(a) *Calculated using between-sequence information*

	(1)	(2)	(3)	(4)	(5)	(6)
(1)	315·38					
(2)	0·37	379·32				
(3)	0·43	0·52	286·67			
(4)	0·37	0·46	0·01	306·89		
(5)	0·21	0·54	0·28	0·52	305·29	
(6)	−0·02	0·14	0·25	0·33	0·40	235·60
	(1)	(2)	(3)	(4)	(5)	(6)

(b) *Calculated from the standard ANOVA analysis with fixed subject effects*

	(1)	(2)	(3)	(4)	(5)	(6)
(1)	314·48					
(2)	0·52	334·66				
(3)	0·45	0·44	313·55			
(4)	0·31	0·31	0·10	476·07		
(5)	0·08	0·30	0·16	0·48	462·71	
(6)	0·11	0·04	0·30	0·42	0·44	434·06
	(1)	(2)	(3)	(4)	(5)	(6)

Table 7.4(b), because the four variances are effectively averaged in the ANOVA calculations. However, in spite of the very large differences among the variances and correlations in $\tilde{\Sigma}$, the unbiased estimate of the dispersion matrix is still not greatly different from the ANOVA-based estimate. One might conjecture that since this design is close to balance in the Williams sense, this observation should be expected from the results of Kunert (1987a) mentioned above. Arguably the differences are large enough though for the matrix in Table 7.4(a) to be considered preferable in this case.

7.5   Empirical generalized least squares (EGLS) estimation

If Σ were known then the GLS estimator defined in (7.5) would have minimum variance among unbiased estimators and an analysis based on it would be the appropriate one to use. In practice of course Σ is not known, but we have seen in the previous section how it can be estimated from the data. When the uniform error assumption is not appropriate we could use such an estimate in place of the true Σ in (7.5) in an attempt to improve over the precision of the OLS estimators used above and in Section 5.9. It should be noted, however, that there is no guarantee that such an EGLS estimator will be more precise than the corresponding OLS estimator. The relative precision of the two estimators depends on the design of the trial, the model fitted and on Σ. The precision with which Σ is estimated is critical and in small trials it is the additional variation introduced by this that can on occasion lead to a decrease in precision in comparison with ordinary least squares. One problem with the EGLS approach at the moment is the current lack of knowledge about the behaviour of such estimators in small trials, making assessment of their comparative value rather difficult. Once again, however, the two-treatment dual-sequence designs form a special case, and for these we are able to provide a complete EGLS analysis. We consider such trials first before moving on to the general case.

7.5.1 Two-treatment designs

For the two-treatment designs we shall change the notation slightly. We divide the parameters in the linear model into two sets, (1) those defining effects which are constant across-sequences (overall constant and period effects), $\boldsymbol{\beta}_1$ say, and (2) those that make comparisons between the sequences (direct treatment, carry-over, sequence, and so on), $\boldsymbol{\beta}_2$ say. By symmetry we can then write

$$E[\bar{\mathbf{y}}_{(1)}] = [\mathbf{X}_1, \mathbf{X}_2] \begin{bmatrix} \boldsymbol{\beta}_1 \\ \boldsymbol{\beta}_2 \end{bmatrix} \quad \text{and} \quad E[\bar{\mathbf{y}}_{(2)}] = [\mathbf{X}_1, -\mathbf{X}_2] \begin{bmatrix} \boldsymbol{\beta}_1 \\ \boldsymbol{\beta}_2 \end{bmatrix}$$

for suitable choices of the design matrices $\mathbf{X}_1$ and $\mathbf{X}_2$. From this we get, after some manipulation, the GLS estimator of $\boldsymbol{\beta}_2$:

$$\hat{\boldsymbol{\beta}}_{2(\text{GLS})} = (\mathbf{X}_2^T \Sigma^{-1} \mathbf{X}_2)^{-1} \mathbf{X}_2^T \Sigma^{-1} (\bar{\mathbf{y}}_{(1)} - \bar{\mathbf{y}}_{(2)}) \qquad (7.14)$$

Suppose that we have a model with as many independent parameters as there are sequence-by-period means ($2p$ in this case). Such a model can always be constructed, even if some parameters represent effects that are not of direct interest. We shall describe such a model as **saturated**, noting that this term is sometimes also used for models with as many parameters as observations. To simplify the exposition we shall be assuming that the models contain sequence effects rather than fixed subject effects. As shown in the appendix to this chapter, either approach leads ultimately to the same estimates of the direct treatment, carry-over and direct-by-period interaction effects. Since we are including period effects, X_1 will always have maximum rank p. Whether or not a model is saturated will therefore depend on the rank of X_2. (We are assuming as previously that the model is not over-parameterized, that is, the number of columns of the design matrix equals its rank.) A saturated model arises if X_2 is also of rank p. An example is the model for a three-period design which includes sequence, direct treatment and first-order carry-over effects. It is clear from (7.14) that OLS and GLS estimators of β_2 coincide under a saturated model.

To obtain the EGLS estimator from (7.14) we simply replace Σ by the within-sequence dispersion matrix S defined in Section 7.4. Using a standard matrix equality (Rao, 1967, Lemma 2b) we can rewrite the resulting estimator in the form

$$\hat{\beta}_{2(EGLS)} = (X_2^T X_2)^{-1} X_2^T (\bar{y}_{(1)} - \bar{y}_{(2)}) \\ - (X_2^T X_2)^{-1} X_2^T SQ (Q^T SQ)^{-1} Q^T (\bar{y}_{(1)} - \bar{y}_{(2)}) \quad (7.15)$$

where Q is any $p \times (p - r)$ matrix of full rank that satisfies $Q^T X_2 = 0$, for r the rank of X_2. In particular, if we obtain X_2 by dropping parameters from a saturated model, defined by X_{2S} say, then the rows of Q can be chosen as the rows of $(X_{2S})^{-1}$ that correspond to the dropped parameters. We can then give a direct interpretation to the components on the right-hand side of (7.15). The first component,

$$(X_2^T X_2)^{-1} X_2^T (\bar{y}_{(1)} - \bar{y}_{(2)})$$

is the OLS estimator of β_2, $\hat{\beta}_{2(OLS)}$ say, from the original model. Denoting the parameters dropped from the saturated model by β_d, it can be seen that in the second component, $Q^T (\bar{y}_{(1)} - \bar{y}_{(2)})$ is the OLS (and GLS) estimator of β_d from the saturated model. Denote this by $\hat{\beta}_{dS}$. Finally, the term $Q^T SQ$ ($= S_{22}$ say) is the sample dispersion matrix of $\hat{\beta}_{dS}$ and the elements of $(X_2^T X_2)^{-1} X_2^T SQ$ ($= S_{12}$ say), are the sample covariances between the elements of $\hat{\beta}_{2(OLS)}$ and $\hat{\beta}_{dS}$. Hence $\hat{\beta}_{2(EGLS)}$ can be recognized as a covariate-adjusted estimator with regression coefficients $S_{12} S_{22}^{-1}$. That is,

$$\hat{\beta}_{2(EGLS)} = \hat{\beta}_{2(OLS)} - S_{12} S_{22}^{-1} \hat{\beta}_{dS}$$

This result means that we can use standard analysis-of-covariance procedures to construct an EGLS analysis of data from a two-sequence, two-treatment trial. The dependent variate for each effect is defined by the contrast among each subject's observations that corresponds to that particular effect. These are just the variates used in Sections 4.7 and 4.9. To define the covariates it is necessary to add parameters to the model in order to achieve saturation. Often there will be an obvious choice for these, although any selection will serve. The contrasts corresponding to the least squares estimates of these additional parameters are then calculated from each subject and the resulting $p - r$ sets of values constitute the covariates. The EGLS estimator $\hat{\beta}_{2(\text{EGLS})}$, its standard error, and associated tests and confidence intervals are then obtained through an orthodox analysis of covariance comparing the two sequence groups.

As an illustration we take the 2×2 cross-over with baseline measurements and, using the results in Kenward and Jones (1987b), we give the EGLS alternative to the analysis described in Section 2.9. In this case $p = 4$ and, including the direct treatment, first- and second-order carry-over and sequence effects, we have a saturated model. As in Section 2.9 we can fit a sequence of models, omitting terms in order as they are found to be negligible. The models used in Section 2.9 also included sequence effects. One reason for this is to ensure that the other elements of β_2 are estimated within subjects, eliminating between-subject variation. When we move to EGLS estimation this role for the sequence (or subject) effects is no longer necessary. Implicitly we are weighting the between- and within-subject components according to their observed comparative variability. However, there is another reason for including the sequence effects. In small trials it is possible to get effects associated with sequence purely through bad luck with the randomization. Provided that the other effects do not interact with the sequence

Table 7.5 *Variates needed for the EGLS analyses of the 2×2 cross-over with baseline measurements (for a definition of the parameters see Section 2.9)*

Parameter	Other parameters in addition to β_2	Dependent variate	Covariate
θ	τ, λ	$\frac{1}{2}X_2$	X_1
λ	τ	$\frac{1}{2}(Y_1 + Y_2)$	X_1, X_2
τ		$\frac{1}{4}(Y_2 - Y_1)$	$X_1, X_2, Y_1 + Y_2$
λ	τ, sequence	$\frac{1}{2}(X_1 - Y_1 + X_2 - Y_2)$	$X_1 - X_2$
τ	sequence	$\frac{1}{4}(Y_2 - Y_1)$	$(X_1 - Y_1 + X_2 - Y_2), (X_1 - X_2)$

Run-in (X_1), first treatment (Y_1), wash-out (X_2) and second treatment (Y_2) measurements.

Table 7.6 *EGLS and OLS estimates from Example 2.1 (for a definition of the parameters see Section 2.9)*

Parameter	OLS estimate (s.e.)	EGLS estimate (s.e.)
θ	−0·045 (0·092)	0·004 (0·096)
λ	0·071 (0·140)	0·094 (0·143)
τ	0·088 (0·044)	0·082 (0·034)

differences, the analysis remains valid if the sequence effects are included in the model. Hence with EGLS we can choose either to include or to omit the sequence effects. Each choice leads to a different set of EGLS estimators. In Table 7.5 are listed the contrasts that define the dependent variate and covariate(s) for various EGLS estimators that might be used in the analysis of data from a 2×2 cross-over trial with baseline measurements. Note that there is some ambiguity in the definition of the covariates because any nonsingular linear combination of them will lead to effectively the same analysis.

We summarize the results of the EGLS analysis (without sequence effect) for Example 2.1 in Table 7.6 where the various EGLS estimates are listed together with their standard errors. As a comparison we also include the OLS estimates with standard errors as calculated in Section 2.9. We note a few points from these results. In this case the use of EGLS changes the estimates very little from the previous OLS values. Two standard errors are slightly larger (for $\hat{\theta}_{EGLS}$ and $\hat{\lambda}_{EGLS}$) while the third (for $\hat{\tau}_{EGLS}$) is about 21% smaller than that of the OLS estimate. This underlines the point that the use of EGLS does not necessarily improve the precision of an estimate. As with the use of any covariate, the sizes of correlations between the dependent variate and covariates are critical. It might be argued that the estimate with the smallest standard error should be chosen. However, as Kenward (1985) shows, this can lead, although not necessarily, to a large underestimate of the true standard error of the resulting choice of estimate. Such bias increases with increasing numbers of covariates and decreasing residual degrees of freedom. Typically the two-sequence cross-over designs that we are considering here will not have many periods, rarely more than four or five. Since the number of covariates involved in EGLS estimation can be at most $p - 1$, such bias will probably not be too serious.

If we have a two-treatment trial which consists of more than one dual pair of sequences then, for effects that can be estimated separately from each dual pair, we can apply the same *ad hoc* technique used in Section 4.9 to obtain EGLS estimates from the whole trial: the EGLS estimates from each dual pair are combined using the inverses of their estimated variances as weights.

As a final point, the sequence of analysis of covariance tests for the p parameters that are associated with the columns of X_{2S} constitute a partition into statistically independent components of the overall normal-based likelihood ratio test for the combined sequence main effect and sequence-by-period interaction.

7.5.2 Higher-order designs

We now consider EGLS estimation for higher-order designs. For any estimate, $\hat{\Sigma}$ say, of Σ we can simply write down the corresponding EGLS estimate of ξ by substituting the estimate for Σ in (7.5). An obvious estimate to use is S, but we could also attempt to model the structure of Σ. If an appropriate model is chosen then the resulting estimate should in some sense be more 'precise' than S and this in turn should lead to a more precise estimate of ξ. The modelling of covariance structures constitutes an entire subject of its own: Jöreskog (1981) provides an introductory survey, and given the limitations of space we can do little more than mention it in passing. Commonly, models for covariance structures are fitted using maximum likelihood procedures and we include some examples in the next section under the general heading of likelihood methods. We note that the covariance models fitted later could also be used here.

As an illustration we can use S to obtain EGLS estimates of the effects from Example 5.1, the three-period trial used in the previous section, for which S is given in Table 7.3(a). Substituting this estimate for Σ in the formula for the GLS estimator we obtain the values given in Table 7.7, with the OLS estimates for comparison.

Table 7.7 *EGLS and OLS estimates from Example 5.1*

Effect	OLS estimate	EGLS estimate
$\hat{\tau}_2 - \hat{\tau}_1$	$-25{\cdot}01$	$-21{\cdot}93$
$\hat{\tau}_3 - \hat{\tau}_1$	$-12{\cdot}05$	$-9{\cdot}49$
$\hat{\lambda}_2 - \hat{\lambda}_1$	$3{\cdot}89$	$2{\cdot}58$
$\hat{\lambda}_3 - \hat{\lambda}_1$	$0{\cdot}35$	$-0{\cdot}17$

In this case the difference between the two sets of estimates does not appear to be important, given the standard errors of the OLS estimates, but clearly we also need reliable standard errors for the EGLS estimates to be able to make a useful comparison. Unfortunately there is no finite-sample formula for these, and this leads us to the main problem with EGLS in higher-order cross-over trials: the estimation of standard errors in 'small' trials.

It is not difficult to see that for any consistent estimator of Σ that is independent of the sequence-period means, the corresponding EGLS estimator has an asymptotic multivariate normal distribution with the dispersion matrix V_ξ defined in (7.6). Furthermore, a consistent estimator of V_ξ is obtained by substituting $\hat{\Sigma}$ for Σ in these expressions. The EGLS estimator and its estimated asymptotic dispersion matrix are asymptotically independent and so standard asymptotic procedures can be used for drawing inferences. In particular, S or any consistent estimator calculated wholly from it, can be used in this way. (It is not so clear, however, whether $\tilde{\Sigma}$, defined in the previous section, can similarly be used, because it is not independent of the sequence-period means.) If, in the example, we substitute S for Σ we get the estimated asymptotic dispersion matrix of the four effects, in the same order as above:

$$
\begin{array}{llll}
22 \cdot 98 & & & \\
0 \cdot 48 & 22 \cdot 76 & & \\
0 \cdot 28 & 0 \cdot 16 & 35 \cdot 71 & \\
0 \cdot 09 & 0 \cdot 30 & 0 \cdot 51 & 38 \cdot 36
\end{array}
$$

Comparing this with the unbiased estimate of the dispersion matrix of the OLS estimates (Table 7.3(a)) we see little difference. The EGLS variances above are slightly smaller, although even this small difference disappears if we take the other estimated OLS dispersion matrix in Table 7.3(c). However, it is not clear how close an approximation the asymptotic result provides in this case, so comparing the precision of the OLS and EGLS estimates in this way may not be very meaningful.

If a trial is large enough to justify the use of asymptotic results then the EGLS procedure presents few problems. The questions remaining then are how to define 'large' in this context, and how to obtain reliable estimates of the precision of EGLS estimators from 'small' trials. We are able to obtain finite-sample results for the two-sequence designs because the symmetry between the two sequences allows the application of standard results from repeated-measurement analysis. For these designs we can write down the unconditional dispersion matrix of $\hat{\boldsymbol{\xi}}$, that is, after taking expectations over the 'covariates'. It is

$$\frac{n-3}{n-3-p+r}\mathbf{V}_\xi,$$

(Kenward, 1985, p. 23). We see that the asymptotic dispersion matrix $\mathbf{V}_\xi$ is biased downwards in finite samples, but not greatly so, considering that $p-r$ will rarely be larger than 3. It is plausible that such underestimation will be carried over to the higher-order designs. Unfortunately the symmetry that allows the calculation of this result is lost in higher-order designs and so, at the moment, there are no clear guidelines concerning the finite-sample behaviour of EGLS estimators or on the appropriate calculation of their precision.

7.6 Likelihood methods

We have already made use of likelihood methods in earlier chapters. Maximum likelihood (ML) estimators and likelihood ratio (LR) tests were used explicitly with the log-linear models for categorical data. Also, given a uniform error structure, the OLS methods used in earlier chapters can be included in the class of likelihood methods. The methods are very flexible and are used in most areas of statistical analysis. However, their advantageous properties are, in general, asymptotic (the OLS methods used earlier are an exception to this) and in this section we must resort to asymptotic results to derive appropriate techniques. This leaves open the question of the behaviour of the following procedures in small samples. Apart from computation, this is their main drawback at the moment.

We begin by writing down the log likelihood for a set of data from a cross-over trial in which each subject supplies a complete set of measurements. We are assuming that the observations have a joint normal distribution.

$$\log l = \text{constant} - \tfrac{1}{2}n\log|\mathbf{\Sigma}|$$

$$- \tfrac{1}{2}\sum_{i=1}^{s}\sum_{k=1}^{n_i}(\mathbf{y}_{(i)k} - \boldsymbol{\pi} - \mathbf{A}_{(i)}\boldsymbol{\xi})^{\mathrm{T}}\mathbf{\Sigma}^{-1}(\mathbf{y}_{(i)k} - \boldsymbol{\pi} - \mathbf{A}_{(i)}\boldsymbol{\xi})$$

We can maximize this to obtain estimates of the parameters, both associated with the design (π and ξ) and with the dispersion matrix Σ. A structure can be imposed on Σ or alternatively all $\frac{1}{2}p(p+1)$ dispersion parameters can be estimated. The properties of maximum likelihood estimators in general are discussed in Kendall, Stuart and Ord (1979, Chapter 18). Given certain regularity conditions there will exist a unique maximum to the likelihood, with corresponding unique parameter estimates, and these conditions are likely to hold in practice for the types of model considered here unless a particularly awkward structure is chosen for Σ. Hence the problem of obtaining ML estimates is largely a matter here of computational technique.

Some authors have considered the problem of the maximization of the likelihood above for certain specific designs. Almost invariably some form of iterative procedure is required. Patel (1985) uses ML estimators of effects for the 2×2 cross-over trial with missing values (see Section 2.11) and derives both large- and small sample-procedures based on these. Taka and Armitage (1983) and Gill and Shukla (1987) both obtain maximum likelihood estimates for their autoregressive models, while Bora (1984, 1985) writes down expressions that could be used to obtain estimates for the designs and autoregressive models that he considers (see Section 7.3). These authors have tended to use modifications of the Newton–Raphson algorithm, which involves the calculation of second-order derivatives of the log likelihood, and typically these procedures are computationally efficient. Although this can be tedious, it is not particularly difficult and could be done in principle for any model and design. However, this is not really feasible for routine work for which one would like to be able to take any design and compare the fit of different models without having to make large computational modifications for each change of design or model. For this an adaptable and flexible approach is needed. A simple method which allows this, but which is less efficient with respect to computer time, is **repeated substitution**. This method is used by Patel (1986), who considers likelihood methods under an unconstrained covariance structure, for a class of problems containing the cross-over trial as one important special case.

We can conveniently and naturally separate the parameters in the log likelihood above into those associated with the design (defining the means) and those associated with the covariance structure (defining Σ). We shall denote these by $\boldsymbol{\beta} = (\beta_1, \ldots, \beta_u)^T$ and $\boldsymbol{\phi} = (\phi_1, \ldots, \phi_v)^T$ respectively. The latter can be regarded as nuisance parameters: we would like to fit a parsimonious model to the co-variance structure, but the actual parameters of the structure are unlikely to be of great interest in themselves. The other parameters $\beta_1, \ldots, \beta_u$ comprise $\pi_1^*, \ldots, \pi_p^*$ and $\xi_1, \ldots, \xi_g$, the ξ_i representing the effects of direct interest.

The iterative routine to be used maximizes the likelihood with respect to each of these parameters in turn, the other set being held constant. Each of the two stages of this cycle takes a particularly simple and familiar form. The method can be regarded as a generalization of iteratively reweighted least squares. If Σ were known, the ML estimator of ξ would be the GLS estimator $\hat{\xi}$ defined in (7.5). The associated ML estimator of π_j^* would be

$$\hat{\pi}_j^* = n^{-1} \sum_{i=1}^{s} \sum_{k=1}^{n_i} y_{ijk} - n^{-1} \mathbf{A}_j \hat{\xi} \tag{7.16}$$

On the other hand, for given β the MLE of Σ is obtained by minimizing

$$\log|\Sigma^{-1}| - \operatorname{tr} \mathbf{S}_\beta \Sigma^{-1} \tag{7.17}$$

with respect to ϕ, where

$$\mathbf{S}_\beta = n^{-1} \sum_{i=1}^{s} \sum_{k=1}^{n_i} (\mathbf{y}_{(i)k} - \pi - \mathbf{A}_{(i)}\xi)(\mathbf{y}_{(i)k} - \pi - \mathbf{A}_{(i)}\xi)^{\mathrm{T}} \tag{7.18}$$

The function (7.17) can be recognized as that arising from the likelihood of a Wishart distribution on n degrees of freedom, with the Wishart matrix replaced by $n\mathbf{S}_\beta$. The corresponding equations that need to be solved to obtain the MLE of ϕ are

$$\frac{\partial \Sigma^{-1}}{\partial \phi_i}(\Sigma - \mathbf{S}_\beta), \qquad i = 1, \ldots, s \tag{7.19}$$

Many standard routines exist for solving these equations for par-ticular structures; see Jöreskog (1981) for a discussion of the general problem and Kenward (1981), Jennrich and Schluchter (1986) and Kenward and Jones (1987b) for routines and structures that are particularly appropriate in the present context. If no structure is imposed on Σ then its estimate is just $\mathbf{S}_\beta$.

The overall procedure is as follows. A starting value for β is obtained. An obvious choice is the OLS estimate. Using this, $\mathbf{S}_\beta$ is calculated from (7.18) and an estimate of ϕ obtained from the solutions to (7.19). The Σ corresponding to the current estimate of

ϕ is substituted into (7.5) and (7.16) to obtain an updated estimate of β. The process is repeated until the estimates of both β and ϕ converge to some required degree of accuracy. The advantage of this method is the separation of the two types of estimation. It is simple to change the model for the means, for example to drop carry-over parameters, or to change the covariance structure, without changing the overall form of the routine. In practice convergence has been acceptably fast.

The use of maximum likelihood estimates leads naturally to the construction of LR tests (Kendall, Stuart and Ord, 1979, Chapter 24). For a model defined by a subset of parameters, β_0 and ϕ_0 say, of β and ϕ we have the log LR statistic

$$\Lambda = -2n[\log l(\hat{\beta}, \hat{\phi}) - \log l(\hat{\beta}_0, \hat{\phi}_0)]$$

where $\log l(\hat{\alpha})$ is the maximized log likelihood for the model defined by the parameters α. Assuming that the model defined by β_0 and ϕ_0 is adequate, Λ has asymptotic χ_w^2 distribution, where w is the number of parameters omitted from β and ϕ to obtain β_0 and ϕ_0. In practice of course we may well have either $\beta = \beta_0$ or $\phi = \phi_0$. The small-sample χ^2 approximation could perhaps be improved through the use of an appropriate Bartlett correction factor (Bartlett, 1954).

The log LR takes a particularly simple form in the current situation. It can be shown that, for covariance structures that are reasonably well behaved, at the maximum of the likelihood

$$\text{tr}\,\hat{\Sigma}^{-1}S_{\hat{\beta}} = p$$

(Bock and Bargmann, 1966, p. 521; Kenward, 1981), where $S_{\hat{\beta}}$ is S_β evaluated at $\hat{\beta}$. It follows that

$$\Lambda = -n[\log l[|\hat{\Sigma}_0^{-1}|] - \log l[|\hat{\Sigma}^{-1}|]]$$

Likelihood ratios can also be used to construct confidence intervals for parameters; see for example, Cox and Hinkley (1974, Section 7.2).

From the form of the likelihood and the asymptotic properties of ML estimators it can also be shown that, for an adequate model, $\hat{\beta}$ and $\hat{\Sigma}$ are asymptotically independent and $\hat{\xi}$ has asymptotic dispersion matrix given by the GLS dispersion matrix V_ξ defined in (7.6). This means that alternative tests and confidence intervals (or regions) can be constructed for a set of elements of ξ using the corresponding estimated submatrix of V_ξ (sometimes called **Wald** statistics; see for example, Wald, 1943). For a subset $\hat{\xi}_1$ ($w \times 1$) of $\hat{\xi}$

with corresponding estimated asymptotic dispersion matrix $\hat{\mathbf{V}}_{\xi 1}$,

$$(\hat{\boldsymbol{\xi}}_1 - \boldsymbol{\xi}_1)^{\mathrm{T}} \hat{\mathbf{V}}_{\xi 1}^{-1} (\hat{\boldsymbol{\xi}}_1 - \boldsymbol{\xi}_1)$$

has an asymptotic χ_w^2. The test statistic obtained by setting $\boldsymbol{\xi}_1 = \mathbf{0}$ is asymptotically equivalent to the LR statistic defined earlier for $\boldsymbol{\xi} = (\boldsymbol{\xi}_0^{\mathrm{T}}, \boldsymbol{\xi}_1^{\mathrm{T}})^{\mathrm{T}}$ and $\boldsymbol{\phi}_0 = \boldsymbol{\phi}$.

Patel (1986) considers both these types of statistic with unconstrained $\boldsymbol{\Sigma}$ and attempts to improve on the simple asymptotic χ^2 approximation for certain particular tests. He works by analogy with the MANOVA case and supposes that particular transformations of $\mathbf{S}_{\hat{\beta}}$ are approximately proportional to Wishart matrices. This is certainly plausible, and it allows Patel to derive F-approximations for certain classes of hypothesis test. At the moment these approximations are conjectural and it would be interesting to assess their accuracy from a simulation study. If found to perform adequately they could prove to be very useful.

We now apply these likelihood methods to the two examples used in Sections 7.4 and 7.5. Recall that the first, Example 5.1, is a three-period, three-treatment cross-over trial with 23 subjects and with systolic blood pressure as the measurement under analysis. In Section 7.4 the within-sequence dispersion matrix $\mathbf{S}$ was used to check for uniformity of the covariance structure of these data, and the null hypothesis was not rejected. We can now test the same hypothesis using a LR test based on all the information. We include both direct treatment and carry-over effects in $\boldsymbol{\beta}$ (in this case $\boldsymbol{\beta} = \boldsymbol{\beta}_0$) and compare the fit of the unconstrained covariance structure ($\boldsymbol{\phi}$ of dimension 6) with the uniform structure ($\boldsymbol{\phi}_0$ of dimension 2). By maximizing the likelihood under the two alternative covariance structures we get the log LR statistic

$$\Lambda = -23[18 \cdot 0563 - 18 \cdot 2378] = 4 \cdot 49$$

on $6 - 2 = 4$ degrees of freedom. As before, there is no reason to reject the null hypothesis; the uniform structure appears adequate in this case. As a comparison with $\mathbf{S}$ and $\tilde{\boldsymbol{\Sigma}}$ we give the unconstrained ML estimate of $\boldsymbol{\Sigma}$:

$$
\begin{array}{lll}
540 \cdot 28 & & \\
0 \cdot 41 & 629 \cdot 04 & \\
0 \cdot 64 & 0 \cdot 70 & 680 \cdot 61
\end{array}
$$

The correlations are similar to those of both $\mathbf{S}$ and $\tilde{\boldsymbol{\Sigma}}$, and the variances are somewhat smaller. It is known that in saturated models the unconstrained ML estimate of Σ is $\mathbf{S}$ with expectation $[(n-s)/n]\Sigma$. It is reasonable to suppose that the ML estimate from unsaturated models will also be biased downwards to some extent, but we cannot at the moment say by how much. If ξ is set to zero, the ML estimator has expectation $[(n-1)/n]\Sigma$ and so an approximate correction for the bias might be found between the two ratios $n/(n-s)$ and $n/(n-1)$. It is not to be expected, however, that the expectation of $\hat{\Sigma}$ will be exactly proportional to Σ, as in these two special cases.

Having accepted the uniform covariance structure for these data, the OLS/ANOVA analysis of Section 5.9 is appropriate. However, it is interesting to see how the ML estimates of the effects differ from those obtained previously. We can obtain these under an unconstrained or uniform covariance structure. We do not include sequence effects in the model, so the latter will not coincide with the OLS estimates obtained previously. The estimates of the effects are presented in Table 7.8, together with their estimated standard errors, the latter being asymptotic for the ML estimates. The OLS and uniform ML estimates are very similar indeed, indicating the minimal contribution in this case of the between-subject information. The standard errors of the ML estimates are a little lower, and arguably this difference can largely be attributed to small-sample bias of the asymptotic estimates. The differences both in the estimates of the effects and their associated standard errors are larger with the ML estimates based on the unconstrained covariance structure. Recall that there are two potential sources of bias in the error estimates. The asymptotic dispersion matrix $\mathbf{V}_\xi$ will be biased to some degree (possibly small) in finite samples, and the estimate of $\mathbf{V}_\xi$ obtained

Table 7.8 *Maximum likelihood and OLS (within-subject) estimates of effects from Example 5.1 (estimated standard errors in parentheses)*

Effect	OLS (within-subjects)	Maximum likelihood Uniform Σ	Maximum likelihood Unconstrained Σ
$\hat{t}_2 - \hat{t}_1$	$-25\cdot01\,(5\cdot57)$	$-25\cdot27\,(5\cdot17)$	$-21\cdot60\,(4\cdot49)$
$\hat{t}_3 - \hat{t}_1$	$-12\cdot05\,(5\cdot60)$	$-12\cdot00\,(5\cdot20)$	$-8\cdot49\,(4\cdot45)$
$\hat{\lambda}_2 - \hat{\lambda}_1$	$3\cdot89\,(7\cdot41)$	$3\cdot16\,(6\cdot75)$	$3\cdot66\,(5\cdot44)$
$\hat{\lambda}_3 - \hat{\lambda}_1$	$0\cdot35\,(7\cdot67)$	$0\cdot52\,(6\cdot98)$	$0\cdot97\,(5\cdot65)$

through $\hat{\Sigma}$ may itself be biased. The apparent reduction in the standard errors compared with the OLS and other ML values is probably associated with both sources of bias.

We turn now to the second example, Example 5.2. Using the likelihood procedures we are now able to test formally for a uniform covariance structure, a test that we were unable to make in Section 7.4 because of the absence of within-sequence replication. Including both direct treatment and first-order carry-over effects in ξ we obtain the likelihood ratio test statistic for uniformity:

$$\Lambda = -14[28\cdot5467 - 30\cdot2158] = 23\cdot37$$

on 8 degrees of freedom. The corresponding probability is 0·003 and clearly we must reject the hypothesis of uniformity. The ML estimate of Σ is

$$
\begin{array}{llll}
7796\cdot0 & & & \\
0\cdot69 & 1929\cdot6 & & \\
0\cdot42 & 0\cdot72 & 4437\cdot0 & \\
0\cdot54 & 0\cdot54 & 0\cdot54 & 1284\cdot4
\end{array}
$$

This is close to the estimate $\tilde{\Sigma}$ obtained in Section 7.4 and it would appear to be the large differences among the variances that are the cause of the rejection of uniformity. Given this, the stationary autoregressive structure defined in Section 7.3 is unlikely to offer any improvement over the uniform structure and this is indeed the case: we have $\Lambda = 22\cdot331$ on 7 degrees of freedom for the comparison of the autoregressive and unconstrained structures. There is no other obvious structure to use which might lead to a worthwhile reduction in the dimension of ϕ so we shall continue with the unconstrained structure.

Next we examine the ML estimates of the elements of ξ. These are given in Table 7.9 with their associated asymptotic standard errors, together with the OLS estimates for comparison. As might be expected from the clear non-uniformity of the dispersion matrix there are notable differences between the ML and OLS estimates and between the corresponding standard errors. The ML standard errors are about 30% smaller, but again we would expect these to be biased downwards.

In the absence of uniformity, the OLS analysis in Section 5.9 is not valid and we need to use alternatives to the ANOVA tests, in particular for the overall tests for first-order carry-over and direct

Table 7.9 *Maximum likelihood and OLS (within-subject) estimates of the effects from Example 5.2 (estimated standard errors in parentheses)*

Effect	OLS (within-subjects)	ML (unconstrained Σ)
$\hat{t}_2 - \hat{t}_1$	$-41.79\,(17.73)$	$-38.88\,(12.76)$
$\hat{t}_3 - \hat{t}_1$	$-13.19\,(18.29)$	$-22.61\,(14.12)$
$\hat{t}_4 - \hat{t}_1$	$-64.79\,(17.71)$	$-59.40\,(12.10)$
$\hat{\lambda}_2 - \hat{\lambda}_1$	$25.32\,(21.82)$	$21.41\,(13.66)$
$\hat{\lambda}_3 - \hat{\lambda}_1$	$22.73\,(21.51)$	$38.56\,(13.94)$
$\hat{\lambda}_4 - \hat{\lambda}_1$	$5.39\,(20.83)$	$5.66\,(12.90)$

treatment effects. The log LR statistic for the former is

$$\Lambda = -14[29.3335 - 29.8477] = 7.20$$

on 3 degrees of freedom, with corresponding probability 0·07. Again we note that without a correction factor the χ^2 approximation may not be good in such a small sample. Taking the test at face value, however, there is some weak evidence for a carry-over effect. Similarly, the statistic for direct treatment effects, not adjusted for carry-over effects, is

$$\Lambda = -14[30.6397 - 29.3335] = 18.29$$

on 3 degrees of freedom, with corresponding probability close to 10^{-5}. The evidence of a direct treatment effect is overwhelming, and we can interpret this result through the effects given in Table 7.9 or alternatively from estimates obtained after dropping the carry-over effects from the model.

So far we have assumed that each subject provides a complete set of measurements. This allows us to use standard, and comparatively straightforward, estimating procedures within each stage of the iterative cycle described earlier. However, within the likelihood approach, we can generalize the model used in several ways. We can write, for the (i, k)th subject,

$$\mathbf{y}_{(i)k} \sim N(\mathbf{X}_{(i)k}\boldsymbol{\theta}; \boldsymbol{\Sigma}_{ik})$$

where $\mathbf{y}_{(i)k}$ has dimension q_{ik}, that is the (i, k)th subject provides q_{ik} measurements. The terms $\mathbf{X}_{(i)k}$ and $\boldsymbol{\theta}$ are respectively the subject's design matrix and a set of unknown parameters. Since each subject is associated with a particular design matrix the model can accommodate incomplete sequences of measurements, and covariates that are associated with each treatment period ('time-varying covariates'). There can also be additional repeated measurements within periods, which is just the situation considered in Chapter 6. Again these sequences can be incomplete and through $X_{(i)k}$ it is possible to model these repeated measurements with a linear function. The model can be generalized further to allow a nonlinear function to be used. In the same way as above we can also impose some structure on Σ_{ik}. However, to make progress in the estimation of the parameters in this model we require one of two conditions. Either there must be a complete set of measurements, possibly hypothetical, for which we have a parameterized dispersion matrix Σ. Each subject provides a subset of these measurements and consequently Σ_{ik} is constructed by removing rows and columns from Σ. In other words, the times of measurement are fixed although a subject may not have measurements from all times. Clearly there is also some limit to the number of parameters on which Σ may depend. Alternatively, if times of measurement are not fixed then both θ and Σ_{ik} must be functions of time.

The model can also be generalized to incorporate random effects. A subset of the parameters in θ are assumed to be random variables drawn from a further multivariate normal distribution. Such 'two-stage' models can lead to a more parsimonious representation of the covariance structure and provide a natural framework for prediction. There are also strong links between the use of these models and Bayesian analysis.

There has recently been much work on these types of general model, although only Patel (1986) refers directly to cross-over trials. For an introduction to the literature the reader is referred to Ware (1985), Jennrich and Schluchter (1986), Goldstein (1986), Berk (1987) and Louis (1988). There are also generalizations that can be used for categorical data; see for example Ware *et al.* (1988) and the references given there. Many of these authors deal with large sets of data from complex sociological and epidemiological studies and clearly a main concern is to provide manageable and efficient computing methods for obtaining ML estimators. The large size of the data sets can be used to justify the asymptotic results, the validity of which are consequently of less concern. In a cross-over trial the situation can be rather different and the small-sample behaviour of the procedures much more relevant. As the models become more complicated it becomes harder to derive useful finite-sample results and as yet there is little information available on these. We therefore echo the conclusions reached above, that the likelihood methods have great potential but at the moment cannot be recommended for routine use with modestly sized cross-over trials.

7.7 Discussion

We finish this chapter with a brief discussion of the points raised in the preceding sections. At the moment routine cross-over design and analysis ignores the repeated-measurements aspect of the data. Obviously the main question we need to answer is whether or not this matters.

For design, we have seen that the same arrangements, for example Williams squares, tend to have the more desirable properties both under uniform and under autoregressive error structures, at least when the latter have a positive autocorrelation. Under more general covariance structures it appears difficult to draw general conclusions about the comparative merits of designs and, as yet, no one has produced such results. The only sensible course of action would appear to be to continue using these same designs, which we know are good choices in certain circumstances and which are not known to be bad choices in any other circumstances (excepting perhaps some very extreme and arguably pathological cases). Of course, we may have to modify this view if practically relevant results can be found.

We know that an analysis based on OLS can be questionable if the covariance structure is not uniform, and the four-period, fourteen-sequence trial used as an illustration in this chapter is an example of this. We can, however, conjecture on the basis of Kunert's (1987a) results that, provided the design is at least approximately balanced with respect to direct treatments and carry-overs, the OLS analysis will not be wildly misleading. Standard repeated-measurement procedures can be used to test for uniformity if there is a moderate amount of replication within sequence groups. Otherwise more general likelihood ratio methods can be used. For the two trials we have considered in this section one appeared to conform to the uniformity assumption, and the other clearly did not. It is interesting that we were able to reject the uniformity assumption with great confidence even with a trial involving only 14 subjects.

We have examined the covariance structure in other trials and found similar results. The uniform structure can be a reasonable approximation, but is rejected occasionally and this does cast some doubt on the automatic use of ANOVA methods for analysis. A small study is reported in Kenward and Jones (1987b, Section 3) which involved the examination of the covariance structure of the sets of four measurements from 2×2 cross-over designs with baseline measurements. Out of 15 sample dispersion matrices, four were compatible with the uniform structure and one of the remainder was compatible with the stationary first-order autoregressive structure. The others displayed no obvious pattern that could be modelled in a parsimonious way. This agrees with another more general finding of our own: when the uniform structure is rejected the autoregressive structure rarely appears to provide an acceptable alternative. In conclusion, it appears very difficult to predict what will happen in general, but the uniform and the unconstrained structures are perhaps the two most practically useful alternatives to consider for the analysis. We doubt whether it is worth constructing analyses around the more stringent covariance structures such as the stationary autoregressive and moving average unless it can be shown that these do in fact provide reasonable approximations to the observed structures in a non-negligible proportion of cross-over trials.

If the uniform structure is rejected then there is a choice of analyses that can be used, and we have considered these in Sections 7.4 to 7.6. Straightforward analyses are possible for the two-sequence designs and these have known small-sample properties. The same is not true at the moment for the higher-order designs, although there are several alternatives which can be used with asymptotic results. We would argue, however, that one should not use these methods routinely as a way of ensuring robustness to non-uniformity. When the uniform assumption holds the orthodox ANOVA methods are considerably more powerful, they make use of familiar techniques and their properties are well understood. We have also seen that the uniform assumption need not be inappropriate in spite of the lack of justification through randomization.

Appendix   Least squares estimation for a general cross-over design

In the preceding chapters we have generally been concerned with inference about effects associated with treatments, that is, with direct treatment, carry-over, direct-by-period interaction effects, and so on. On those occasions when we need explicit expressions for estimators of these effects, to be able to compare designs for example, it is convenient to obtain them by the simplest route. In this appendix we show how the correct expressions can be derived in several ways using different models for the expectations of cross-over data. In this context the use of different models is an artifice to obtain simple derivations of estimators of effects; it does not imply that analyses based on the different models would be equivalent. In particular, it is easier to manipulate models with sequence (group) effects rather than subject effects, and we show below how each leads to equivalent estimators, but analyses based on the two types of model would not lead to the same estimates of error. We demonstrate equivalences for the following three cases:

1. a model which contains a different parameter for each subject (fixed subject effects);
2. a model with sequence effects but no subject effects;
3. a model for the contrasts between the means for each period in each sequence group.

We will be deriving expressions for GLS estimators under a general dispersion matrix Σ for the observations from each subject. This contains as a special case OLS estimation and, under Case 1 below, includes the models and analyses described in Chapters 4 and 5.

It is assumed that we have a general cross-over design with s sequence groups, p periods and n_i subjects in each group, $n_1 + n_2 + \cdots + n_s = n$, and we use the notation and definitions defined in Section 7.2.

Case 1

Let ϕ_{ik} denote the subject parameter for subject k in group i and set $\boldsymbol{\phi}_i = [\phi_{i1}, \phi_{i2}, \ldots, \phi_{in_i}]^T$ and $\boldsymbol{\phi} = [\boldsymbol{\phi}_1^T, \boldsymbol{\phi}_2^T, \ldots, \boldsymbol{\phi}_s^T]^T$. Further, let $\mathbf{y}_{(i)} = [\mathbf{y}_{(i)1}^T, \mathbf{y}_{(i)2}^T, \ldots, \mathbf{y}_{(i)n_i}^T]^T$ and $\mathbf{y} = [\mathbf{y}_{(1)}^T, \mathbf{y}_{(2)}^T, \ldots, \mathbf{y}_{(s)}^T]^T$. We can then write

$$E[\mathbf{y}] = [\mathbf{I}_n \otimes \mathbf{j}_p, \mathbf{X}] \begin{bmatrix} \boldsymbol{\phi} \\ \boldsymbol{\beta} \end{bmatrix} = \mathbf{X}_+ \boldsymbol{\psi}_1, \qquad \text{say}$$

where $\otimes$ is the right Kronecker product and the $(v \times 1)$ vector

$\boldsymbol{\beta} = [\boldsymbol{\pi}^\mathrm{T}, \boldsymbol{\xi}^\mathrm{T}]^\mathrm{T}$. Without loss of generality we assume that sufficient constraints have been applied to the parameters to ensure that $\mathbf{X}$ is of full rank.

If $\mathbf{X}_i$ is the $(p \times v)$ design matrix that applies to each subject in group i, then we can write

$$\mathbf{X} = [\mathbf{j}_{n_1}^\mathrm{T} \otimes \mathbf{X}_1^\mathrm{T}, \ldots, \mathbf{j}_{n_s}^\mathrm{T} \otimes \mathbf{X}_s^\mathrm{T}]$$

Also we have

$$V[\mathbf{y}] = \mathbf{V} = \mathbf{I}_n \otimes \boldsymbol{\Sigma}$$

Now in this case the GLS estimator of $\boldsymbol{\psi}_1$ is

$$\hat{\boldsymbol{\psi}}_1 = \begin{bmatrix} \hat{\boldsymbol{\phi}} \\ \hat{\boldsymbol{\beta}}_1 \end{bmatrix} = (\mathbf{X}_+^\mathrm{T} \mathbf{V}^{-1} \mathbf{X}_+)^{-1} \mathbf{X}_+^\mathrm{T} \mathbf{V}^{-1} \mathbf{y}$$

$$= \begin{bmatrix} \mathbf{A}_1 & \mathbf{B}_1 \\ \mathbf{B}_1^\mathrm{T} & \mathbf{C} \end{bmatrix}^{-1} \begin{bmatrix} \mathbf{Q}_1 \\ \mathbf{P} \end{bmatrix}$$

where

$$\mathbf{A}_1 = \mathbf{j}_p^\mathrm{T} \boldsymbol{\Sigma}^{-1} \mathbf{j}_p \mathbf{I}_n$$

$$\mathbf{B}_1^\mathrm{T} = [\mathbf{j}_{n_1}^\mathrm{T} \otimes \mathbf{X}_1^\mathrm{T} \boldsymbol{\Sigma}^{-1} \mathbf{j}_p, \ldots, \mathbf{j}_{n_s}^\mathrm{T} \otimes \mathbf{X}_s^\mathrm{T} \boldsymbol{\Sigma}^{-1} \mathbf{j}_p]^\mathrm{T}$$

$$\mathbf{C} = \sum_{i=1}^{s} n_i \mathbf{X}_i^\mathrm{T} \boldsymbol{\Sigma}^{-1} \mathbf{X}_i$$

$$\mathbf{Q}_1 = [\mathbf{j}_p^\mathrm{T} \boldsymbol{\Sigma}^{-1} \mathbf{y}_{(1)1}, \ldots, \mathbf{j}_p^\mathrm{T} \boldsymbol{\Sigma}^{-1} \mathbf{y}_{(s)n_s}]^\mathrm{T}$$

and

$$\mathbf{P} = \sum_{i=1}^{s} n_i \mathbf{X}_i^\mathrm{T} \boldsymbol{\Sigma}^{-1} \bar{\mathbf{y}}_{(i)}$$

We are directly interested in the estimator $\hat{\boldsymbol{\beta}}_1$. Using standard matrix results we have

$$\hat{\boldsymbol{\beta}}_1 = (\mathbf{C} - \mathbf{B}_1^\mathrm{T} \mathbf{A}_1^{-1} \mathbf{B}_1)^{-1} (\mathbf{P} - \mathbf{B}_1^\mathrm{T} \mathbf{A}_1^{-1} \mathbf{Q}_1)$$

$$= \left(\sum_{i=1}^{s} n_i \mathbf{X}_i^\mathrm{T} \mathbf{H}_\Sigma \mathbf{X}_i \right)^{-1} \sum_{i=1}^{s} n_i \mathbf{X}_i^\mathrm{T} \mathbf{H}_\Sigma \bar{\mathbf{y}}_{(i)} \tag{7.20}$$

where

$$\mathbf{H}_\Sigma = \boldsymbol{\Sigma}^{-1} - \boldsymbol{\Sigma}^{-1} \mathbf{j}_p (\mathbf{j}_p^\mathrm{T} \boldsymbol{\Sigma}^{-1} \mathbf{j}_p)^{-1} \mathbf{j}_p \boldsymbol{\Sigma}^{-1}$$

Using a standard matrix equality we can also write

$$\mathbf{H}_\Sigma = \mathbf{K}(\mathbf{K}^\mathrm{T} \boldsymbol{\Sigma} \mathbf{K})^{-1} \mathbf{K}^\mathrm{T} \tag{7.21}$$

where $\mathbf{K}$ is any $p \times (p-1)$ matrix of rank p satisfying $\mathbf{K}^T \mathbf{j}_p = 0$. In other words, the rows of $\mathbf{K}^T$ define a complete set of contrasts.

Case 2
To obtain the appropriate model we replace ϕ_{ik} by the corresponding sequence parameter γ_i. We then have

$$E[\mathbf{y}] = \mathbf{X}_G \boldsymbol{\psi}_2$$

where $\mathbf{X}_G = [\text{diag}(\mathbf{j}_{pn_1}, \ldots, \mathbf{j}_{pn_s}), \mathbf{X}]$ and $\boldsymbol{\psi}_2 = [\boldsymbol{\gamma}^T, \boldsymbol{\beta}^T]^T$, for $\boldsymbol{\gamma} = [\gamma_1, \ldots, \gamma_s]^T$. The GLS estimator of $\boldsymbol{\psi}_2$ is

$$\hat{\boldsymbol{\psi}}_2 = \begin{bmatrix} \hat{\boldsymbol{\gamma}} \\ \hat{\boldsymbol{\beta}}_2 \end{bmatrix} = (\mathbf{X}_G^T \mathbf{V}^{-1} \mathbf{X}_G)^{-1} \mathbf{X}_G^T \mathbf{V}^{-1} \mathbf{y}$$

$$= \begin{bmatrix} \mathbf{A}_2 & \mathbf{B}_2 \\ \mathbf{B}_2^T & \mathbf{C} \end{bmatrix}^{-1} \begin{bmatrix} \mathbf{Q}_2 \\ \mathbf{P} \end{bmatrix}$$

where

$$\mathbf{A}_2 = \text{diag}\,[n_1 \mathbf{j}_p^T \boldsymbol{\Sigma}^{-1} \mathbf{j}_p, \ldots, n_s \mathbf{j}_p^T \boldsymbol{\Sigma}^{-1} \mathbf{j}_p]$$
$$\mathbf{B}_2 = [n_1 \mathbf{X}_1^T \boldsymbol{\Sigma}^{-1} \mathbf{j}_p, \ldots, n_s \mathbf{X}_s^T \boldsymbol{\Sigma}^{-1} \mathbf{j}_p]^T$$

and

$$\mathbf{Q}_2 = [n_1 \mathbf{j}_p^T \boldsymbol{\Sigma}^{-1} \bar{\mathbf{y}}_{(1)}, \ldots, n_s \mathbf{j}_p^T \boldsymbol{\Sigma}^{-1} \bar{\mathbf{y}}_{(s)}]^T$$

From this we obtain

$$\hat{\boldsymbol{\beta}}_2 = \left(\sum_{i=1}^s n_i \mathbf{X}_i^T \mathbf{H}_\Sigma \mathbf{X}_i \right)^{-1} \sum_{i=1}^s n_i \mathbf{X}_i^T \mathbf{H}_\Sigma \bar{\mathbf{y}}_{(i)}^T$$

the same expression as in (7.20) above, that is $\hat{\boldsymbol{\beta}}_1 = \hat{\boldsymbol{\beta}}_2$.

Case 3
Instead of modelling the raw data, $\mathbf{y}$, we now obtain GLS estimators directly from sets of within-subject contrast means defined by $\mathbf{K}^T \bar{\mathbf{y}}_{(i)}$, where $\mathbf{K}$ is as defined above in Case 1. Since $\mathbf{K}^T \mathbf{j}_p = 0$, we have $E[\mathbf{K}^T \bar{\mathbf{y}}_{(i)}] = \mathbf{K}^T \mathbf{X}_i \boldsymbol{\beta}$ under either of the models in Cases 1 and 2 above. Also, we have $V[\mathbf{K}^T \bar{\mathbf{y}}_{(i)}] = n_i^{-1} \mathbf{K}^T \boldsymbol{\Sigma} \mathbf{K}$.

Defining

$$\mathbf{X}_K = \begin{bmatrix} \mathbf{K}^T \mathbf{X}_1 \\ \mathbf{K}^T \mathbf{X}_2 \\ \ldots \\ \mathbf{K}^T \mathbf{X}_s \end{bmatrix}, \quad \mathbf{V}_K = \text{diag}\,[n_1^{-1} \mathbf{K}^T \boldsymbol{\Sigma} \mathbf{K}, n_2^{-1} \mathbf{K}^T \boldsymbol{\Sigma} \mathbf{K}, \ldots, n_s^{-1} \mathbf{K}^T \boldsymbol{\Sigma} \mathbf{K}]$$

and

$$\bar{\mathbf{y}}_{\mathrm{K}} = \begin{bmatrix} \mathbf{K}^{\mathrm{T}}\bar{\mathbf{y}}_1 \\ \mathbf{K}^{\mathrm{T}}\bar{\mathbf{y}}_2 \\ \cdots \\ \mathbf{K}^{\mathrm{T}}\bar{\mathbf{y}}_s \end{bmatrix}$$

we can write the GLS estimator of $\boldsymbol{\beta}$ as

$$\hat{\boldsymbol{\beta}}_3 = (\mathbf{X}_{\mathrm{K}}^{\mathrm{T}}\mathbf{V}_{\mathrm{K}}^{-1}\mathbf{X}_{\mathrm{K}})^{-1}\mathbf{X}_{\mathrm{K}}^{\mathrm{T}}\mathbf{V}_{\mathrm{K}}^{-1}\bar{\mathbf{y}}_{\mathrm{K}}$$
$$= \left(\sum_{i=1}^{s} n_i \mathbf{X}_i^{\mathrm{T}}\mathbf{K}(\mathbf{K}^{\mathrm{T}}\boldsymbol{\Sigma}\mathbf{K})^{-1}\mathbf{K}^{\mathrm{T}}\mathbf{X}_i \right)^{-1} \sum_{i=1}^{s} n_i \mathbf{X}_i^{\mathrm{T}}\mathbf{K}(\mathbf{K}^{\mathrm{T}}\boldsymbol{\Sigma}\mathbf{K})^{-1}\mathbf{K}^{\mathrm{T}}\bar{\mathbf{y}}_{(i)}$$

which is equivalent to the expression for $\hat{\boldsymbol{\beta}}_1$ in (7.20) with $\mathbf{H}_{\Sigma}$ as expressed in (7.21). We could have also obtained the same estimator by modelling the contrasts from each subject, $[\mathbf{I}_n \otimes \mathbf{K}^{\mathrm{T}}]\mathbf{y}$, with dispersion matrix $\mathbf{I}_n \otimes \mathbf{K}^{\mathrm{T}}\boldsymbol{\Sigma}\mathbf{K}$.

References

Abeyasekera, S. and Curnow, R.N. (1984) The desirability of adjusting for residual effects in a crossover design. *Biometrics*, **40**, 1071–8.

Afsarinejad, K. (1983) Balanced repeated measurements designs. *Biometrika*, **70**, 199–204.

Agresti, A. (1984) *Analysis of Ordinal Categorical Data*. Wiley, New York.

Altham, P.M.E. (1971) The analysis of matched proportions. *Biometrika*, **58**, 561–76.

Anscombe, F.J. and Tukey, J.W. (1963) The examination and analysis of residuals. *Technometrics*, **5**, 141–60.

Armitage, P. and Berry, G. (1987) *Statistical Methods In Medical Research*. Blackwell Scientific Publications, Oxford.

Armitage, P. and Hills, M. (1982) The two-period crossover trial. *The Statistician*, **31**, 119–31.

Atkinson, G.F. (1966) Designs for sequences of treatments with carry-over effects. *Biometrics*, **22**, 292–309.

Azzalini, A. and Giovagnoli, A. (1987) Some optimal designs for repeated measurements with autoregressive errors. *Biometrika*, **74**, 725–34.

Balaam, L.N. (1968) A two-period design with t^2 experimental units. *Biometrics*, **24**, 61–73.

Balmer, D.W. (1988) Recursive enumeration of $r \times c$ tables for exact likelihood evaluation. *Applied Statistics*, **34**, 290–301.

Barker, N., Hews, R.J., Huitson, A. and Polonieki, J. (1982) The two period cross over trial. *Bulletin in Applied Statistics*, **9**, 67–116.

Bartlett, M.S. (1954) A note on multiplying factors for various chi-squared approximatations. *Journal of the Royal Statistical Society*, B, **16**, 296–8.

Behrens, W.V. (1929) Ein Beitrag zur Fehlerberechnung bei weniger Beobachtungen. *Landwirtschaftl. Jahrb.*, **68**, 807–37.

Bennett, B.M. (1971) On tests for order and treatment differences in a matched 2×2. *Biometrical Journal*, **3**, 95–9.

Berenblut, I.I. (1964) Change-over designs with complete balance for first residual effects. *Biometrics*, **20**, 707–12.

Berenblut, I.I. (1967a) The analysis of change-over designs with complete balance for first residual effects. *Biometrics*, **23**, 578–80.

Berenblut, I.I. (1967b) A change-over design for testing a treatment factor at four equally spaced levels. *Journal of the Royal Statistical Society*, B, **29**, 370–3.

Berenblut, I.I. (1968) Change-over designs balanced for the linear component of first residual effects. *Biometrika*, **55**, 297–303.

Berenblut, I.I. and Webb, G.I. (1974) Experimental design in the presence of autocorrelated errors. *Biometrika*, **61**, 427–37.

Berk, K. (1987) Computing for incomplete repeated measures. *Biometrics*, **43**, 385–98.

Bishop, S.H. and Jones, B. (1984) A review of higher-order cross-over designs. *Journal of Applied Statistics*, **11**, 29–50.

Bishop, Y.M.M., Fienberg, S.E. and Holland, P.W. (1975) *Discrete Multivariate Analysis*. MIT Press, Cambridge, Mass.

Blaisdell, E.A. (1978) Partially balanced residual effects designs. PhD dissertation, Temple University, Philadelphia, Pa.

Blaisdell, E.A. and Raghavarao, D. (1980) Partially balanced change-over designs based on m-associate class PBIB designs. *Journal of the Royal Statistical Society*, B, **42**, 334–8.

Bock, R.D. and Bargmann, R.E. (1966) Analysis of covariance structures. *Psychometrika*, **31**, 507–34.

Bonney, G.E. (1987) Logistic regression for dependent binary observations. *Biometrics*, **43**, 951–73.

Bora, A.C. (1984) Change-over designs with errors following a first order autoregressive process. *Australian Journal of Statistics*, **26**, 179–88.

Bora, A.C. (1985) Change-over design with first order residual effects and errors following a first order autoregressive process. *The Statistician*, **34**, 161–73.

Bose, R.C. and Shimamoto, T. (1952) Classification and analysis of partially balanced incomplete block designs with two associate classes. *Journal of the American Statistical Association*, **47**, 151–84.

Boulton, D.M. and Wallace, C.S. (1973) Occupancy of a rectangular array. *Computer Journal*, **16**, 57–63.

Box, G.E.P. and Tiao, G.C. (1973) *Bayesian Inference in Statistical Analysis*. Addison–Wesley, Reading, Mass.

Bradley, J.V. (1958) Complete counterbalancing of immediate sequential effects in a Latin square design. *Journal of the American Statistical Association*, **53**, 525–8.

Brandt, A.E. (1938) Tests of significance in reversal or switchback trials. *Research Bulletin No. 234*, Iowa Agricultural Experimental Station.

Broemeling, L.D. (1985) *Bayesian Analysis of Linear Models*. Marcell Dekker, New York.

Broster, W.H. and Broster, V.J. (1984) Long term effects of plane of nutrition on the performance of the dairy cow. *Journal of Dairy Research*, **51**, 149–96.

Broster, W.H., Broster, V.J., Clements, A.J. and Smith, T. (1981) The relationship between yield of dairy cows and response to change in plane of nutrition. *Journal of Agricultural Science*, **104**, 535–57.

Brown, W.B. (1980) The crossover experiment for clinical trials. *Biometrics*, **36**, 69–79.

Castle, M.E. and Watson, J.N. (1984) Silage and milk production: a comparison between concentrates containing different amounts of protein as supplements for silage of high digestibility. *Grain Forage Science*, **39**, 93–9.

Chassan, J.B. (1964) On the analysis of simple cross-overs with unequal numbers of replicates. *Biometrics*, **20**, 206–8.

Chassan, J.B. (1970) A note on relative efficiency in clinical trials. Letter to the editor. *Journal of Clinical Pharmacology*, **10**, 359–60.

Chatfield, C. and Collins, A.J. (1980) *Introduction to Multivariate Analysis*. Chapman and Hall, London.

Cheng, C.S. and Wu, C.F. (1980) Balanced repeated measurements designs. *Annals of Statistics*, **8**, 1272–83. Corrigendum (1983), **11**, 349.

Ciminera, J.L. and Wolfe, R.K. (1953) An example of the use of extended cross-over designs in the comparison of NPH insulin mixtures. *Biometrics*, **9**, 431–46.

Clatworthy, W.H. (1973) *Tables of Two-associate Partially Balanced Designs*. National Bureau of Standards Applied Mathematics Series No. 63, US Department of Commerce.

Clayton, D. and Hills, M. (1987) A two-period crossover trial, in *The Statistical Consultant in Action* (eds D.J. Hand and B.S. Everitt). Cambridge University Press.

Cochran, W.G. (1939) Long-term agricultural experiments (with discussion). *Journal of the Royal Statistical Society*, B, **6**, 104–48.

Cochran, W.G., Autrey, K.M. and Cannon, C.Y. (1941) A double change-over design for dairy cattle feeding experiments. *Journal of Dairy Science*, **24**, 937–51.

Conover, W.J. and Iman, R.L. (1981) Rank transformations as a bridge between parametric and non-parametric statistics. *The American Statistician*, **35**, 124–9.

Cook, R.D. and Weisberg, S. (1982) *Residuals and Influence in Regression*. Chapman and Hall, New York.

Cornell, R.G. (1980) Evaluation of bioavailability data using non-parametric statistics, in *Drug Absorption and Disposition: Statistical Considerations* (ed. K.S. Albert). American Pharmaceutical Association, pp. 51–7.

Cornish, E.A. (1954) The multivariate *t*-distribution associated with a set of normal sample deviates. *Australian Journal of Physics*, **7**, 531–42.

Cotter, S.C., John, J.A. and Smith, T.M.F. (1973) Multi-factor experiments in non-orthogonal designs. *Journal of the Royal Statistical Society*, B, **35**, 361–7.

Cox, D.R. (1970) *The Analysis of Binary Data*. Chapman and Hall, London.

Cox, D.R. (1972) The analysis of multivariate binary data. *Applied Statistics*, **21**, 113–20.

Cox, D.R. (1984) Interaction. *International Statistical Review*, **52**, 1–31.

Cox, D.R. and Hinkley, D.V. (1974) *Theoretical Statistics*. Chapman and Hall, London.

Cox, M.A.A. and Plackett, R.L. (1980) Matched pairs in factorial experiments with binary data. *Biometrical Journal*, **22**, 697–702.

Davis, A.W. and Hall, W.B. (1969) Cyclic change-over designs. *Biometrika*, **56**, 283–93.

Diggle, P.J., Donnelly, J.B. and Kirkby, A. (1985) CSIRO Department of Mathematics and Statistics Report No. ACT 85/18.

Dunnett, C.W. and Sobel, M. (1954) A bivariate generalization of Student's *t*-distribution with tables for certain special cases. *Biometrika*, **41**, 135–69.

Dunsmore, I.R. (1981a) Growth curves in two-period change-over models. *Applied Statistics*, **30**, 575–8.

Dunsmore, I.R. (1981b) Analysis of preferences in two-period cross-over designs. *Biometrics*, **37**, 223–9.

Ebbutt, A.F. (1984) Three-period crossover designs for two treatments. *Biometrics*, **40**, 219–24.

Everitt, B.S. (1977) *The Analysis of Contingency Tables*. Chapman and Hall, London.

Farewell, V.T. (1985) Some remarks on the analysis of cross-over trials with a binary response. *Applied Statistics*, **34**, 121–8.

Faulder, C. (1985) *Whose body is it? The Troubling Issue of Informed Consent*. Virago, London.

Fava, G.M. and Patel, H.I. (1986) A survey of crossover designs used in industry. Unpublished manuscript.

Federer, W.T. (1955) *Experimental Design – Theory and Application*. Macmillan, New York.

Federer, W.T. and Atkinson, G.F. (1964) Tied-double-change-over designs. *Biometrics*, **20**, 168–81.

Fidler, V. (1984) Change-over clinical trial with binary data: mixed-model-based comparison of tests. *Biometrics*, **40**, 1063–70.

Fidler, V. (1987) Log-linear mixed models for categorical data. *Statistica Neerlandica*, **41**, 45–57.

Fieller, E.C. (1940) The biological standardization of insulin (with discussion). *Supplement to the Journal of the Royal Statistical Society*, **7**, 1–64.

Finney, D.J. (1956) Cross-over designs in bioassay. *Proceedings of the Royal Society*, B, **145**, 42–60.

Finney, D.J. and Outhwaite, A.D. (1955) Serially balanced sequences. *Nature*, **176**, 748.

Finney, D.J. and Outhwaite, A.D. (1956) Serially balanced sequences in bioassay. *Proceedings of the Royal Society*, B, **145**, 493–507.

Fisher, R.A. (1941) The asymptotic approach to Behrens integral, with further tables for the *d* test of significance. *Annals of Eugenics.*, **11**, 141–72.

Fleiss, J.L. (1986a) *The Design and Analysis of Clinical Experiments*. Wiley, New York.

Fleiss, J.L. (1986b) On multiperiod crossover studies. Letter to the editor. *Biometrics*, **42**, 449–50.

Fletcher, D.J. (1987) A new class of change-over designs for factorial experiments. *Biometrika*, **74**, 649–54.

Fletcher, D.J. and John, J.A. (1985) Changeover designs and factorial structure. *Journal of the Royal Statistical Society*, B, **47**, 117–24.

Fluehler, H., Grieve, A.P., Mandallaz, D., Mau, J. and Moser, H.A. (1983) Bayesian approach to bioequivalence assessment: an example. *Journal of Pharmaceutical Sciences*, **72**, 1178–81.

Freeman, G.H. and Halton, J.L. (1951) Note on an exact treatment of contingency, goodness of fit and other problems of significance. *Biometrika*, **38**, 141–9.

Freeman, P.R. (1988) The performance of the two-stage analysis of two-treatment crossover trials. Submitted for publication.

Friedman, L.M., Furberg, C.D. and Demets, D.L. (1981) *Fundamentals of Clinical Trials*. Wright, Boston.

Gabriel, K.R. (1962) Ante-dependence analysis of an ordered set of variables. *Annals of Mathematical Statistics*, **33**, 201–12.

Gart, J.J. (1969) An exact test for comparing matched proportions in crossover designs. *Biometrika*, **56**, 75–80.

Gentleman, J.F. (1975) Generation of all C_r^n combinations by simulating nested Fortran DO loops. *Applied Statistics*, **24**, 374–6.

Gentleman, J.F. and Wilk, M.B. (1975) Detecting outliers in a two-way table: I. Statistical behavior of residuals. *Technometrics*, **17**, 1–14.

George, S.L. and Desu, M.M. (1973) Testing for order effect in a crossover design. *Biometrical Journal*, **15**, 113–16.

Gibbons, J.D. (1985) *Nonparametric Statistical Inference*. Marcel Dekker, New York.

Gill, P.S. and Shukla, G.K. (1985) Efficiency of nearest neighbour block designs with balance for residual effects. *Biometrika*, **72**, 539–44.

Gill, P.S. and Shukla, G.K. (1987) Autoregressive models for repeated measurements: design and analysis. Submitted for publication.

Goldstein, H. (1986) Multilevel mixed model analysis using iterative generalized least squares. *Biometrika*, **73**, 43–56.

Gore, S.M. and Altman, D.G. (1982) *Statistics in Practice*. British Medical Association, London.

Gould, A.L. (1980) A new approach to the analysis of clinical drug trials with withdrawals. *Biometrics*, **36**, 721–7.

Greenhouse, S.W. and Geisser, S. (1959) On methods in the analysis of profile data. *Psychometrika*, **24**, 95–112.

Grieve, A.P. (1982) The two-period changeover design in clinical trials. Letter to the editor. *Biometrics*, **38**, 517.

Grieve, A.P. (1985) A Bayesian analysis of the two-period crossover design for clinical trials. *Biometrics*, **41**, 979–90.

Grieve, A.P. (1986) Corrigenda to Grieve (1985). *Biometrics*, **42**, 459.

Grieve, A.P. (1987a) A note on the analysis of the two-period crossover design when the period-treatment interaction is significant. *Biometrical Journal*, **29**, 771–5.

Grieve, A.P. (1987b) Applications of Bayesian software: two examples. *The Statistician*, **36**, 282–8.

Grieve, A.P. (1989) Crossover versus parallel designs, in *Statistical Methodology in the Pharmaceutical Sciences* (ed. D.A. Berry). Marcell Dekker, New York.

Grizzle, J.E. (1965) The two-period change-over design and its use in clinical trials. *Biometrics*, **21**, 467–80.

Grizzle, J.E. (1974) Corrigenda to Grizzle (1965). *Biometrics*, **30**, 727.

Grizzle, J.E., Starmer, C.F. and Koch, G.G. (1969). Analysis of categorical data by linear models. *Biometrics*, **25**, 489–504.

Haberman, S. (1979) *Analysis of Frequency Data*, Volume 2, New Developments. Academic Press, New York.

Hedayat, A. and Afsarinejad, K. (1975) Repeated measures designs, I, in *A Survey of Statistical Design and Linear Models* (ed. J.N. Srivastava). North-Holland, Amsterdam.

Hedayat, A. and Afsarinejad, K. (1978) Repeated measures designs, II. *Annals of Statistics*, **6**, 619–28.

Hews, R.J. (1981) Further note on the interpretation of results from the two-period cross-over clinical trial. *PSI Newsletter*, No. 2.

Hills, M. and Armitage, P. (1979) The two-period cross-over clinical trial. *British Journal of Clinical Pharmacology*, **8**, 7–20.

Hoekstra, J.A. (1987) Design of milk production trials. *Livestock Production Science*, **16**, 373–84.

Hollander, M. and Wolfe, D.A. (1973) *Nonparametric Statistical Methods*. Wiley, New York.

Huitson, A. (1981) A note on the interpretation of results from the two-period cross-over clinical trial. *PSI Newsletter*, No.2.

Hunter, K.R., Stern, G.M., Laurence, D.R. and Armitage, P. (1970) Amantadine in Parkinsonism. *Lancet*, **i**, 1127–9.

Jennrich, R.I. and Schluchter, M.D. (1986) Unbalanced repeated-measures models with structured covariance matrices. *Biometrics*, **42**, 805–20.

John, J.A. (1973) Generalized cyclic designs in factorial experiments. *Biometrika*, **60**, 55–63.

John, P.W.M. (1971) *Statistical Design and Analysis of Experiments*. Macmillan, New York.

Jones, B. (1985) Using bricks to build block designs. *Journal of the Royal Statistical Society*, B, **47**, 349–56.

Jones, B. and Kenward, M.G. (1987) Modelling binary data from a three-period cross-over trial. *Statistics in Medicine*, **6**, 555–64.

Jones, B. and Kenward, M.G. (1988) Modelling binary and categorical cross-over data. *Proceedings of the American Statistical Association Joint Meetings*, New Orleans, August.

Jöreskog, K.G. (1981) Analysis of covariance structures. *Scandinavian Journal of Statistics*, **8**, 65–92.

Keen, A., Thissen, J.T.N.M., Hoekstra, J.A. and Jansen, J. (1986) Successive measurements experiments. *Statistica Neerlandica*, **40**, 205–23.

Kempthorne, O. (1983) *The Design and Analysis of Experiments.* Krieger, Florida.

Kendall, M.G., Stuart, A. and Ord, J.K. (1979) *The Advanced Theory of Statistics*, Volume 2, *Inference and Relationship* (4th edn). Griffin, London.

Kenward, M.G. (1981) Unpublished PhD thesis, University of Reading, UK.

Kenward, M.G. (1985) The use of fitted higher-order polynomial coefficients as covariates in the analysis of growth curves. *Biometrics*, **40**, 19–28.

Kenward, M.G. (1987) A method for comparing profiles of repeated measurements. *Applied Statistics*, **36**, 296–308.

Kenward, M.G. and Jones, B. (1987a) A log-linear model for binary cross-over data. *Applied Statistics*, **36**, 192–204.

Kenward, M.G. and Jones, B. (1987b) The analysis of data from 2 × 2 cross-over trials with baseline measurements. *Statistics in Medicine*, 911–26.

Kershner, R.P. and Federer, W.T. (1981) Two-treatment crossover designs for estimating a variety of effects. *Journal of the American Statistical Association*, **76**, 612–18.

Kiefer, J. (1975) Construction and optimality of generalised Youden designs, in *A Survey of Statistical Design and Linear Models* (ed. J.N. Srivastava). North-Holland, Amsterdam.

Kiefer, J. and Wynn, H.P. (1981) Optimum balanced block and Latin square designs for correlated observations. *Annals of Statistics*, **9**, 737–57.

Kirkwood, T.B.L. (1981) Bioequivalence testing – a need to rethink. *Biometrics*, **37**, 589–94.

Koch, G.G. (1972) The use of non-parametric methods in the statistical analysis of the two-period change-over design. *Biometrics*, **28**, 577–84.

Koch, G.G., Amara, I.A., Stokes, M.E. and Gillings, D.B. (1980)

Some views on parametric and non-parametric analysis for repeated measurements and selected bibliography. *International Statistical Review*, **48**, 249–65.

Koch, M. (1987) A refined nomenclature for interaction effects in crossover trials: emphasis on treatment-by-carryover interactions. Submitted for publication.

Kunert, J. (1984) Optimality of balanced uniform repeated measurements designs. *Annals of Statistics*, **12**, 1006–17.

Kunert, J. (1985) Optimal repeated measurements designs for correlated observations and analysis by least squares. *Biometrika*, **72**, 375–89.

Kunert, J. (1987a) On variance estimation in cross-over designs. *Biometrics*, **43**, 833–45.

Kunert, J. (1987b) Nearest neighbour designs for correlated errors. *Biometrika*, **74**, 717–24.

Lachin, J.M. (1981) Introduction to sample size determination and power analysis for clinical trials. *Controlled Clinical Trials.*, **2**, 93–113.

Larson, H.J. and Bancroft, T.A. (1963) Biases in prediction by regression for certain incompletely specified models. *Biometrika*, **50**, 391–402.

Laska, E. and Meisner, M. (1985) A variational approach to optimal two-treatment crossover designs: applications to carryover-effect models. *Journal of the American Statistical Association*, **80**, 704–10.

Laska, E.M., Meisner, M. and Kushner, H.B. (1983) Optimal crossover designs in the presence of carryover effects. *Biometrics*, **39**, 1089–91.

Law, M.G. (1987) A Bayesian analysis of higher-order cross-over designs. Unpublished MSc dissertation, University of Kent at Canterbury.

Lawes, J.B. and Gilbert, J.H. (1864) Report of experiments on the growth of wheat for twenty years in succession on the same land. *Journal of the Agricultural Society of England*, **25**, 93–185, 449–501.

Le, C.T. (1984) A new test for cross-over clinical trials with order effects. *Biometrical Journal*, **5**, 583–7.

Lewis, S.M., Fletcher, D.J. and Matthews, J.N.S. (1988) Factorial cross-over designs in clinical trials, in *Optimal Design and Analysis of Experiments* (eds Y. Dodge, V. Fedorov and H.P. Wynn). North-Holland, Amsterdam.

Liebig, J. (1847) *Chemistry in its Application to Agriculture and*

Physiology (4th edn). (In English; eds L. Playfair and W. Gregory.) Taylor and Walton, London.

Linnerud, A.C., Gates, C.E. and Donker, J.D. (1962) Significance of carryover effects with extra period Latin square change-over design (abstract). *Journal of Dairy Science*, **45**, 675.

Louis, T.A. (1988) General methods for analysing repeated measures. *Statistics in Medicine*, **7**, 29–45.

Louis, T.A., Lavori, P.W., Bailar, J.C. and Polansky, M. (1984) Crossover and self-controlled designs in clinical research. *The New England Journal of Medicine*, **310**, 24–31.

Lucas, H.L. (1951) Bias in estimation of error in change-over trials with dairy cattle. *Journal of Agricultural Science*, **41**, 146.

Lucas, H.L. (1957) Extra-period Latin-square change-over designs. *Journal of Dairy Science*, **40**, 225–39.

Lund, R.E. (1975) Tables for an approximate test for outliers in linear models. *Technometrics*, **17**, 473–6.

McCullagh, P. (1980) Regression models for ordinal data (with discussion). *Journal of the Royal Statistical Society*, B, **42**, 109–42.

McCullagh, P. and Nelder, J.A. (1983) *Generalized Linear Models*. Chapman and Hall, London.

MacKenzie, G. and O'Flaherty, M. (1982) Direct simulation of nested Fortran DO-LOOPS. *Applied Statistics*, **31**, 71–4.

McNemar, Q. (1947). Note on the sampling error of the difference between correlated proportions or percentages. *Psychometrika*, **12**, 153–7.

Machin, D. and Campbell, M.J. (1987) *Statistical Tables for the Design of Clinical Trials*. Blackwell Scientific Publications, Oxford.

Mainland, D. (1963) *Elementary Medical Statistics* (2nd edn). Saunders, Philadelphia, Pa.

Mandallaz, D. and Mau, J. (1981) Comparison of different methods for decision-making in bioequivalence assessment. *Biometrics*, **37**, 213–22.

Marks, H.P. (1925) The biological assay of insulin preparations in comparison with a stable standard. *British Medical Journal*, **ii**, 1102–4.

Matthews, J.N.S. (1987) Optimal crossover designs for the comparison of two treatments in the presence of carryover effects and autocorrelated errors. *Biometrika*, **74**, 311–20.

Matthews, J.N.S. (1988a) Recent developments in crossover designs. *International Statistical Review*, **56**, 117–27.

Matthews, J.N.S. (1988b) Optimal dual-balanced two treatment crossover designs. Submitted for publication.

Matthews, J.N.S. (1988c) The analysis of data from crossover designs: efficiency of ordinary least squares. Submitted for publication.

Morrison, D.F. (1986) *Multivariate Statistical Methods* (2nd edn). McGraw-Hill, New York.

Moses, L.E. (1963) Rank tests of dispersion. *Annals of Mathematical Statistics*, **34**, 973–83.

Nam, J. (1971) On two tests for comparing matched proportions. *Biometrics*, **27**, 945–59.

Namboodiri, K.N. (1972) Experimental design in which each subject is used repeatedly. *Psychological Bulletin*, **77**, 54–64.

Oman, S.D. and Seiden, E. (1988) Switch-back designs. *Biometrika*, **75**, 81–9.

Pagano, M. and Halvorsen, K.T. (1981) An algorithm for fitting the exact significance levels for $r \times c$ contingency tables. *Journal of the American Statistical Association*, **76**, 931–4.

Parkes, K.R. (1982) Occupational stress among student nurses: a natural experiment. *Journal of Applied Psychology*, **67**, 784–96.

Patefield, M. (1981) An efficient method of generating random $r \times c$ tables with given row and column totals. *Applied Statistics*, **30**, 91–7.

Patel, H.I. (1983) Use of baseline measurements in the two-period cross-over design. *Communications in Statistics – Theory and Methods*, **12**, 2693–712.

Patel, H.I. (1985) Analysis of incomplete data in a two-period crossover design. *Biometrika*, **72**, 411–18.

Patel, H.I. (1986) Analysis of repeated measures designs with changing covariates in clinical trials. *Biometrika*, **73**, 707–15.

Patel, H.I. and Hearne, E.M. (1980) Multivariate analysis for the two-period repeated measures crossover design with applications to clinical trials. *Communications in Statistics – Theory and Methods*, **A9**, 1919–29.

Patterson, H.D. (1950) The analysis of change-over trials. *Journal of Agricultural Science*, **40**, 375–80.

Patterson, H.D. (1951) Change-over trials. *Journal of the Royal Statistical Society*, B, **13**, 256–71.

Patterson, H.D. (1952) The construction of balanced designs for experiments involving sequences of treatments. *Biometrika*, **39**, 32–48.

Patterson, H.D. (1970) Non-additivity in change-over designs for a quantitative factor at four levels. *Biometrika*, **57**, 537–49.

Patterson, H.D. (1971) Unbiased estimation of error in the analysis of change-over trials. *Bulletin of the International Statistical Institute*, **44**, 320–4.

Patterson, H.D. (1973) Quenouille's change-over designs. *Biometrika*, **60**, 33–45.

Patterson, H.D. and Lucas, H.L. (1962) Change-over designs, North Carolina Agricultural Experiment Station, Tech. Bull. No. 147.

Pigeon, J.G. (1984) Residual effects designs for comparing treatments with a control. PhD dissertation, Temple University, Philadelphia, Pa.

Pigeon, J.G. and Raghavarao, D. (1987) Crossover designs for comparing treatments with a control. *Biometrika*, **74**, 321–8.

Plackett. R.L. (1981) *The Analysis of Categorical Data*. Griffin, London.

Pocock, S.J. (1983) *Clinical Trials*. Wiley, New York.

Poloniecki, J. and Daniel, D. (1981) Further analysis of the Hills and Armitage enuresis data. *The Statistician*, **30**, 225–9.

Poloniecki, J.D. and Pearce, A.C. (1983) Interaction in the two-way crossover trial. Letter to the editor. *Biometrics*, **39**, 798.

Preece, D.A. (1982) Balance and design: another terminological tangle. *Utilitas Mathematica*, **21C**, 85–186.

Prescott, R.J. (1979) On McNemar's and Gart's tests for cross-over trials. Letter to the editor. *Biometrics*, **35**, 523–4.

Prescott, R.J. (1981) The comparison of success rates in cross-over trials in the presence of an order effect. *Applied Statistics*, **30**, 9–15.

Quenouille, M.H. (1953) *The Design and Analysis of Experiments*. Griffin, London.

Racine, A., Grieve, A.P. Flühler, H. and Smith, A.F.M. (1986) Bayesian methods in practice: experiences in the pharmaceutical industry (with discussion). *Applied Statistics*, **35**, 93–150.

Raghavarao, D. (1971) *Constructions and Combinatorial Problems in Design of Experiments*. Wiley, New York.

Raghavarao, D. (1989) Crossover designs in industry, in *Design and Analysis of Experiments, With Applications to Engineering and Physical Sciences* (ed. S. Gosh), Marcell Dekker, New York.

Rao, C.R. (1967) Least squares theory using an estimated dispersion matrix and its application to measurement of signals. *Proceedings of the Fifth Berkeley Symposium on Mathematical Statistics and Probability*, **I**, 359–73.

Richards, W.A. (1980) Randomization analysis of covariance and change-over designs. PhD dissertation, Iowa State University.

Rowell, J.G. and Walters, R.E. (1976) Analysing data with repeated observations on each experimental unit. *Journal of Agricultural Science Cambridge*, **87**, 423–32.

Russell, K.G. and Eccleston, J.A. (1987) The construction of optimal balanced incomplete block designs when adjacent observations are correlated. *Australian Journal of Statistics*, **29**, 91–100.

Salsburg, D. (1981) Development of statistical analysis for single dose bronchodilators. *Controlled Clinical Trials*, **2**, 305–17.

Sampford, M.R. (1957) Methods of construction and analysis of serially balanced sequences. *Journal of the Royal Statistical Society*, B, **19**, 286–304.

Satterthwaite, F.E. (1946) An approximate distribution of estimates of variance components. *Biometrics Bulletin*, **2**, 110–14.

Saunders, I.W. (1984) Enumeration of $r \times c$ tables with repeated row totals. *Applied Statistics*, **33**, 340–52.

Seath, D.M. (1944) A 2×2 factorial design for double reversal feeding experiments. *Journal of Dairy Science*, **27**, 159–64.

Seeger, P. (1980) The two-period changeover design applied to dairy cows. *Swedish Journal of Agricultural Research*, **10**, 175–80.

Selwyn, M.R., Dempster, A.R. and Hall, N.R. (1981) A Bayesian approach to bioequivalence for the 2×2 changeover design. *Biometrics*, **37**, 11–21.

Selwyn, M.R. and Hall, N.R. (1984) On Bayesian methods for bioequivalence. *Biometrics*, **40**, 1103–8.

Selwyn, M.R. and Hall, N.R. (1985). On testing for bioequivalence. Letter to the editor. *Biometrics*, **41**, 561.

Sen, M. and Mukerjee, R. (1987) Optimal repeated measurements designs under interaction. *Journal of Statistical Planning and Inference*, **17**, 18–91.

Shapiro, S.S. and Wilk, M.B. (1965) Analysis of variance test, for normality and complete samples. *Biometrika*, **52**, 592–611.

Sheehe, P.R. and Bross, I.D.J. (1961) Latin squares to balance immediate residual and other effects. *Biometrics*, **17**, 405–14.

Shen, C.D. and Quade, D. (1983) A randomization test for a three-period three-treatment crossover experiment. *Communications in Statistics – Theory and Methodology*, **12**, 183–99.

Simpson, T.W. (1938) Experimental methods and human nutrition (with discussion). *Journal of the Royal Statistical Society*, B, **5**, 46–69.

Taka, M.T. and Armitage, P. (1983) Autoregressive models in clinical trials. *Communications in Statistics – Theory and Methods*, **12** (8), 865–76.

Taylor, W.B. and Amstrong, P.J. (1953) The efficiency of some experimental designs used in dairy husbandry experiments. *Journal of Agricultural Science*, **43**, 407–12, 386–93.

Vartak, M.N. (1955) On an application of Kronecker product of matrices to statistical designs. *Annals of Mathematical Statistics*, **26**, 420–38.

Wald, A. (1943) Tests of statistical hypothesis concerning the general parameters when the number of observations is large. *Transactions of the American Mathematical Society*, **54**, 426–82.

Wallenstein, S. (1979) Inclusion of baseline values in the analysis of crossover designs (abstract). *Biometrics*, **35**, 894.

Wallenstein, S. and Fisher, A.C. (1977) Analysis of the two-period repeated measurements crossover design with application to clinical trials. *Biometrics*, **30** 261–9.

Ware, J.H. (1985) Linear models for the analysis of longitudinal studies. *The American Statistician*, **39**, 95–101.

Ware, J.H., Lipsitz, S. and Speizer, F.E. (1988) Issues in the analysis of repeated categorical outcomes. *Statistics in Medicine*, **7**, 95–107.

Westlake, W.J. (1974) The use of balanced incomplete block designs in comparative bioavailability trials. *Biometrics*, **30**, 319–27.

Westlake, W.J. (1975) Statistical problems in interpreting comparative bioavailability trials. *International Journal of Clinical Pharmacology*, **11**, 342–5.

Westlake, W.J. (1976) Symmetrical confidence intervals for bioequivalence trials. *Biometrics*, **32**, 741–4.

Westlake, W.J. (1979a) Statistical aspects of comparative bioavailability trials. *Biometrics*, **35**, 272–80.

Westlake, W.J. (1979b) Design and statistical evaluation of bioequivalence studies in man, in *Principles and Perspectives in Drug Bioavailability* (eds J. Blanchard, R.J. Sawchuk and B.B. Brodie). Karger, Basel.

Whitehead, J. and Ezzet, F. (1988) Random effects linear models for binary, ordinal and grouped survival data. Submitted for publication.

Willan, A.R. (1988) Using the maximum test statistic in the two-period crossover clinical trial. *Biometrics*, **44**, 211–18.

Willan, A.R. and Pater, J.L. (1986a) Carryover and the two-period crossover design. *Biometrics*, **42**, 593–9.

Willan, A.R. and Pater, J.L. (1986b) Using baseline measurements in the two-period crossover clinical trial. *Controlled Clinical Trials*, **7**, 282–9.

Williams, E.J. (1949) Experimental designs balanced for the estimation of residual effects of treatments. *Australian Journal of Scientific Research*, **2**, 149–68.

Williams, E.J. (1950) Experimental designs balanced for pairs of residual effects. *Australian Journal of Scientific Research*, **3**, 351–63.

Yates, F. (1938) The gain in efficiency resulting from the use of balanced designs. *Journal of the Royal Statistical Society*, B, **5**, 70–4.

Yates, F. (1982) Regression models for repeated measurements. *Biometrics*, **38**, 850–3.

Yates, F. (1984) Tests of significance for 2×2 contingency tables (with discussion) *Journal of the Royal Statistical Society*, B, **147**, 426–63.

Zimmerman, H. and Rahlfs, V. (1978) Testing hypotheses in the two-period change-over with binary data. *Biometrical Journal*, **20**, 133–41.

Author index

Subject index